The World Turned Upside Down: The Second Low-Carbohydrate Revolution

Illustrations and Jacket Design Robin A. Feinman


ISBN-13: 978-0-9792018-2-0
ISBN-10: 0-9792018-2-9

Published by NMS Press, Brooklyn, NY, http://www.nmsociety.org
And Duck in a Boat LLC, Snohomish, WA, http://www.carbwarscookbook.com

Also by NMS Press and Duck in a Boat LLC:

Judy Barnes Baker - Nourished - A Cookbook for Health, Weight Loss and Metabolic Balance.
Judy Barnes Baker - Carb Wars - Sugar is the New Fat.



For information about permissions or about discounts for bulk orders or to book an event with the author or his colleagues or any other matter, please write to feinman@mac.com.

Disclaimer:
This book contains the opinions and ideas of the author and is offered for information purposes only. It is sold with the understanding that the author and publisher do not engage in rendering health services. The reader should consult his or her own medical and health providers as appropriate before adopting any of the ideas discussed in this book or drawing any inferences from it.

The author and publisher specifically disclaim responsibility for any liability loss or risk personal or otherwise, which is incurred as a consequence, directly or indirectly, of the use and application of any of the contents of this book.

# The World Turned Upside Down: The Second Low-Carbohydrate Revolution

*How the science of carbohydrate restriction arising from a rag-tag collection of popular diets defeated the powerful low-fat army and became the default approach to health.*

Richard David Feinman, Ph. D.

Illustrations by Robin Feinman

In the American Revolution, when Cornwallis surrendered at Yorktown (1781), the British supposedly marched out playing the popular song " The World Turned Upside Down." (http://www.contemplator.com/england/ worldtur.html). Probably too good to be true — the greatest army in the world had lost a war to a bunch of guerillas — it was a popular song and there are several versions (http://www.contemplator.com/scotland/kingjoy.html). In America the song was also known as Derry Down and The Old Women Taught Wisdom.

If buttercups buzz'd after the bee,  
If boats were on land, churches on sea,  
If ponies rode men and if grass ate the cows,  
And cats should be chased into holes by the mouse,  
If the mamas sold their babies  
To the gypsies for half a crown;  
If summer were spring and the other way round,  
Then all the world would be upside down.

CONTENTS

---

## Part 2

### Policy And The Mess In Nutrition

---

## Part 3

### Food And Eating



## Part 4

### The World Turned Upside Down

# INTRODUCTION

I've always had a weight problem. From old photographs, I would rarely have been considered fat but I was always trying to lose weight. When I was eight years old, I wanted to get thinner in order to look really sharp in my Brooklyn Dodgers uniform to impress Barbara Levy who was pretty obviously the most beautiful girl in the world. I don't recall having any great success and it was only fairly recently that I found out that Barbara Levy is now Barbara Boxer, Senator from California. In any case, I always knew that starch made me fat — oddly, I was less afraid of sugar because I thought, mistakenly, that there wasn't that much in Coca-Cola and other sodas, my major source. I probably grew up with what is usually called a poor self-image and, as the old joke goes, inside of every Botero is a Giacometti trying to get out.

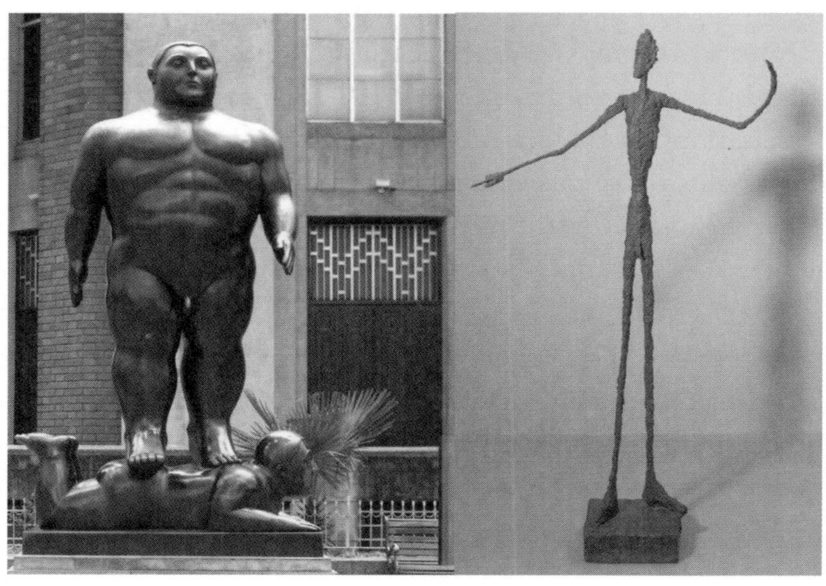

I did know to cut out starch and obvious solid sugar, however, and I made other observations, e.g., that cold cereal for breakfast made me slightly sick although I can't remember what I did eat. At least some of the time, it was bacon and eggs which, in those days, was just one of the things that people ate. Nobody recoiled in horror at bacon. The only dietary advice was to eat from the different food groups and there were graphics of pie charts with little symbols in each piece of the pie. The bottle of milk was one that stuck in my mind. I felt early on that it was not interesting. I knew that you didn't need an "expert" to tell you what to eat. When the USDA (United States Department of Agriculture) food pyramid appeared, I knew it was a crock and I assumed that everybody else did too. Everybody knows that, if you have a weight problem, bread will make you fat. And if you don't have a weight problem, why do you need the USDA. I assumed everybody was in agreement on that. That was not so. I am not sure why people went along. After all, it was about food. Everybody has experience of food. We all do three experiments in "nutritional science" each day. It probably had to do with the history of medicine. Among the turning points in that history was the discovery of vitamins. Unlike poisons and microorganisms, this was stuff that if you didn't have, made you sick. Another stimulus was the identification of cigarette smoke as a causal agent in lung disease. There, even though there was a toxic agent, the associations were more subtle and one needed statistics or other expert insights to see the connection. This may have given people the idea that there were experts who could see harm where we didn't.

In my youth, I simply ignored the problem. I thought that I knew what to eat (I was mostly right) and obesity was a personal rather than a professional question. Decades later, teaching metabolism, I had to confront the interaction of science and nutrition. It proved to be more difficult than I would have guessed. This book is the story of nutrition, a story of biochemistry and metabolism — how you process the food that you eat. It is an interesting story of the application of science to daily life. If you know a little chemistry, you can appreciate the way that evolution reached into the mixing pot of chemical reactions to obtain energy from the environment. Even if you don't know chemistry, you can see the beauty in the life machine.

But there is another side. As you might guess from the contentious and continually changing stories in the media, it is also a rather discouraging tale of the limitations of human behavior in facing truth and preventing harm. It is an almost unbelievable story of very poor and irresponsible science from the medical community, the most highly respected part of our society.

## THE PROBLEM OF EXPERTS AND EATING TO THE METER

However hard it is for scientists not to trust experts, it is harder for the general population. I was still astounded when I saw a question on an online diabetes site that said "My morning oatmeal spikes my blood glucose. How much carbohydrate should I have?" The answer from the experts was waffling and tedious but never included the advice "Don't eat any more oatmeal than that which *doesn't* spike your blood glucose."

So early on there was my interest in food and it remained an undercurrent. Later in life, it resurfaced in my professional life. There was also chemistry.

## CHEMISTRY

When I was eight years old, my father taught me about atoms — I have one of those memories that may or may not be accurate: sitting in my father's car, he is telling me that the whole world was made of atoms in the same way that the apartment house across the street was made of bricks. Whether or not the scene really took place, it was a major influence in my life and chemistry was a defining feature of my life. (Other vivid memories of my early life in Brooklyn, being at Ebbetts Field and seeing Jackie Robinson hit an inside-the-ballpark home run, turn out to not be true. He had hit only one, in 1948 before I had ever seen a live game).

The point of atomic theory, the thing that captures everybody's imagination when they are first exposed to it, is that it is a global and absolute theory; it explains everything that was done in the laboratory or even in the kitchen. Various fields of chemistry have that universal feeling with different degrees of intellectual rigor but eventually I recognized that biochemistry was a good place to be if you weren't sure what you wanted to be when you grow up. You can do drug design or theoretical chemistry or animal behavior or nutrition and still call yourself a biochemist.

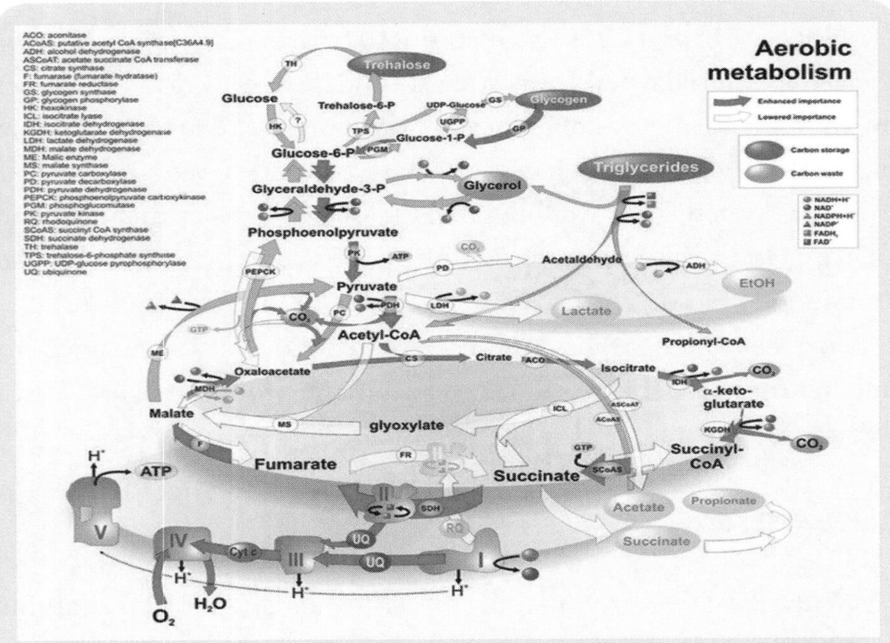


FIGURE 1-1. from Braeckman *et al.* Intermediary metabolism (February 16, 2009), WormBook, ed. The C. *elegans* Research Community, WormBook, doi/10.1895/wormbook.1.146.1, http://www.wormbook.org, distributed under terms of the Creative Commons Attribution License.

## TEACHING NUTRITION

I have worked in a number of fields in biochemistry but at SUNY Downstate Medical Center, where I have been for many years, it was teaching metabolism to medical students that led me into nutrition in a professional way.

Metabolism is the study of the processing of food and the biochemical reactions that control life functions. It is a fairly complicated subject, those parts that we understand. There are the numerous individual biochemical reactions and students tend to see the subject the way somebody described the study of history: just one damn thing after another. There are general principles and big concepts but you do have to know the details. Not all the details. Not all the stuff on the scary metabolic chart (**Figure 1-1**). At the end of the book, it'll be less scary.

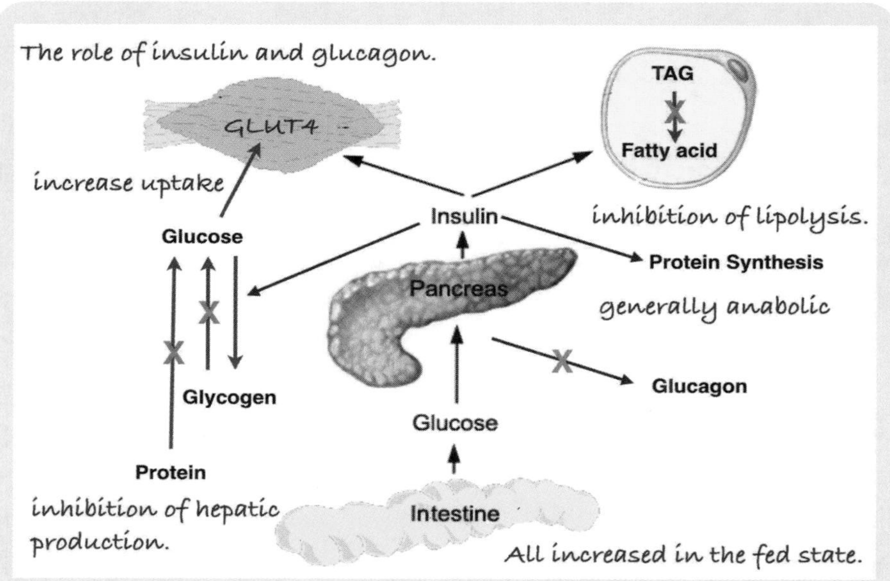


FIGURE 1-2. Insulin as a master controller of metabolism. In the fed state, stimulation of insulin secretion by the pancreas leads to protein synthesis, fat storage and maintenance of glycogen stores.

I used low-carbohydrate diets — at the time primarily a weight loss diet — as a heuristic device, that is, teaching method. Control of blood glucose and insulin (the hormone whose release is controlled by glucose) is really central to many different processes in biochemistry. The main idea is that in the complicated network of biochemical reactions, insulin stands out as a major point of regulation. **Figure I-2** shows how we describe it to medical students and this is how we will describe it here. The ups and downs of insulin are what we try to control in the use of dietary carbohydrate restriction as a therapeutic method. So, low-carbohydrate diets provided some unifying theme in teaching. I still teach it that way although now we emphasize diabetes where impaired ability to handle dietary carbohydrate is the salient feature. Low-carbohydrate diets are also popular — periodically very popular. It is likely that the current revolution can't be turned back. I and other people who use this teaching method have described how the real world can help learn the chemistry [1-3].

Around 2000, one of our medical students who had been a dietitian — we have several second career students — had a suggestion for our course. Her recommendation was to include formal nutrition in the biochemistry course and she provided subject matter from standard nutritional practice. I cannot really describe what it was about — probably, even at the time, it was so vacuous that it could not be retained in memory. Anyway, at first I objected because whatever it was, it wasn't about biochemistry. Criticizing how lectures are given is, of course, like complaining about how the dishes are done: everybody sees an immediate solution. I wound up having to give formal lectures in nutrition. I really didn't know the literature. I had long-ago found that carbohydrate restriction was best for me and, while low-carbohydrate diets provided me with a good framework for teaching metabolism, therapies do not always have a close relation to theories so it all involved a certain amount of background study.

My first lectures on nutrition were pretty much neutral. I simply tried to cover some aspects of low-carbohydrate and low-fat diets (these really are the two main choices) presenting the pros and cons of the different approaches in a simple way. Low-fat diets are not based substantially on biochemical mechanisms. They follow, mostly from observations, correlations between the presence of cholesterol or other lipids in the blood and cardiovascular disease — at least initially this was the main focus — or, as it morphed into a recommendation on obesity, it started emphasizing the point that fat has more calories per gram than other things and the obvious assumption that the more calories, the greater the effect on body weight — the ill-fated idea that "you are what you eat" which hangs over everything. Because metabolism explained, in some way, the apparent benefits of a low-carb diet, that did not mean that I could document the effects with established information from published science. So, my lectures were rather simple and straight-forward while I tried to get a grip on the scientific literature. It didn't take long to see that something was terribly wrong. In simply trying to get some of the facts, I stepped into a world of bad science, self-deception and a scandal equal to any in the history of medicine.

## THE NURSES HEALTH INITIATIVE

Science is very specialized. Although I had been doing research on blood coagulation, obviously related to cardiovascular disease (CVD), I did not pay much attention to the diet-heart hypothesis — the idea that fat and cholesterol in the diet raises blood cholesterol which, in turn, leads to CVD. I *was* suspicious of such a theory because biology tends to run on hormones and enzymes, that is, control mechanisms, not on mass action (the principle that chemical processes are determined by how much reactants are put into them). The grand principle in biochemistry is that there is hardly anything that is not connected with feedback.

If you try to lower your dietary cholesterol, the liver will respond by making more. So simply adding more or less is not guaranteed to give much change at all and I was skeptical if not well-informed.

Whatever my misgivings about diet-heart, however, I didn't question it very deeply. When I went back to the original literature to find the evidence supporting low-fat recommendations, as I had to do for preparing my lectures, it was a rude awakening. My assumption that there was at least a grain of truth in the diet-heart hypothesis was overly optimistic. If it is not a total sham, it is pretty close. One of the first papers that I came across in my literature survey was a report from the Nurses Health Study (NHS). As described by Wikipedia,

> "established in 1976 ... [the NHS] and the Nurses' Health Study II, established in 1989 by Dr. Walter Willett, are the most definitive long-term epidemiological studies conducted to date on women's health.... 121,700 female registered nurses since 1976 and 116,000 female nurses since 1989 to assess risk factors for cancer and cardiovascular disease....Participating organizations ... include the Harvard Medical School, Harvard School of Public Health, and several Harvard-affiliated hospitals...."

Willett and his associate Frank Hu [4] examined the risk of cardiovascular disease from substitution of different kinds of fat. Obviously, important stuff for my lectures. The study also asked about substituting carbohydrate. I found the result astounding. **Figure I-3**, redrawn from the paper, shows the effects of substituting one type of fat for another or of substituting carbohydrate for fat.

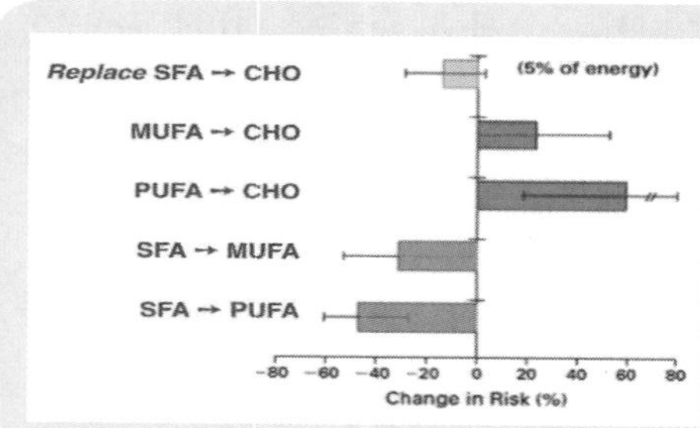


FIGURE I-3. Estimated Changes in Risk of Coronary Heart Disease Associated with Isocaloric Substitutions (error bars show 95% confidence interval). Redrawn from Hu, et al. [4]

The effect of these substitutions — whether risk went up (right side of the graph, red bars) or down (left, green bars) was surprising. Replacing saturated fat with either polyunsaturated fat (vegetable oils) or with monounsaturated fat (olive or canola oil) reduced risk substantially. That's what they've been saying so no surprise there. However, if the polyunsaturated fat was replaced with carbohydrate, Hu, *et al.* found an average 60 % increase in risk. What? Carbohydrate is worse than fat for cardiovascular risk? That's not how it was supposed to be. What about saturated fat? Surely, that's the bad guy.

Replacing saturated fat with carbohydrate does provide some benefit according to the figure but there is something else.

In this kind of figure, the (horizontal) error bars show the spread of individual values which, in this case, was pretty large. In other words, regardless of the average benefit of substituting monounsaturated fat for saturated, some people had much more and some, much less. Some, in fact, were going the other way. How bad could saturated fat be, if some people get worse when they substitute carbohydrate for saturated fat? It's worse. Without going into the details of the statistics, the rule is that if the (horizontal) error bars cross the zero line then there is no significant effect of the substitution (tan bar). Substituting carbohydrate in place of saturated fat was at best neutral, or more precisely, was as likely to increase risk as to lower it. And the same for monounsaturated fat. Looking at **Figure I-3**, it is hard to see a risk of fat — the authors were explicit about that — but hasn't risk from fat been the message all along? Certainly the idea that carbohydrate is a risk is not brought out in the media or the pronouncements of health agencies. And then there was the authors' summary of the paper:

> Our data provide evidence in support of the hypothesis that a higher dietary intake of saturated fat ... is associated with an increased risk of coronary disease, whereas a higher intake of monounsaturated and polyunsaturated fats is associated with reduced risk. These findings reinforce evidence from metabolic studies that replacing saturated

> fat...with unhydrogenated monounsaturated and polyunsaturated fats favorably alters the lipid profile, but that reducing overall fat intake has little effect.

That's the concluding paragraph of their paper. No mention of carbohydrate. The most striking thing to me was that if you looked at the risk from carbohydrates in comparison to the risk from saturated fat, that is, the risk of substituting one for the other, it didn't make any difference. And worse. Substituting carbohydrate for other fats *increased* risk. How could this be? Fat out. Carbohydrate in. Wasn't that the clear recommendation for improved health from just about every health agency and every expert. The data said it didn't matter. Was it dishonest not to bring that out in the discussion in the paper? At best, it was an error of omission. The authors from the Harvard School of Public Health were, and still are, the more modest among those vilifying fat, insisting that it is only the type of fat that we need worry about. I was probably not alone, but I invented the term "lipophobes" for proponents of low-fat. It's a wise guy term and since I was still something of an inside player in the science world, I was reluctant to put it into print until Michael Pollan started using it without any sense of irony [5].

This is the field that I was now professionally involved in. I did not adequately attend to the sense of being sucked into a whirlpool from which it would be hard to escape. And anyway, the data was there for all to see. It is the author's choice to play down the strongest result. I suspect that they thought that "reducing overall fat intake has little effect" was the major conclusion. It would still be surprising to many people even without knowing that substituting carbohydrate for fat raises risk.

A trip to the supermarket tells you that these results from the Nurses' Health Initiative had little effect; the low-fat story is still with us. More striking is that two meta-analyses — a questionable statistical procedure of trying to average many different studies — came to the same conclusion. [6-8]. Siri-Tarino, *et al.*, in particular, concluded that "...there are few epidemiologic or clinical trial data to support a benefit of replacing saturated fat with carbohydrate" [8] although they neglected to cite the low-carbohydrate studies that supported the position. In March of 2014, yet another meta-analysis came to the same conclusion. What will turn out to be most remarkable about all of these studies is that they present a re-analyses of studies that had found no effect of saturated fat to begin with. One has to ask why the results were not accepted when first published. Some of them are twenty years old.

*...from what we know now, from the current state of research, with the exception of well-defined genetic abnormalities...there may be no predictable effect on heart disease from your diet.*

How is it possible that, in this most scientific period in history, our society runs on incorrect scientific information? That's one of the questions that I will try to answer in this book — or at least describe. I am not sure that there is an answer. Looking ahead, I will introduce the revolutionary idea that, from what we know now, from the current state of research, with the exception of well-defined genetic abnormalities like familial hypercholesterolemia, there is no predictable effect of your diet on heart disease. It is a hypothesis and we may know more as we understand the genetics but the diet-heart hypothesis remains only a conjecture without experimental support. It will be one of the themes in this book and one of the battle grounds for the second-revolution.

## ABOUT THIS BOOK -WHO IT'S FOR -WHY I WROTE IT

Two big influences in my life: food and chemistry. Food is close to biochemistry. The beauty of biochemistry is that it relates the movement of electrons to what's on your plate and I thought I could explain it. I like writing about biochemistry. Sometimes we can see it all fit together and if we take a lot of the things that we know for granted, thinking about what we don't know can make us curious, the defining feature of the scientific life. If you want to know how it works, you are the person I had in mind when I started the book.

This is a book for scientists. Not particularly for guys with an atomic-force microscope in their lab, but for people who want to look at nutrition from a scientific point of view. Science is less about sophisticated measurements, than it is about basic honesty. It is true that scientific fields can be very mathematical or intellectually profound — the warning that if you think you understand quantum mechanics you are already on the wrong track has been attributed to many physicists, probably because most of them have actually said it — but all sciences, even quantum mechanics, are tied to logic and common sense, and are frequently directly accessible. Part of the game, most researchers feel, is to make the results easy to understand. Einstein is widely quoted as saying that we want to make it simple but not too simple. Modern medicine, despite its reliance on technology, explicitly accepts an obligation to explain things logically to the patient. It doesn't always fulfill this obligation well but that is the goal.

I will try to fill some of the gaps and define words. For the tough spots, you have to read it like a scientist. How do we read? We're all specialists and most of us can't read a technical article, sometimes even in our own field, without some bumps. Skip over the bumps and see if you can get the big picture and maybe come back to it later. And a lot of the details are just a Google away.

If you write a book about biochemistry, it's about chemistry but if you write a book about nutrition, it's about everything. So, not every chapter in this book is for everybody. I have tried to provide a continuous thread but different subjects require different kinds of discussion. The goal was to make the individual discussions self-contained and to provide technical background as we go but some topics are necessarily technical and I include those that are important. You can skip them but I suggest giving them a shot.

And you can't escape the sociology and politics of medicine. Establishment medical journals and the private and government health agencies have insisted on low-fat, low-calorie dogma in the face of all its failures. This breakdown in scientific practice is deeply discouraging to me and was an additional motivation for my writing this book.

Beyond the corruption of science is the harm to the patient. A major focus of this book is the concept of the metabolic syndrome. The idea that superficially different physiologic states — overweight, high blood pressure, the so-called atherogenic dyslipidemia (the lipid markers that are assumed to contribute to cardiovascular disease) — are tied together and in combination indicate risk of disease is, in my view, a great intellectual insight. That the common effector is likely the hormone insulin, points to the importance of controlling dietary carbohydrate, the major stimulus for insulin secretion.

The resistance of the medical profession to dietary carbohydrate restriction in the treatment of metabolic syndrome and, more important, to its most obvious risk, diabetes, I find incomprehensible. Everybody knows somebody with diabetes. Echoes of the early days in Brooklyn made it very upsetting to see pictures of Jackie Robinson taken shortly before his death from diabetes complications at age 52. Because it is progressive, the disease is an under-appreciated source of suffering. Clinicians will tell you that it is like cancer in its devastating effects. Diabetes is the major cause of amputations after accidents and the major cause of acquired blindness. That is a motivation for writing this book and why you may find it important.

It is a scandal at the level of Semmelweis, an early nineteenth century Viennese physician. To reduce the incidence of puerperal fever (infection after childbirth), Semmelweis suggested that physicians wash their hands after performing autopsies and before delivering babies. They refused; it was too much trouble. But it was the nineteenth century before the germ theory was established and that's some kind of excuse. It's hard to know how we will describe the actions of the American Diabetes Association (ADA) who believe that for people with diabetes:

> "Sucrose-containing foods can be substituted for other carbohydrates in the meal plan or, if added to the meal plan, covered with insulin or other glucose-lowering medications." [9]

The most difficult part of writing this book is understanding, or again, at least describing — I don't think it is possible to understand — how the whole field of medical nutrition could be wrong. Way wrong. Not in detail but totally off the mark. As misguided as the alchemists' pursuit of creation of gold. And, however bizarre the distance from science in this most scientific of ages, there is the real harm to patients. It is hard to explain because the esteem in which medicine is held is based on real accomplishment and expertise and it is hard to see why they would go so wrong in nutrition. For me, having precedents makes it real if not completely comprehensible. Here's one that I keep in mind. It's about the Israeli Defense Forces and Intelligence on the days before the Yom Kippur War (1973):

> The intelligence chiefs believed they knew a deeper truth...that rendered irrelevant all the cries of alarm going up around them. Zeira and his chief aides were to demonstrate the ability of even brilliant men to adhere to an *idée fixe* in the face of mountains of contrary evidence .... They clung to their view even though the Egyptian

> deceptions were contradicted by evidence of war preparations that AMAN's [military intelligence] own departments were daily gathering.... But the deception succeeded beyond even Egypt's expectations because it triggered within Israel's intelligence arm and senior command a monumental capacity for self-deception.
>
> — Rabinovitch, The Yom Kippur War

They could have lost it all. They could have lost the whole country. They were largely saved by a couple of field commanders (notably Ariel Sharon) who were wild and crazy guys. (Audacity and not following orders may be what saves nutrition as well).

Finally, this book is for the person (and those for whom she spoke) who posted this on my blog.

> How does one know if a study is 'flawed'? I see a lot of posts on here that say a lot of major studies are flawed. How? Why? What's the difference if I am gullible and believe all the flawed studies, or if I (am hopefully not a sucker) believe what the Fat Heads [a low-carb site] are saying and not to believe the flawed studies — eat bacon.
>
> Where are the true studies that are NOT flawed.... and how do I differentiate? : /

She was right to be suspicious. It is not always easy. There are so many nutrition papers that try to snow you with technical detail and, in fact, those are the ones to be suspicious of. There are technical parts of scientific papers but you need to be sure that they aren't making it harder than it needs to be. And, some of the papers are simply not true. Most researchers know that if you make up the data on a federally-funded grant, you can go to jail, but in interpreting things, you can say just about any damned thing. I will try to explain how to interpret these papers. In particular, I will try to explain what the statistics mean. What they mean for somebody who doesn't know much about statistics.

## THE SECOND LOW-CARB REVOLUTION

The killer-app is still the treatment of diabetes with a low-carbohydrate diet. Intuitively obvious, proved in many experimental trials and widely used anecdotally and clinically, there are virtually no contra-indications. Resistance to its use appears to rest entirely with pressure from political organizations, primarily the American Diabetes Association (ADA) which, while looking for a way to save face, still refuses to endorse low-carbohydrate strategies. The latest guidelines emphasize "individualization" presumably as a way of softening their previous opposition to low-carbohydrate. The word is used 21 times in their position paper [10]. However, what principles are to be used for each individual are not stated. The foolishness of recommending carbohydrates for people with a disease whose most salient manifestation is an inability to adequately metabolize carbohydrates is not disowned. "Individualization" is correctly called a cop-out. According to http://www.merriam-webster.com/ "an excuse for not doing something; something that avoids dealing with a problem in an appropriate way."

We also have, at the same time, a constant flow of blogposts and books that show the low-fat-diet-heart hypothesis for the intellectual and clinical disaster that it really was (or is). The most recent, most complete, *The Big Fat Surprise* [11] is surprising in its description of the depths of self-delusion if not dishonesty in keeping low-fat alive. While the pace of criticism is increasing, these exposés document that the diet-heart hypothesis has been debunked since its inception. What is new is that the efficacy of statins, the last hope, the big bail-out for the lipophobes, is now seriously in question.

If you step back and look at the data, the "concerns," the voices on the Huffington post or the numerous blogs belonging to dietitians who have set up a business, it shines through that the easiest way to lose weight is to go on a low-carbohydrate diet. The "concerns," voiced for forty years, have never materialized and the tests of carbohydrate restriction come out in its favor, however poorly they are cited. There are now dozens of implementations, although the Atkins name has attained a somewhat generic status like Kleenex®. Silence is, in fact, the most widely used tactic of the naysayers although they are surprisingly aggressive when they do say something.

At the same time, there is a frantic effort to seek out an alternative, Mediterranean diets, low-glycemic (GI) index diets, low-sugar diets or whatever Dr. Oz is pushing when you read this. This book has been sometime in the writing, and when I wrote the previous sentence, I meant "Dr. Oz" in the generic sense of the latest cure-all, not knowing what he actually thought but, by May of 2014, Dr. Oz was, in fact, pushing a low-carbohydrate diet, or at least running alongside it. The interview with a proponent of dietary carbohydrate restriction can be seen at http://bit.ly/1uOoL1D under the headline "...Dr. Peter Attia and Dr. Oz on Saturated Fat. Oz Admits He's Been Wrong." This has to be taken as an important sign of the progress in the second low-carb revolution although I am not sure what Dr. Oz will be pushing when this book is in front of your eyes.

## METABOLIC SYNDROME -METABOLIC CONTROL

There is almost nothing in biology that is not connected with feedback. This fundamental idea is widely ignored but it is pervasive. If you reduce your intake of cholesterol, your body will respond by synthesizing cholesterol. If you stop eating carbohydrate, your body will respond by synthesizing glucose and making other fuels available. This grand idea puts severe limitations on what you can do (as in the case of cholesterol) but can point to some opportunities (as in the case of carbohydrate reduction) but generally, it suggests caution in jumping to conclusions.

The paradox is that, given the first principle, there is a global effect of the hormone insulin. We can get very far simply by regulating this hormone. While not free from feedback, the effects of manipulating insulin can be highly predictable, the main theme of this book. Always in the background is the metabolic syndrome (MetS). The observation, generally credited to Gerald Reaven, endocrinologist and currently Professor Emeritus at Stanford, was that a collection of seemingly different physiologic effects — overweight, high blood pressure, high blood glucose, high insulin and the collection of blood lipid markers referred to as atherogenic dyslipidemia (high triglycerides, low HDL) — were all tied together by a common causal thread, the disruption in the metabolic response to insulin [12]. The physiologic markers of MetS predict progression to the associated disease states (obesity, diabetes, hypertension and cardiovascular disease) but all respond to dietary carbohydrate restriction. That is the big pitch. This observation provides evidence that it really is a syndrome (has a common underlying cause) and simultaneously points us to the most effective treatment. No dietary approach is better and no drug will target all of the markers.

There are, in fact, critics of MetS who doubt that it is a syndrome at all, but what they really mean, is that the effects have to be treated with a collection of drugs, drugs for diabetes, drugs for heart disease, drugs for high blood pressure. A low-carb diet which is widely accepted as effective for weight loss is likely a strategy for general health for most people. Acceptance of such a notion is the goal of the revolution.

Oddly enough, the bright light on the horizon is the ketogenic diet for cancer. Oddly, because carbohydrate-restriction for diabetes is a slam-dunk and that should have been the crystallizing point for change. As a therapy, it virtually guarantees results insofar as there is anything like a guarantee in this business. Carbohydrate restriction follows from basic biochemistry and there are a large number of very strong tests. Yet there is extensive resistance to its use for people with diabetes.

Against this background, treatment of cancer is not encountering the same obstinacy despite the fact that we have very little solid evidence at all. We do see a close connection of cancer with obesity and diabetes and the role of insulin which seems to carry the day as it couldn't for obesity and diabetes. I describe work by my colleague, Eugene Fine, targeting insulin in the treatment of cancer. I describe this work and its acceptance, despite its small size as a research project, as the sign of future progress [13]. If it turns out that we learn to treat diabetes by learning to treat cancer, it would not be the strangest thing that ever happened in science.

## ORGANIZATION

If we had ham, we could have ham and eggs, if we had eggs.

— *Old American idiom*

It's all tied together. The science is not divorced from the politics. The Framingham study [14], the first very large population trial would test not only a scientific principle — whether dietary fat and cholesterol are related to risk of cardiovascular disease (they were not) — but also whether the recommendations of health agencies were a rush to judgment (they were). The study had such a large political component that, striking as the scientific outcome was — there was no effect of dietary fat, saturated fat or cholesterol on cardiovascular disease — it just couldn't be seen to fail. The results were not published and were buried for years until rediscovered by a statistician who had it published. This intertwining of the political and the science is a pattern that persists and I try to tell both stories and the effect of their mixture.

I have opted for loose organization and some degree of repetition. Put another way, because everything is tied together, regardless of what kind of organization I chose, the output will be loose. My main principle, however, is that basic science comes first. I give preference to the demonstrations in nutritional and medical practice that come out of the fundamental results of biochemistry, of hard science. Big clinical trials have to be judged on their inherent strength but, if they contradict basic science, they have an obligation to explain why. And science is continuous with common sense. It doesn't matter how many statistical tests you have, if the results violate common sense, it is unlikely to be science.

The poor research published by prestigious people and prestigious institutions means the nature of science itself has to be investigated. So, we will have to define scientific principles and explain how to read a scientific paper and decide if peer review has done its job. Finally, I will provide information on cooking and eating.

But first, the answer. In **Chapter 1**, I give you the bottom line, the practical consequences of the science. The rest of the book will try to justify the statements and recommendations.

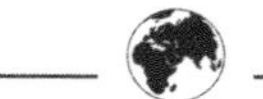

# Part 1

## Nutrition And Metabolism

---

## The Stuff You Eat
## And What Happens To It

---

# Chapter 1

# The Summary In Advance

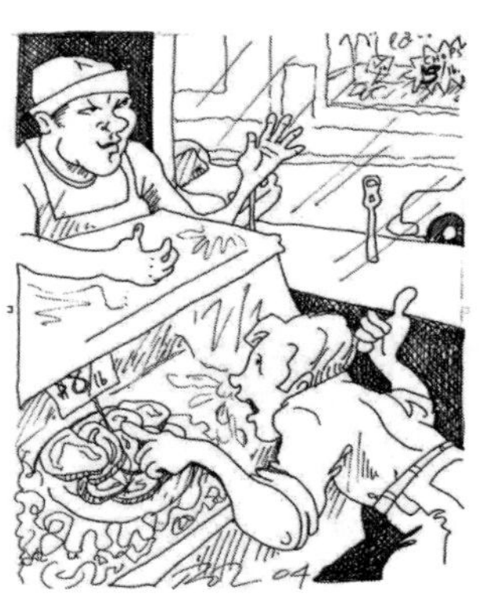

What should I eat?" That's the question that I invariably get at my lectures to medical students or presentations at a scientific meeting or even in a private conversation about scientific experiments. The level of technical detail that I discuss varies with the audience but people always want to know the bottom line. It is not unreasonable to ask for practical advice.

Sometimes the question is framed as "What's the best diet?", which I can answer with the old joke about the guy who goes to the butcher and sees that pork chops are $8 a pound.

Customer: "Why so much? Across the street, he is selling them for $5 a pound."

Butcher: "Why don't you buy them there?"

Customer: "Today, he's all out."

Butcher: "When I'm all out, they're only $2 a pound."

The best diet is the one that works. It doesn't matter how "scientific" it is or how "healthy" your physician thinks it is. If you gain weight, or if your fasting blood sugar goes up, it's useless or worse. It would be hard to say that the diet recommended by government and private health agencies has provided much help for the current widespread obesity and diabetes. Defenders usually tell you that it is because people are not really following the guidelines. They don't say *how* they know that the recommendations are good if nobody follows it. So here are three rules that I propose as a good guide. Also, a few principles that will help you follow them. These are different from what your doctor may say and the rest of the book will justify these principles.

## THE THREE RULES FOR GETTING CONTROL OF YOUR DIET

**RULE 1.** If you're OK, you're OK.

**RULE 2.** If you want to lose weight: Don't eat. If you have to eat, don't eat carbs. If you have to eat carbs, eat low-glycemic index carbs.

**RULE 3.** If you have diabetes or metabolic syndrome, carbohydrate restriction is the "default" approach, that is, the one to try first.

**RULE 1** is actually surprising to many people: If you don't have a weight problem, if you feel OK, if you are healthy and if you do not have a family history of disease, there is no compelling reason to change your diet. You may want to find out more about nutrition and biochemistry but the idea that there was once a Garden of Eden diet that we all ate until somebody brought high fructose corn syrup into the world and all our woe seems unlikely.

Not everybody has this view. There is the idea, not always said explicitly, that, analogous to Freud's *The Psychopathology of Everyday Life*, we are all doing something wrong and life is a continuous battle between what our bodies really need and the pressures of civilization. It's not like that. We evolved to be adaptable. Lots of dietary approaches work and none of us are going to get out of this alive.

And then there's the Nutritional Guidelines for Americans from the USDA (Department of Agriculture) – the Department is specifically charged by congress with providing advice to people who are healthy, that is, people who don't need advice, or, as we say in Brooklyn, fixing something that ain't broke. Like psychoanalysts, they feel endowed by their creator with the intuitive power to penetrate unspoken, unmeasured, deep truths and are able to tell us that we are not eating the right thing and that we are at risk for some future disease. They are, however, quick to take offense if you suggest that their inability to control the epidemic of obesity and diabetes makes it very unlikely that they know what the right thing is.

**Rule 2.** If you want to lose weight: Don't eat. If you have to eat, don't eat carbs. If you have to eat carbs, eat low-GI carbs.

I said this as a joke at a conference but there is much truth in it. Not that starvation is a good long-term strategy — the danger is that you will lose muscle mass along with your fat — but frequently we think that it is important to eat all the time. That is not true and intermittent fasting, which is garnering a certain amount of interest, may be a very useful strategy for weight loss. There are exceptions; some medical conditions, diabetes in particular, may require individual variation. Calorie reduction is beneficial for diabetes but the need to avoid ups and downs means that there are other considerations. We tend to think that hunger is some kind of physiologic signal telling us that our body needs food. We think that this is a signal that must be answered immediately. It's not like that. Chapter 13 will make the argument that hunger only means that you are in a situation where you are used to eating. It may be a situation, like the business lunch or the tail-gate party that has little to do with your state of nourishment. The hunger pangs that you feel may be real enough but you are not compelled to answer them.

Calories are a measure of the total energy available from burning food. The less food you eat, the less energy you will have. Not all calories are the same though. Many experiments that show success with calorie reduction, on analysis, reveal that the effect was due to the *de facto* reduction in carbohydrate. Some dietary strategies will waste more energy than others (as heat and other unproductive effects). That's what the second part of **Rule 2** says, but it is still true that if you don't eat, you will get thin.

## CARBOHYDRATE RESTRICTION

Calories count but the advice by experts, that *only* calories count, is wrong. There are great advantages to diet strategies that go beyond calories.

For most people the best long-term (or short-term) strategy for weight loss will be to reduce carbohydrate intake. There are extensive data in the medical literature to support this idea but the best evidence may be anecdotal. In the field of weight-loss, anecdotal evidence is pretty good. Everybody knows somebody who lost a lot of weight on the Atkins diet. Some report that the pounds seem to "melt away." There is no guarantee that you will have the same experience and everybody hits a plateau but it is still your best bet. People who are on low-carbohydrate diets — and they usually are the people who have had trouble with other kinds of diets — will tell you that they are easy to stay on. Those who quit, may or may not gain weight but rarely gain back all of the lost weight. People who give dire warnings about low-carb diets almost always are people who have not tried them and when they tell you that patients can't stay on low-carb diets, it turns out they have never actually recommended them to their patients. Even these people sometimes change their mind. My experience, also, is that it is a ratchet. People rarely go back to low-fat. And contrary to the *kvetching* on TV, there are many things to eat. Chapter 25 will give you some recipes to get you started.

Low-carb diets follow from basic biochemistry. The key factor is improved control of insulin, the anabolic (building up) hormone that is most reliably controlled by carbohydrate. They are consistently successful and that is what keeps it going. As in any diet, people may quit at a certain point — we have 600 million years of evolution and a lifetime of behavioral conditioning telling us to eat anything that tastes good — but once successful, even if we fall off the wagon, it is usually to a low-carb diet that we go back to. Nutritionists will tell you that "yo-yo dieting" has some risk but there is no evidence for that and, of course, we are happy for the period where we are thin, however long that is.

Whatever is good or bad about low-carbohydrate strategies, for most people, low-fat diets are worse than doing nothing. Some people can do well on them — there is an advantage in feeling hungry — but most of us can't. If you can get yourself into the frame of mind where you like the "lean and hungry" feel, then anything that reduces calories will be okay. All diets have recidivism but most people on low-fat, calorie-restricted diets don't even get the opportunity to fall off the wagon — if you don't lose weight, there is no wagon. That the experts tell you, it is better to lose weight slowly, should be a tip-off. Everything else we do in life we try to do as quickly and efficiently as possible. We recognize that it may take longer than we want. Only psychoanalysis and conventional low-calorie weight loss set out to go slowly by design.

The scientific literature backs up the anecdotal evidence. Jeff Volek, one of the major researchers in carbohydrate restriction put this spin on it: "Nutrition research is hard. Too many things change and it's easy to come up with nothing. When you study low-carb diets, people lose weight. Put people on a low-carb diet and you get real data." As I finish this book, the long-standing refusal of the nutritional establishment to face the data is finally falling away. It will be increasingly easy to follow a low-carbohydrate approach. It will be more common to have the support of physicians. Experimentally, carbohydrate restriction has better compliance than anything else possibly due to the greater satiety of protein and fat or, more likely, the poor satiety in most carbohydrates. Current fashion is to say that sugar is addictive which trivializes the serious, sometimes life-threatening consequence of real addictions, like alcohol and narcotics but, for whatever reason, people on low-carbohydrate diets reduce food intake spontaneously and, in addition, benefit from an inherent efficiency in weight lost calorie-for-calorie. The doctrine that only calories count is not true however vehement its defense. You can test for yourself, at least at the level of perception. You can find out if, on a low-carbohydrate diet you *seem* to be eating more even while losing weight.

Later chapters will describe experimental studies that support these conclusions about low-carbohydrate strategies but there is one truly remarkable phenomenon that tells you about the edge low-carbohydrate diets have in satiety. When diet comparisons are carried out experimentally, most often the protocol is to allow the low-carbohydrate group freedom to eat *ad lib* as long as they follow the restrictions on carbohydrate. Low-fat controls, on the other hand, are restricted to a fixed number of calories. The rationale is that many popular low-carbohydrate diets, like the Atkins Diet, put no limit on consumption — the idea is that fat and protein intake is self-limiting when carbohydrate is low. Setting up the experiment this way is poor experimental design in that you are now testing two things; the ability of a low-carbohydrate diet to limit caloric intake as well as the proposed difference in physiologic effects of the type of diet. (It also raises the stakes on the carbohydrate-restricted diet). Nonetheless, the fact that the low-carbohydrate diet almost always wins in such comparisons tells you that, as advertised, you don't have to count calories in a diet based on carbohydrate restriction. (Again, not that calories don't count, but rather that they take care of themselves).

The greatest virtue of carb restriction is its fail-safe feature. If you are not rapidly losing weight or seem to hit the wall, it is a way of eating (WOE) that gives you freedom from the sense of fighting a war against fat. You will almost never gain weight and you will escape that overbearing feeling that every meal is a battle. The real threat of overweight is not health. Mortality correlates with weight only at the very extremes. The real threat is the sense of loss of control. I am not a health care provider but I get emails from executives, officers in the military, people who hold dominion over their professional world but who have trouble controlling their own body mass. For the average person, it can take over their life. It can be a tremendous psychological burden. Cut out most of the carbs in your life and life is better.

The glycemic index (GI) follows from the same principle as carbohydrate restriction, control of insulin effects, but the approach focuses on the predicted effect of dietary carbohydrate on your blood glucose. Numbers are assigned to different foods based on the increase in blood glucose for the two hours following ingestion of fixed amounts of carbohydrate. This number, the GI, is relative to the effect of the same amount of pure glucose or, following nutritionists' seeming penchant for imprecision, to the same amount of white bread. In the end, a low-GI diet is a weak form of low-carbohydrate diet. It never does as well as real low-carbohydrate diets in experimental trials and it is easier to simply reduce carbohydrate because you know what you're doing whereas low-GI has all kinds of practical limitations. Because it is fundamentally an experimental, as opposed to theoretical, parameter the average of the GI of the different individual foods in a meal is not guaranteed to be the GI of the actual meal. (And, of course, it involves counting and calculation which is just how diets maintain control over your life). For many nutritionists, it is a politically correct *alternative* to low-carbohydrate diets but the point of **Rule 2** is that it is strictly secondary to real reduction in total carbohydrate.

**RULE 3.** If you have diabetes or metabolic syndrome, carbohydrate restriction is the "default" approach, that is, the one to try first.

Almost everyone is now within two degrees of separation of somebody who has diabetes. Diabetes is a disease of carbohydrate intolerance. In type 1, there is a substantially reduced or total inability of the pancreas to produce insulin in response to carbohydrate. Type 2 is characterized by poor response of the cells of the body to the insulin that is produced (insulin resistance) as well as progressive deterioration of the insulin-producing cells of the pancreas. The defining symptom and major cause of the pathology is high blood sugar. The idea for treatment is simple. If diabetes is a disease of carbohydrate intolerance, it seems reasonable that adding dietary carbohydrate would make things worse. This expectation is generally borne out. It may seem odd to appeal to common sense in an age when the CEO of a failed public company can pay himself a hundred million dollars, but that's how it is. There are people with diabetes who can tolerate greater or lesser amounts of carbohydrate but, for most people, it works exactly as it is supposed to and dietary carbohydrate restriction may even be best for those people who can tolerate higher carbohydrate. And there are no experimental or clinical data that show a contradiction. I will make the case that diabetes, because of its ties to insulin, represents a kind of extreme case of other metabolic conditions like obesity.

It is amazing that anyone would suggest anything other than carbohydrate restriction for people with diabetes, but the low-fat propaganda is very pervasive. Many "diabetes educators" still recommend reducing fat rather than reducing carbohydrates for people with diabetes, a testament to the triumph of politics over science.

If you are on medication, you have to do a low-carbohydrate diet with your physician: Carbohydrate restriction will have the same effect in lowering blood glucose as many medications and you need to avoid hypoglycemia (low blood sugar). Some people see this as the single best argument for carbohydrate restriction; in most diseases, reduction in medication is considered a sign of success. Generally, your physician, if he or she has any experience with carbohydrate restriction, will reduce or eliminate your medication before putting you on a low-carbohydrate diet.

## Doing It: Eat to the Meter

This is the principle used by people with diabetes. The meter is the glucometer which does what it sounds like. It measures blood glucose. If the food you just ate causes a spike in blood sugar, it is a sign to avoid that food. Oddly, diabetes educators may tell you that if the food spikes your blood glucose, that means you need more insulin to deal with that food.

Those of us with a weight problem might sensibly eat to what I call the ponderometer, the bathroom scale. More generally, eat for results as in the butcher, above, who is not out of pork chops. If the experts tell you to eat more whole grains and they seem to be making you fat, stop!

## Doing It: The Best Exercise Is One That You Do

The nutrition world agrees on very few things but there are few detractors from the principle that exercise is inherently beneficial. It is not really good for weight loss by itself unless you're a professional athlete or in basic training, but it does enhance the benefits of dieting.

Some of the effects are vascular, that is physiologic rather than biochemical, so it is hard to pin down the relation to nutrition but finding any agreement in any field is always a good thing.

The best exercise, like the best diet, is the one that you can get yourself to do regularly. That may be an individual thing. Proponents of each type of exercise think that the others are no good but you can find one that fits your style or, more important, one that you get in the habit of doing, even if it is not your style. I am personally a believer in slow-burn (slow repetition with heavy weights) [15]. It is probably best for people who think that they are entering old age, in that it is efficient; you can get perceptible benefit from one set of 90 seconds.

An encouraging development in exercise physiology is the technique that they call "periodization," a pretentious way of saying that it is good to mix up different types of exercise on different days. You now have official sanction for switching between different types of exercise because you are bored.

## DOING IT: PREPARE FOR BATTLE. PREPARE FOR VICTORY

Even the easiest diet has problems, ups and downs and temptations. You do have to think about what you are going to do in different situations. If you know that the celebratory business meeting will be serving pizza, go in with a plan. (Eat beforehand, decide if you are comfortable enough with the group to eat the top off the pizza, etc.) There are techniques for staying on your diet and dealing with hunger, but you also have to prepare for success, that is, what to do, if you actually aren't hungry. If you decide to do a low-carbohydrate diet and you sit down to the recommended broccoli and steak and you are full after eating one quarter of what you usually eat, you should be prepared to stop. In restaurants, doggie-bags are good unless it is your first date but then you'll probably be on your best behavior anyway.

What should you do if the birthday cake looks disgusting and you don't *want* to eat it? It is, after all, your boss's birthday. There are many techniques. Put the birthday cake on your plate. Walk around the room stabbing at it with your fork. After a while you can put in on the sideboard with all the other half-eaten pieces of cake.

## DOING IT: MINISTER TO YOURSELF -CROSS-EXAMINE EXPERTS

Doctors don't study nutrition. Nutritionists don't study medicine. Neither studies much science. It is a stereotype, or at least an exaggeration — there are many great scientists trained as MDs — but stereotypes come from someplace. There are no special requirements for being able to do a good scientific experiment. Having an MD, however, is not sufficient to qualify you as an expert on anything except your medical specialty. You have to learn a lot yourself and you have to ask the experts to justify their opinions. In the end, you are your own expert. Go for results rather than experts. Isn't this the same as **Rule 4** "Eat to the Meter"? Let's call it a corollary.

Perhaps the hardest thing to deal with is the idea that the whole field of professional nutrition might be fundamentally flawed. It is genuinely hard to understand that the progression of warnings about how red meat or white rice will kill you might not only be contrary to your own intuition but might actually be scientifically meaningless. It is hard to accept the idea that the dozens of publications coming out of the Harvard School of Public Health and published in *The New England Journal of Medicine* are of extremely poor scientific quality. Where's peer review? Where's expert training? All we can say is that there are many precedents in medicine and you have to be open to the possibility.

## DOING IT: THE LOW-CARBOHYDRATE PRINCIPLES

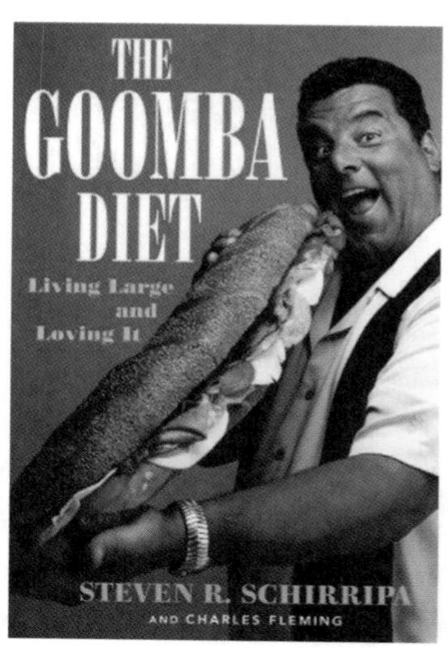


My personal preference is for principles over formal "diets." However, if you like diets, that is, something with formal instructions, there are millions: The American Diabetes Association diet (they deny that they have one but they do), The Russian Air Force Diet which is very effective if you don't go AWOL; typical breakfast is a cup of coffee. (Undoubtedly better than during WWII but it is not a good idea to go AWOL in the Russian Armed Forces). There is also *The Goomba Diet*, by and for Italian-Americans (could I have made this up?). The paleo diets are like the Mediterranean diet in that nobody really knows what they are but they are generally low-carb. Numerous books and websites will give you precise instructions.

For low-carb diets, *The New Atkins for a New You* [16], *Protein Power* [17] and *The Art and Science of Low-Carbohydrate Living* [115] are a good start. Numerous books and web-sites give you excellent recipes. If your MO is to just fit the general strategy to your own lifestyle, these are the big principles:

## DOING LOW-CARB: YOUR CARBS COME FROM VEGETABLES

The simplest way to break into carbohydrate restriction is by brute force; no rice, no potatoes, no bread and no pasta... and, of course, no dessert beyond small amount of fruit. As above, if you normally eat a steak with potatoes and broccoli, leave out the potatoes. This may be all you have to do. If you are now full on this lower amount of food, put the rest in the refrigerator, or throw it out (if you're worried about starving people, give money to the appropriate charity). If you want to add something back, you can have more steak but, in fact, most people don't want more steak even if they can afford it. So, it's usually more broccoli. Vegetables contain some carbohydrate but the important thing is that you don't really have to count anything. You are likely to have real success with this simple approach. If you have diabetes or metabolic syndrome, you are virtually guaranteed to get better although, again, if you are taking medication, you have to do this with a physician.

To go beyond the basic principles you need to understand that there is both a graded response —— the benefit is roughly proportional to the amount of carbohydrate that you remove from your eating —— as well as a breakpoint. The breakpoint, where there is enhanced weight loss, is generally considered to be marked by the presence of ketone bodies in the blood (ketosis) and urine.

Strictly speaking, the presence of ketone bodies in the urine is called ketonuria (although frequently taken as a sign of ketosis). The ketone bodies indicate a significant switch from reliance on carbohydrate as an energy source to a new predominantly fat-based metabolism. At this point, you will have to attend more precisely to how much carbohydrate you actually ingest. The simple rules will likely get you in the range of 100 g/day which is a big switch for most Americans. To go into ketosis you will have to go below 20-50 g/day (different people have different cut-offs).

The popular Atkins diet recommends that you stay in ketosis for two weeks and then gradually add carbohydrate back presumably for reasons of taste although possibly on the principle that you want to be close to what you are used to but not making yourself fat. Many people stay in ketosis indefinitely but it requires more attention and usually a period of adaptation.

My survey of the Low-Carber Forums (an internet support group) found that most people on low-carb diets eat all the non-root vegetables that they want and don't really count grams of carbohydrate [18] even though most of these people thought that they were on the Atkins diet. At least thinking that you are on a formal diet may not be too restrictive.

If you eat at home a lot it is good to learn how to cook vegetables. Like most such tasks, cooking vegetables involves investing large amounts of time in deep thought and procrastination and a relatively small amount of time actually doing the job. The solution is usually to time yourself. It's always way less time than you think. So, find the appropriate vegetable dishes for, either quick cooking, or for cooking in advance. Cauliflower is a kind of representative of low-carb diets and you can make a steamed cauliflower in a few minutes. Eat it straight or use it later for other very quick recipes. Cooking vegetables has a number of peculiarities described in Chapter 25 which includes a few recipes to get you started.

## DOING LOW-CARB: DON'T BE AFRAID OF FAT

**Fat is what people eat.** The anti-fat campaign has been one of the truly bizarre phenomena in the history of science — in this most scientific of periods, we have simply ignored the failures of the numerous experimental tests of the low-fat idea. Proponents of fat reduction have done all the big, expensive studies. They've put it to the test. The experiments almost always fail, but they keep doing them on the chance that something new will happen, on the chance that some unexpected change in the universe will make the saturated fat that they know is so bad, actually have a bad outcome. It's got to be.

Wherever the idea came from, it was wrong. Fat consumption, if anything, went down during the obesity epidemic — almost all of the increase in calories was in carbohydrates. There is no evidence that there is anything wrong with saturated fat but if you don't like it, there are numerous alternatives. Our understanding of carbohydrate as the control element, and fat as a more passive passenger, suggests that the combination of high carbohydrate *and* high fat will be a bad thing. But you don't want to try to be low-carb and low-fat unless you like feeling hungry. You may like the feeling, and total calorie restriction has general health benefits, but the *de facto* reduction in carbohydrate is probably the controlling factor.

## DOING LOW-CARB: GIVE UP DESSERT AND SWEETS

Reducing sugar is part of reducing carbohydrate. For some people, it may be all you need, or at least enough to get you started. **It will be beneficial if you don't put starch back in place of the sugar that you remove.** The strange collection of bedfellows currently involved in the political movement that I call fructophobia, the attack on sugar, forgot to tell you that sugar is a carbohydrate. If you cut out sugar and replace it with "healthy" high-grain, high-carbohydrate oatmeal, you are stacking the cards against yourself. For many people cutting out sugar is easy but if you have a sweet tooth, you will need some help. One strategy is to imagine that you are conducting an experiment. The hypothesis from anecdotal observation is that cravings for sweets disappear in three days on zero sweets. Your experiment will test whether that is true for you.

If you have to have something sweet, there are several non-nutritive sweeteners, some natural, some artificial. You may want to avoid artificial sweeteners, especially in diet soda since they may sustain your taste for sweets and some people react poorly to them. The scare stories about the artificial sweeteners are not scientifically sound but the possible effect of "sweetness" may be real. Among the simple solutions if you don't mind the artificial sweeteners is sour cream sweetened with sugar-free syrups.

You should do whatever works but I think that, for most people, it is probably better to avoid the mind-set pushed by many nutritionists (reason enough to avoid it) that you are allowed treats, or that you are allowed a "cheat day." You are not "allowed" treats. Nobody's perfect and sweet things do taste good and you will have some. We all screw up periodically and you have to just go back to the plan. Sweets are not really allowed in the sense of being a specific feature of your diet. Consumed sweets are, speaking scientifically, experimental error. There are people who are able to incorporate some sweets as part of their diet and don't deviate from the single ice-cream bar that they have every day as the lone large source of carbs. Some people can get away with it, and if you like food you will certainly find certain foods that are worth the risk to your diet, but they are not "allowed" in the sense of a recommendation. There is a big difference between the attitude that you can't be perfect and you will deviate sometime and the attitude that you deserve an occasional treat. On the other hand, you don't want to indulge in guilt feelings or mentally beat yourself up. The psychologist Alfred Adler always advised: "Do the wrong thing or feel guilty but not both."

The current hysteria about sugar may help you cut back but there is great danger in characterizing things as forbidden fruit, as our very earliest history shows. Especially if they want to ban it. Telling you that you can't have it may make it more appealing and when you see the absurd lengths that the media and researchers alike go to in order to demonize sugar, you may begin to think it is safe. Among lawyers, this is called "The Reverse Mussolini" fallacy: Just because Mussolini made the trains run on time doesn't mean you want them to be unpredictable. (The last time I was in Italy, the trains did run on time, contrary to the Italian stereotype). Just because the USDA says it's bad, doesn't mean it's good.

## Doing Low-Carb: Fruit and Other Tricky Foods

All fruits have sugar and it is best to apply the rule: eat to the meter. If it doesn't interfere with weight loss or blood sugar, or whatever your goal is, then it is okay. I like Suzanne Somers' technique [19]. Unlike many "experts" who may be thin themselves — what does Walter Willett know about fighting fat? — she lost a part in *Starsky and Hutch* because they told her she was "a little too chunky." She recommends eating fruit in pieces; half an apple now, the other half later. The goal is to avoid insulin spikes.

Mike and Mary Dan Eades, authors of *Protein Power* [17] ran a clinic for many years. They had thousands of patients on low-carb diets. Despite generally great success, they had several patients who complained that they had faithfully adhered to the diet but were not losing weight. The Eades found that the three most common foods that caused trouble were cheese, nuts and nut butters; when these were reduced or removed from the diet, patients were able to continue to lose weight. Cheese is probably a simple matter of overconsumption; everything increased during the epidemic of obesity and diabetes — sugar, bread, fruits and vegetables — the only things that went down were red meat and eggs. One anomaly is that cheese consumption was off the chart. So, although apparently safe, moderation must be applied to cheese. Dr. Atkins recommended [20] that you restrict yourself to hard cheese, which pretty much means serious cheese of the type in the gourmet cheese-shop. The greater intensity may be more satisfying but beyond that, it's not obvious why. Almost none of the cheeses in the supermarket qualify as serious cheese. The current price of good cheese, e.g. aged Gouda (2 or 3 years) also insures moderation for most of us.

## DOING LOW-CARB: "NOT LICENSE TO GORGE"

The phrase appears in the original Atkins book several times [20]. The idea is that whereas there are no stated limits on what you can eat if you keep carbohydrate low, overeating is not encouraged. The principle that "a calorie is a calorie" is not correct but calories do count and if you are concerned about your weight, you undoubtedly already know that it is possible to defeat any diet. The nutritionists are actually right about eating slowly (nobody's perfect). Satiety sets in slowly. A possible exception is what to do if you feel that you have the kind of cravings that will set your low-carb diet back. It may be useful to eat something that's allowed even if it seems like overeating. Some high protein, high fat food (if you have an Eastern European butcher, real kielbasa is best). Eventually, your cravings will stabilize. In general, the corollary to **Rule 1** of the General Rules, is that if you have to overeat, don't overeat carbs.

## DEFINITIONS

There are many variations of diets based on carbohydrate restriction. In diabetes, the principle is to keep carbohydrate as low as possible. In less stringent conditions, there may be more room for maneuvering. If specific diets are referred to, **Table 1-1** provides guidelines that should be used because they have been published in more than one peer-reviewed journal by people with the credentials and experience.

- **Low-Carbohydrate diet: less than 130 g/d** or less than **26 %** of a nominal 2000 kcal/d diet. This corresponds to The American Diabetes Association definition of 130 g/d. This is a generally accepted number, likely derived from Cahill's study of the onset of ketosis.

- **Very low-carbohydrate ketogenic diet (VLCKD): 20-50 g/d** or less than **10 %** of the 2000 kcal/d diet. Generally, although not always, accompanied by ketosis, this is the level of the early phases of the plans in many popular low-carbohydrate books.

- **Moderate Carbohydrate Diet: 26-45 %**. The upper limit is chosen as the approximate carbohydrate intake before the obesity epidemic (43 %). Current consumption is about **49 %.**

- **High Carbohydrate Diet:** Greater than 45 %. Recommended target on ADA websites. The 2010 Dietary Guidelines for Americans recommends 45-65 % carbohydrate.

*--for comparison:*

- **Pre-Obesity Epidemic (1971-1974 -NHANES I)**

  Men -42 % carbohydrate (~250 g for 2450 kcal/d)
  Women -45 % carbohydrate (~150 g for 1550 kcal/d)

- **Year 1999 -2000**

  Men 49 % carbohydrate (~330 g for 2600 kcal/d)
  Women 52 % carbohydrate (~230 g for 1900 kcal/d)

Table 1-1. *Operational definitions of carbohydrate restricted diets.*

The definitions are important. Authors in the nutritional literature give themselves license to call anything that they want a low-carbohydrate diet. With a straw man in hand, it is not hard to show that a low-carbohydrate diet is dangerous to your health, but the results do not bear on anything real.

Depending on your goal and who you are, you may find a graded response: The greater the carbohydrate reduction, the greater the weight loss, the greater the improvement in blood glucose, etc. Particularly in weight loss, however, there may be a threshold effect. The onset of ketosis, which for most people occurs at a daily intake of about 30g, will have a more dramatic effect.

## SUMMARY

Three simple rules give you a good guide to action. You are the master of your diet. If you are not fat, if you don't have a health problem or a family history of disease, you probably are doing fine. Low-carbohydrate diets are primarily therapeutic and are the best for diabetes and metabolic syndrome. The evidence, both anecdotal and experimental, says that nothing is better for weight loss. To make it happen, eat to the meter, that is, go for results.

Two reasons for choosing a low-carb diet. First, it works while other stuff fails. After forty years of looking under every rock for risks, nobody can find anything wrong. Second, it makes sense. Directly or *via* insulin, carbohydrates control metabolic matrix. Carbohydrate will determine what happens to the fat that you eat, whether you store it as body fat, or burn it for fuel.

## WHERE WE'RE GOING

Start with the quiz that we give to incoming medical students before they've been exposed to any biochemistry, a test of what they've learned as "citizens." The quiz format provides motivation to learn the material — one student explained that medical students are not happy when they don't know the answer. Chapter 3 looks at the Low-Carbohydrate Revolution of 2002 — how it started, how it was stopped. Chapter 4 provides an overview of metabolism, the principles and how energy is obtained. But first, whaddaya' know?

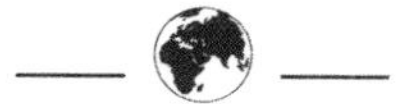

# Chapter 2

# Whaddaya' know?

## TAKE THE QUIZ

We give this questionnaire to first year medical students at the beginning of the course in metabolism before we've taught them anything. Although they are among the most accomplished students in the country, like everybody else, they've been subject to the nutritional information available from rumor and the front of packages in the supermarket. We don't have accurate feedback on the quiz but some of them like the question format and you may too. No particular knowledge is assumed beyond your life as nutritional end-user. The quiz only tests how you were able to sift through all the information that's out there on the internet and in popular books. And it is a teaching device. The answers provide basic information. I list the questions first so you can see how you do. If you don't like quizzes you can skip over to the answers. We also published an early version in the *Nutrition Journal* [3].

1. The most energy dense food (most calories/gram) is:

_______Carbohydrate.
_______Fat.
_______Protein.
_______Alcohol.

2. For a slice of buttered bread, which is more fattening?

_______The butter.
_______The bread.
_______Both are equally fattening.
_______Cannot tell from the information given.

3. During the epidemic of obesity and diabetes, the macronutrient that increased most was:

_______Carbohydrate.
_______Protein.
_______Fat.
_______All about the same. Calories increased across the board.

4. The macronutrient most likely to raise blood glucose in people with type 2 diabetes is:

_______Carbohydrate.
_______Protein.
_______Fat.
_______Alcohol.

5. The dietary requirement for carbohydrate is:

_______approximately 130 g/day
_______approximately 50 % of calories
_______as much as possible
_______there is no dietary requirement for carbohydrate

6. The amount of carbohydrate recommended by the American Diabetes Association and other health agencies:

_______approximately 130 g/day
_______approximately 50 % of calories
_______as much as possible
_______as little as possible.

7. Glycemic Index (GI) measures the increase in blood sugar over 2 hours (per gram of carbohydrate-containing food that is ingested) compared to glucose (=100). For each food indicate the approximate glycemic index as: H, High (70–100), M, Medium (40–70) or L, Low (< 40). You may enter a number if you think you know or can figure it out:

_______White Bread
_______Whole Wheat Bread
_______Ice Cream
_______Carrots
_______Sucrose (Table Sugar)
_______Fructose
_______Bran Muffin
_______Banana

8. A good source of monounsaturated fat is: (check all that apply)

______ Butter
______ Canola Oil
______ Corn Oil
______ Flaxseed Oil
______ Olive Oil
______ Avocado
______ Soybean Oil

9. The diet component that is most likely to raise triglycerides (fat in the blood) is:

______ Fat
______ Carbohydrate
______ Protein

10. In general, what effect does a low-fat diet have on HDL-C (high density lipoprotein cholesterol, "good cholesterol")

______ Increase
______ Decrease
______ No change

11. The dietary change that is most likely to **increase** the risk of cardiovascular disease:

______ unsaturated fat→saturated fat (that is, replace unsaturated fat with saturated fat)
______ unsaturated fat →carbohydrate
______ carbohydrate →unsaturated fat

_______carbohydrate →saturated fat
_______saturated fat →carbohydrate
_______saturated fat →unsaturated fat

## ANSWERS

## THE CALORIE. THE CALORIMETER.

1. The most energy dense food (most calories/gram) is:

_______Carbohydrate.
__X___Fat.
_______Protein.
_______Alcohol.

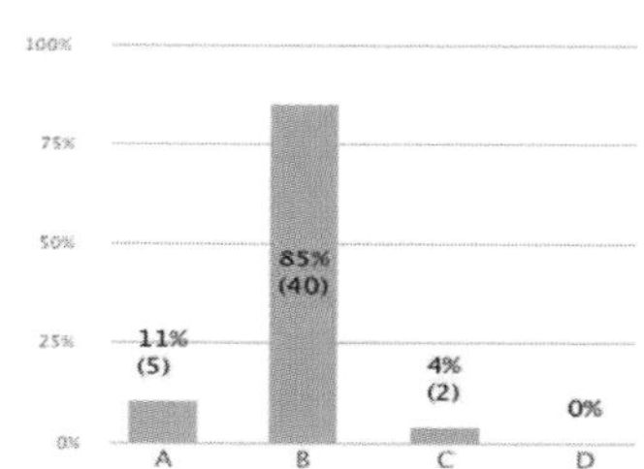


**Student Performance on Question 1.**

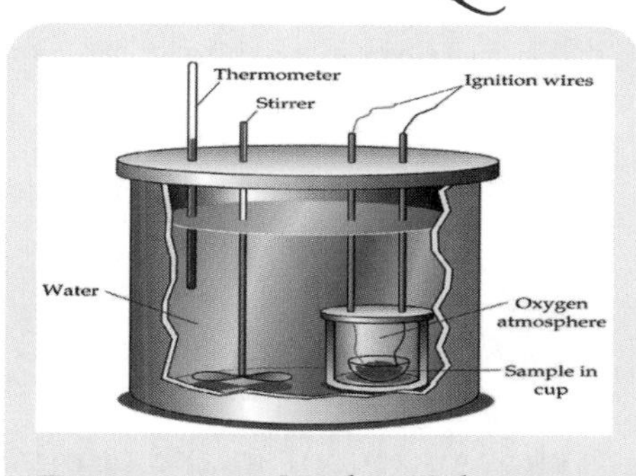


FIGURE 2-1. Modern Calorimeter

Our first year medical students do surprisingly poorly considering that question is so basic.

Typically only 80 % of our incoming class gets this right. Although they have not yet been through the metabolism course, this is a very highly educated group of people and we had assumed that everybody knew that fat was the most energy dense macronutrient. The explanation, which contains some information, is that they were not curious about nutrition because they didn't see it as part of medicine and because they are mostly young, healthy and thin.

The operational numbers in kilocalories/gram are 4, 4, 9 and 7 for carbohydrate, protein, fat and alcohol. Calories are a measure of energy. The definition of energy in physics is not too different from the common idea, it is a measure of the ability to do work. Heat is one form of energy and the calorie is defined in terms of the amount of heat required to raise the temperature of water one degree. Note that the dietary "calorie" is equal to a physical kilocalorie (kcal), that is, 1000 physical calories. Use of "kcal" in nutrition is increasing and in this book we use kcal when actually referring to the quantity. It is one small step to help nutrition become scientific. The calories in food are measured in a device known as a calorimeter. Food is placed in a small container in an atmosphere of oxygen under pressure and then ignited. By measuring the amount of heat generated from the change in temperature in the water bath, we can determine the energy for oxidation which can be assigned to the food. This is the real definition of the nutritional calorie. It all looks obvious but there are a couple of very important points:

> The calories assigned to a food represent the energy for complete combustion of that food in oxygen. Calorie refers to a chemical reaction (not to the food):
>
> Food + oxygen⟶carbon dioxide + water
>
> Food + $O_2 \longrightarrow CO_2 + H_2O$
>
> *(said: "food plus oxygen goes to CO-two and water").*

Heat produced in the calorimeter measures the energy for the specific *reaction*. Again, the energy is in the reaction, *not in the food.* It is not like particle physics where the mass of a particle is given in electron-Volts, a unit of energy (because of $E = mc^2$). We will come back to this point when we consider what is wrong with the idea that a "calorie is a calorie," that the amount of weight you gain or lose on a diet depends only on how many calories without regard to the specific food. It will turn out that the composition of the food is important because, again, the calories associated with a food is the energy obtained in the course of complete combustion of that food as measured in the calorimeter. If you do anything else, make protein, make DNA, make any kind of new cell material, then the calorimeter value does not apply.

Fat is the most energy dense macronutrient at 9 kcal/g and, for that reason, it is considered inherently fattening by nutritionists. This is the basis of traditional recommendations for low-fat diets for obesity. But there is more to the problem than caloric density. And, it turns out that there is more to getting fat than total calories. To see how this all plays out in a real situation, consider the next question.

2. For a slice of buttered bread, which is more fattening?

______ The butter.
______ The bread.
______ Both are equally fattening.
___X__ Cannot tell from the information given.

This is a trick question. It doesn't really have an answer, that is "you cannot tell" is the answer. An argument could be made that 9 kcal/g is inherently more fattening but you really need more information. If you put a lot of butter on the bread it would be more fattening but, in fact, people rarely put more than

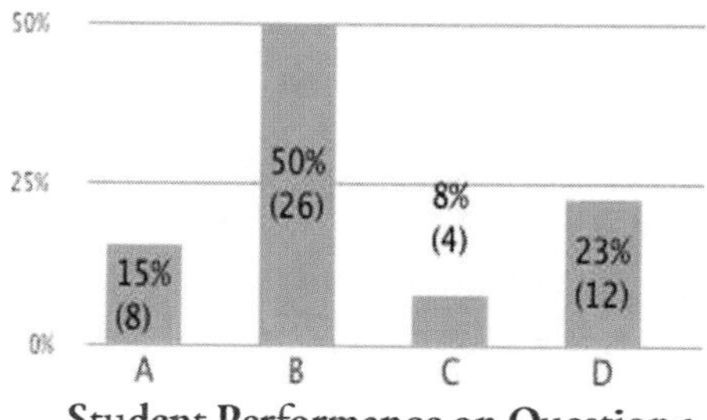

Student Performance on Question 2

100 kcal (tablespoon) on the bread (typically 100 kcal/slice). How fattening food is depends on how much you eat, so the suggestion that you reduce fat because of its caloric density only makes sense if you don't replace it with anything, that is, reduce the calories.

Fat is the most calorically dense food but caloric density, like any density, can be very misleading — density is a measure per amount of material or per unit volume, or per gram, *per* something, so it matters how much of something that you have. Calories per gram is not informative unless you know how many grams. Things like caloric density or any density for that matter are measures of **intensity**, and technically these measurements are called **intensive variables.** Intensive variables are independent of mass; one tablespoon of butter has the same energy *density* (kilocalories per gram) as two tablespoons of butter, but obviously two tablespoons has twice the *total calories* — total calories measures the amount that you have. Such measurements are called extensive variables. Extensive variables depend on how much you have, not the character of the substance. It is the same as the old (updated) riddle: Which is heavier? A pound of uranium or a pound of styrofoam? Of course they are the same. A pound is a pound. Uranium has an extremely high density (about 1.6 times that of lead) so a pound of uranium is only a little bigger than a major league baseball but you would have to fill up the room with styrofoam to equal the same pound.

Fraction, or percent, is another kind of measure of intensity that can be misleading. Looking ahead, this is one reason that recommendations on percent of increase in risk that is always reported in the media is usually meaningless; your odds of winning the lottery are increased by 100 %, that is, doubled, by buying two tickets instead of one. Does that make you want to play? Bottom line: when you hear people say that fat has more calories per grams, you know that that is irrelevant. You have to know how many grams you are actually eating.

## THE OBESITY EPIDEMIC

So, what did we eat during the past thirty or forty years? What kind of macronutrients were in our diet? You may know this better than our students who probably did not attend to the problem.

3. During the epidemic of obesity and diabetes, the macronutrient that increased most was:

___X__Carbohydrate.
_______ Protein.
_______ Fat.
_______ All about the same. Calories increased across the board.

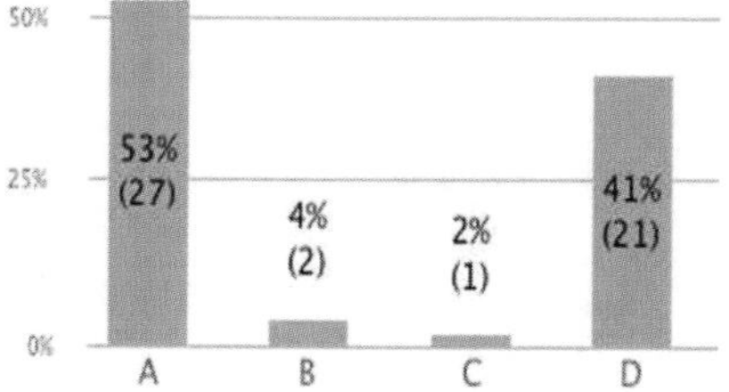

**Student Performance on Question 3**

Many students know at this point where I am coming from and there are probably more votes for carbohydrate than if this were the first question. However, many people, students included, still think that calories were increased across the board.

The epidemic of obesity and diabetes has been accompanied by a substantial *de*crease in the percent fat and, at least for men, the absolute amount also went down slightly.

**FIGURE 2-2** shows data from the National Health and Nutrition Examination Survey (NHANES) which is conducted at the intervals listed in the horizontal axis. The vertical axis is the absolute amount of calories consumed and the large increase in energy consumed appears to be due entirely to a dramatic increase in the consumption of carbohydrate. The percent change shown along the top indicates the expected decrease in fat but, at least for men, the absolute amount of fat (total calories) and, notably, the absolute amount of saturated fat, went down.

There is a lot of error in these kinds of surveys but it is pretty much excluded that there was any *increase* in fat intake. It is also likely that if obesity and diabetes had gotten better, it would have been attributed to the significant fall in saturated fat consumption. The clearest conclusion is that an increase in carbohydrate consumption compared to fat is associated with greater total intake and that a "Western diet," as they call it in the nutrition literature, does not mean a high fat diet.

It is widely said that association does not imply causality. More accurate is that association does not *necessarily* imply causality. Few people would deny that the association of dietary calories and body mass is causal, however non-linear the association might be. Whether the association between increased carbohydrate intake and increased calories is causative is one of the themes in this book.

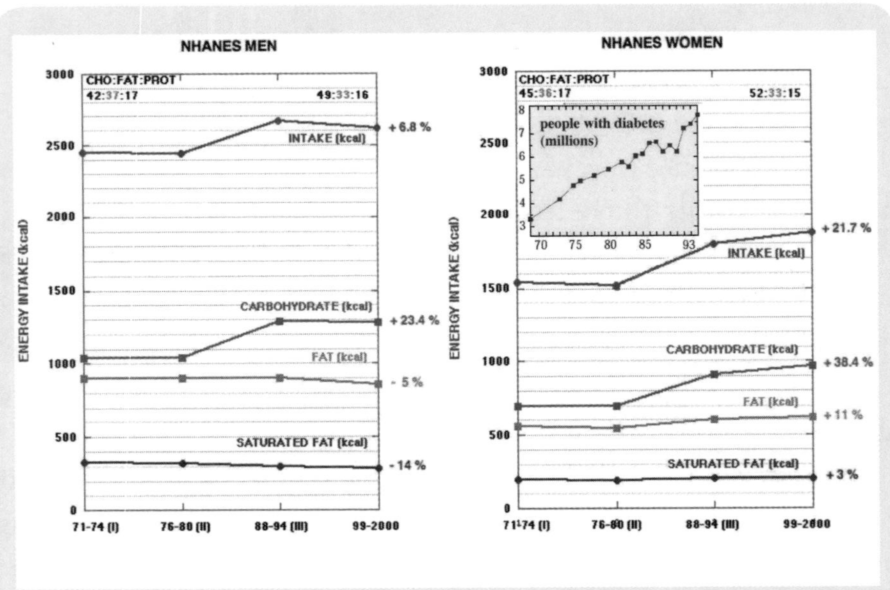


FIGURE 2-2. Consumption of macronutrients during the epidemic of obesity and diabetes. Inset: number of people with diabetes. The horizontal axis represents the period in which NHANES ( National Health and Nutrition Examination Survey) collected data. The left vertical axis is the absolute energy input in kcal. The right axis is the % change in calories. The ratios of macronutrient are shown along the top.

We also ask whether the inset showing the carbohydrate-diabetes association in **Figure 2–2** tells us about what causes what. The argument will be that, given the effectiveness of low-carbohydrate (high-fat) diets as a treatment (sometimes a virtual cure) for diabetes, it would be surprising if carbohydrates were not involved in some way in a causative role.

Finally, there is an obvious association between the official advice of the USDA, the AHA and just about everybody else to reduce fat and increase carbohydrates and what people actually did. They reduced fat, at least as a percentage of calories and they dramatically increased carbohydrates.

Looking ahead, one way to test whether there is a causal link between carbohydrate intake and obesity, is to simply reduce carbohydrates and see if total caloric intake goes down or, in fact whether diabetes incidence goes down. There are some good experiments that test this. The results are as expected and the details of one experiment are described in Chapter 9. Whatever else can be drawn from these data, the association between increased carbohydrate/decreased fat and obesity and diabetes is the single result that makes the largest impact on our medical students and remains an undercurrent in any analysis of the role of macronutrients.

4. The macronutrient most likely to raise blood glucose in people with type 2 diabetes is:

__X__ Carbohydrate.
_____ Protein.
_____ Fat.
_____ Alcohol.

This is, or should be, obvious. The correct answer was chosen by 83 % of our students. The surprise is probably that anybody got it wrong. Diabetes is fundamentally a disease (really several diseases) of carbohydrate intolerance. People with type 1 diabetes cannot produce the hormone insulin in response to blood glucose. People with type 2 have progressive deterioration of the insulin-producing beta cells of the pancreas. They do produce insulin but their cells respond poorly. They are said to show insulin resistance. Insulin has effects on many tissues, particularly adipocytes (fat cells). Diabetes is as much a disease of fat metabolism as of carbohydrate metabolism; the primary effect of insulin is on synthesis and breakdown of fat and a person with type 2 diabetes may have excessive fatty acids in their blood. Nonetheless, the most obvious characteristic and the major risk for other symptoms is the hyperglycemia (high blood glucose). Different carbohydrate-containing foods raise blood glucose to different extents but the general principle holds.

## THE DIETARY REQUIREMENT FOR CARBOHYDRATE

5. The dietary requirement for carbohydrate is:

______approximately 130 g/day
______approximately 50 % of calories
______as much as possible
__X__there is no dietary requirement for carbohydrate

There is no requirement for dietary carbohydrates as there is for the so-called essential amino acids or essential fatty acids. This does not mean that anybody recommends doing without them altogether even if this were possible (even meat has a small amount of carbohydrates).

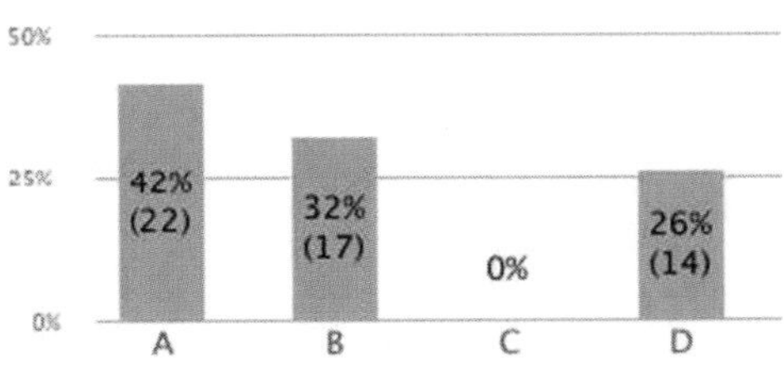

**Student Performance on Question 5**

That there is no dietary requirement for carbohydrate means, in a practical sense, that if you do want to reduce carbohydrate, there is no *biological* limit on how much you can restrict the intake. The extent to which you actually do so will depend on your personal reaction and taste but you do not *need* to consume any at all. It is always emphasized that the brain needs glucose but your body is capable of making glucose from protein from the process known as **gluconeogenesis** and supplying glucose from storage as **glycogen.** There are also alternative fuels in the form of **ketone bodies.** You more or less knew this. If you did need dietary carbohydrate, you would die if you went without food for a week; you store a lot of fat but not much carbohydrate. More on glycogen and gluconeogenesis in Chapter 7.

6. The amount of carbohydrate recommended by the American Diabetes Association (ADA) and other health agencies:

_____approximately 130 g/day
__X__approximately 50 % of calories
_____as much as possible
_____as little as possible

It is hard to believe that a diabetes agency would *recommend* any amount of carbohydrate but this is it. Their 2008 dietary guidelines contain the rather remarkable advice:

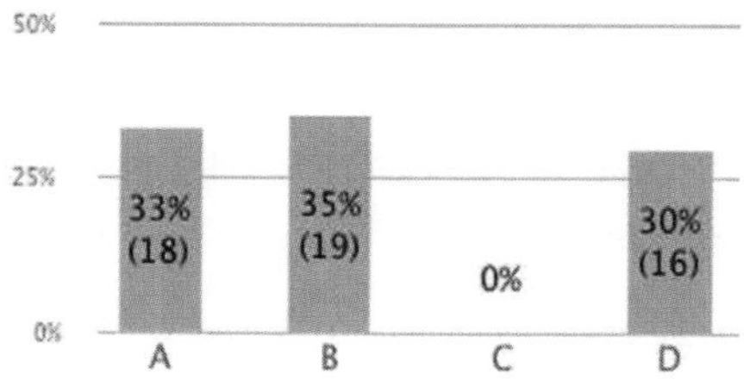

**Student Performance on Question 6**

> Sucrose-containing foods can be substituted for other carbohydrates in the meal plan or, if added to the meal plan, covered with insulin or other glucose-lowering medications. Care should be taken to avoid excess energy intake. (A)

To many people this seems to be saying that it is okay to make things worse so that you can take more drugs. The (A) mark indicates that they consider this advice to be based on their highest level of evidence. They don't cite that evidence but it is surely not experimental. While this book was being written, the ADA quietly dropped this passage from their 2013 guidelines [10] but have not explicitly indicated that it was wrong. It is unknown whether the rank and file of ADA membership ever read those statements, and if so, thought that they were of high quality or simply political statements with which no one has time to fight.

> Although brain fuel needs can be met on lower-carbohydrate diets, long-term metabolic effects of very low-carbohydrate diets are unclear.

In fact, the long term effects *are* clear. Very clear — there are trials going out to one or two years, and internet sites and forums make apparent that it is a way of life for many people with diabetes. Although personal stories are hard to document, we would know if there were any indication of long term problems. More important, there is no reason to suggest that there *would* be any long term effects. In science, you don't start from scratch. You don't assume that there is harm unless there is a reason to. Nothing in reducing carbohydrate suggests harm. And "unclear" implies conflicting data. There is no conflicting data and no reason to expect any. I suggested to a spokesperson for the ADA that they were stronger on what they were opposed to than on anything positive that they had to offer. She admitted that that was a fair criticism. So, why are they opposed to carbohydrate restriction?

> ...such diets eliminate many foods that are important sources of energy, fiber, vitamins, and minerals and are important in dietary palatability.

If "care should be taken to avoid excess energy intake," what would it mean for carbohydrate to be "an important source of energy?" And, does anybody think that taking a vitamin pill is the equivalent of injecting insulin? There is also a subtle switch from "carbohydrate" meaning macronutrient, to using the term to mean carbohydrate-containing food. Finally, I would suggest, as in the future history (see Appendix), that dietary palatability is not their area of expertise.

The guidelines from the ADA, as from other health agencies are supposed to be serious but, in fact, have the character of an infomercial and the standards are those of selling a product rather than presenting a scientific case. It seems that we are supposed to just take it. The ADA is a private organization but they have public support at least in that they are tax-exempt. Their experts are often federally funded as well. Are they really free to say whatever they want? This is the kernel of the second low-carbohydrate revolution.

## Glycemic Index -Politically Correct Low-Carb

7. Glycemic Index measures the increase in blood sugar over 2 hours (per gram of carbohydrate-containing food that is ingested) compared to glucose (=100). For each food indicate the approximate glycemic index as: H, high (70–100), M, Medium (40–70) or L, Low (< 40). You may enter a number if you think you know or can figure it out:

__70__White bread

__50__Whole wheat bread

__57__Ice cream (average)

__38__Ice cream (premium)

__47__Carrots

__60__Sucrose (table sugar)

__20__Fructose

__60__Bran muffin

__60__Banana

In Chapter 1, we had proclaimed Rule 2, the rule for losing weight:

> If you want to lose weight: Don't eat. If you have to eat, don't eat carbs. If you have to eat carbs, eat low-glycemic index carbs.

The value of not eating is obvious and, by now, you should be convinced that something about dietary carbohydrate is important for weight loss, but is there really anything to the glycemic index? Can it help you?

The basic idea is that the effect of carbohydrate on blood glucose will be determined by other factors than simply how much carbohydrate is in a particular food. The glycemic index addresses the old idea, pretty much a dogma when I was in school, that simple sugars would cause a rapid rise in blood glucose, but complex carbohydrate which, at that time, still meant polysaccharides (starch), would not. At some point, though, people asked if this idea was really true and, it turns out, when you actually measure the effect of foods on blood glucose, it's not easily predictable, that is, must be determined experimentally. Glycemic Index (GI) is precisely defined as the area under the blood glucose time-curve during the first 2 hours after consumption of 50 grams of carbohydrate-containing food. In other words, it is total amount of blood glucose for a fixed time period after ingestion (**Figrue 2-3**).

Intellectually, glycemic index was an important idea. The same principle as low-carbohydrate diets, and seemingly of practical value, low-GI diets have evolved to be a politically correct form of carbohydrate restriction and such diets are recommended as an *alternative* to low-carbohydrate diets. Insofar as low-GI diets are really helpful, it is that they are simply a weak form of carbohydrate restriction and, the point of Rule #2, they are strictly secondary to real control of carbohydrate intake. Eric Westman who has experience with both kinds of diets put it well: "If low-GI is good, why not no-GI?"

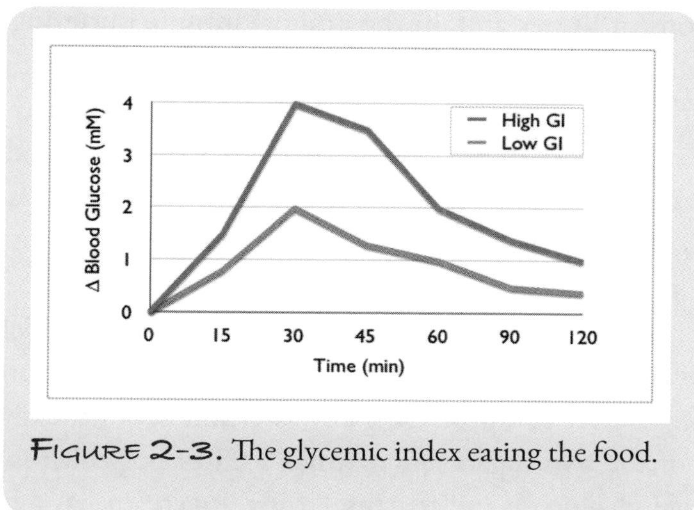


Figure 2-3. The glycemic index eating the food.

GI is mainly influenced by the absolute concentration of glucose in the food, the extent to which glucose appears in the blood (not necessarily from the food itself) and the quantity of other nutrients such as fat or fiber in the carbohydrate-containing food because this may slow the digestion or absorption of carbohydrate. GI diets are complicated and require looking up and calculating values, a feature which may be appealing to some, but is probably annoying to most.

The difference between intensive variables, like calorie density (or any density) and extensive variables, like total carbohydrate eaten, was brought out at the beginning of the quiz. GI is an intensive variable. Two bowls of cereal have the same GI as one. If there is not much carbohydrate (or really much glucose) in a food, it will have a low GI but it could have a large effect if you consume a lot. The **glycemic load** attempts to correct this problem. The glycemic load, or GL, is defined as the GI multiplied by the grams of carbohydrate in a sample of a particular food. Obviously, GL is still an intensive variable. You still have to know how much is consumed.

There is also the overall character of using GI. A slice of white bread has a high GI. The GI will go down if you smear a tablespoon of butter on the bread. It will go down still further if you add two tablespoons of butter and, in the limit of infinite buttering, that is, pure butter, you will have a GI = 0 which is probably not the intent of those people who want to use the GI as a guide to eating.

Overall, low-GI diets may be preferable to high-GI diets but there are many ambiguities. One feature that is of interest is that GI measures blood *glucose*. Fructose, a sugar of great current interest (because it is 50 % of sucrose, that is, table sugar or high fructose corn syrup) is partially converted to glucose in 2 hours which is why the GI of fructose is 20 and not zero. In fact, more is converted after that time, severely compromising any assertion about the differences in effect of the two sugars. Sucrose has a GI of 70 which is roughly the average of glucose and fructose. Thus, ice cream has a lower GI than potatoes. But now we can't recommend ice cream because of the high fructose. Lower GI or lower fructose? How to do both without saying "low-carbohydrate" out loud? This tangled web is woven out of the failure to face scientific fact and must necessarily be unravelled by the low-carbohydrate revolution.

## SUMMARY SO FAR

How did you do? Some critical things were not known to most of our medical students. In summary, whatever you knew before, the stuff that you need to know to pursue what I'm doing here is that:

- Almost all of the increase in calories in the epidemic of obesity and diabetes has been due to a dramatic increase in carbohydrate consumption. The association between the observed pattern of macronutrient consumption and official advice to reduce fat and increase carbohydrates may be causal. How could it be else? It is not, however, a sole cause and the bottom line, that reducing carbohydrate is the best treatment for diabetes, suggests that carbohydrate must have played some role in its origins but this remains unknown. It seems sensible to keep carbohydrates low to avoid diabetes but this is not established. What is established is that the progression of culprits, saturated fat, red meat, white rice that are daily, "proved" by epidemiologic studies to be causes, can probably be excluded.

The crux of the problem in controlling the epidemic of diabetes can be summarized in the following statements:

- Dietary carbohydrates raise blood glucose in people with diabetes more than other macronutrients.

- There is no biological requirement for carbohydrate (for anybody).

- Health agencies recommend high carbohydrates (more than 40 % of total calories).

- The glycemic index (and glycemic load) are a weak form of low-carb strategy. The logical problems and the limited experimental demonstrations of their efficacy make their use questionable as a primary strategy but may be of some use in that they encourage carbohydrate restriction.

- Calories are about processes not substance, and looking ahead, different processes (oxidation in the calorimeter vs. metabolism) make different use of the calories. Also, slightly technical but with direct application, it's good to pay attention to the difference between intensive properties like calorie-density and extensive properties like total calories. When you hear people say that fat is inherently more fattening, you know that doesn't mean anything.

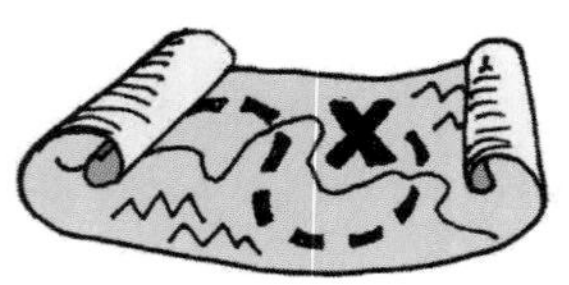

## WHERE WE'RE GOING

The second part of the quiz is about lipids. There's a little more chemistry. Many terms in the popular media are not used correctly and a little precision will help understand the problem. The discussion in this part is somewhat technical if you are unfamiliar with organic chemistry.

**Branch point:** You can skip to Chapter 4 "The First Low-carb Revolution" to follow the narrative and come back to this later. I recommend: plow ahead and look up stuff that is the hardest. You'll usually get another chance on the chemistry.

First, you need to know that the term **lipids** refers to a diverse collection of chemical compounds which have in common the fact that they are sparingly or not at all soluble in water. The group includes fatty acids, fats and oils, cholesterol and derivatives of these compounds. Directly applicable here are the fats and oils and their constituent components, the fatty acids and glycerol. We'll look at fat structure and the meaning of "saturated" and "unsaturated" fat. I'll describe the idea of a lipoprotein, the cholesterol-containing particles, LDL and HDL that are in your lipid work-up. We'll touch on the diet-heart hypothesis and the original idea of the Mediterranean Diet. The big payoff will be to understand how fat interacts with carbohydrate and, looking ahead, we will try to understand how, as we all know too well, carbohydrates can be converted to fat but, to a large extent, fat cannot be converted to glucose. We will want to understand how it is that we cannot use our fat stores to keep glucose at normal levels and how it is that the amount of dietary carbohydrate may be more important than the amount of dietary fat in determining how much body fat we have.

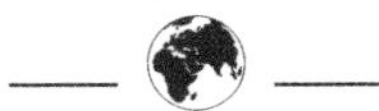

# Chapter 3

# Answers 2. Introduction To Lipid Chemistry

---

## Back to the Quiz

8. A good source of monounsaturated fat is:

_____ Butter
__X__ Canola Oil
_____ Corn Oil
_____ Flaxseed Oil
__X__ Olive Oil
__X__ Avocado Oil
_____ Soybean Oil

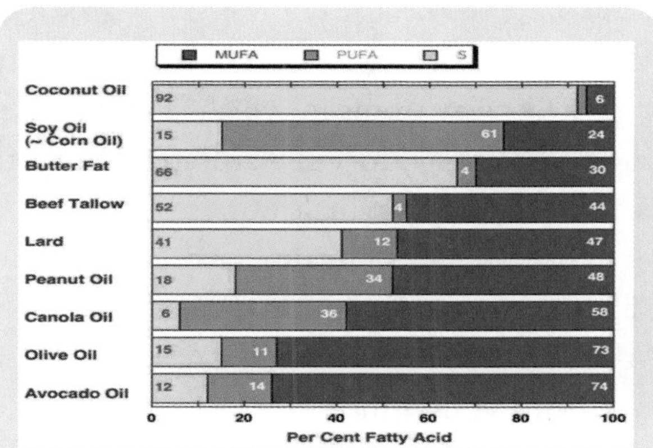


Figure 3-1 Composition of common fats and oils. MUFA = monounsaturated fatty acids. PUFA = polyunsaturated fatty acids.

You hear the terms, "saturated fat" and "polyunsaturated fat" often which are not quite precise; only fatty acids can be unsaturated or saturated. All dietary and body fats and oils are **triglycerides (TG)**, or, more correctly, **triacyl glycerols (TAG)**. The name tells you about the structure: There are three acyl groups (pronounced "ay-seal," ay as in hay). Acyl is the adjective form of acid and the components are **fatty acids** and the three acyl groups are attached to the compound **glycerol**. It is only the fatty acids that can be saturated (SFA) or unsaturated (UFA). "Saturated fat" means that the fat contains a higher proportion of saturated fatty acids. Similarly for unsaturated and its variations, mono-(MUFA), or poly-(PUFA).

Fats have an E-shaped structure. The arms of the E are the fatty acids and the backbone is the compound glycerol. (**Figure 3-2**). The chemical bond that attaches the fatty acid to the glycerol is called an **ester bond**. You only need to know the term ester because when the fatty acids are found alone, especially in blood, they are referred to as **free fatty acids (FFA)** or, because they are no longer attached to the glycerol part by the ester bonds, **non-esterified fatty acids (NEFA)**: FFA and NEFA are the same thing. Fatty acids are long chains of carbon atoms with a carboxylic acid group. The fatty acids provide the real fuel in fat in the long hydrocarbon chains, like gasoline. Fatty acid comprise the arms of the "E." Carbon-carbon double bonds are more chemically reactive and can be converted to single bonds, e.g. with hydrogen atoms in which case they are called saturated, that is saturated with hydrogen. "Saturated" means that all the carbon-carbon chemical bonds are single bonds.

"Saturated fats," again, have a large number of SFAs in the arms of the E structure. Similarly, "unsaturated fats" have high amounts MUFA (monounsaturated fatty acids) and PUFA (polyunsaturated fatty acids). For some fats, however, it is not clear that these terms are useful. One thinks of lard as a kind of pure high saturated fat but it is only 41 % saturated, while it is mostly (47 %) MUFA, predominantly oleic acid, the main fat in olive oil. So it is a question of whether you think that lard is half full of SFA or half empty. Most important, as in the epidemiologic study described in the Introduction, there is no risk for cardiovascular disease associated with consuming saturated fat. This has now been borne out by large population studies and there is simply no correlation — if anything, the studies show that carbohydrate is a greater risk than saturated fat but these kinds of correlations are too weak to attribute any role at all to either. More on this as we go along.

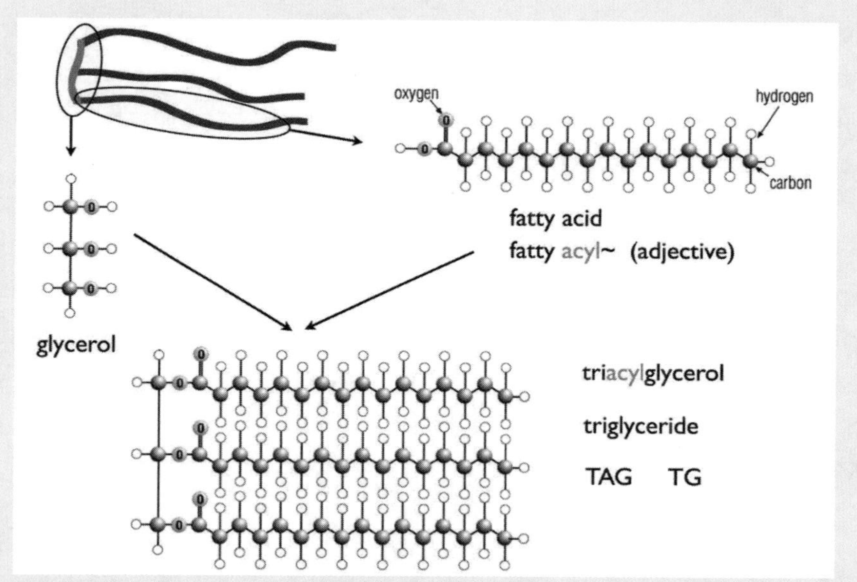


Figure 3-2. Fat structure. Fats and oils are triglycerides (TG), formally triacylglycerol (TAG). There are 3 ester bonds to glycerol.

Butyric Acid-Saturated Fatty Acid

Oleic Acid- Monounsaturated Fatty Acid

Linoleic Acid- Polyunsaturated Fatty Acid

Figure 3-3. Single and double chemical bonds and common fatty acids

The structure of the different kinds of fatty acids are shown in **Figure 3-3.** The major monounsaturated fatty acid is oleic acid. Everybody thinks that monounsaturated fats, those with a high content of MUFA like olive oil are protective of cardiovascular disease but it is not so clear-cut.

Few fats have only SFAs. Coconut oil is the exception but those are medium chain FA (12-16 carbons). Most naturally occurring fats have mixtures of FAs but you can make or isolate from natural sources, a fat that is all stearic acid (called tristearin or just stearin). It is not usually used in food because it is solid and hard but it is used in manufacturing soap and other products.

Saturated fats (again, those with fairly large number of SFAs) tend to be solid while those with more unsaturated fatty acids tend to be liquid — generally, the more unsaturation the higher the melting point. To understand why, we need to look deeper into the structure of fatty acids and the question brings us to the issue of "*trans*-fats."

## WHAT ARE trans-FATS? IN FACT, WHAT IS "trans"?

When vegetable oils are hydrogenated, the process by which some of the unsaturated FAs are turned to saturated, a side-reaction can occur that changes the configuration of some of the unsaturated fatty acids from *cis*-to *trans*-.

Let me explain what *"trans"* means since the Nutritional Murphy's Law dictates that confusion will be introduced wherever possible. The carbon-carbon double bond has rigid geometry, that is, unlike the carbon-carbon single bond, there is no rotation around the bond. So, if you imagine a chain of carbon atoms as in a hydrocarbon like gasoline or the backbone of a fatty acid, if the bonds are all saturated (single) bonds then you can think of the molecule as somewhat floppy because of free rotation around the bonds. If there is a double bond in this chain, there are now two ways to arrange the structure. The two carbons in a double bond can have hydrogen atoms on the same side of the bond (*cis-*) or on opposite sides (*trans-*). **Figure 3-4 shows the geometry around double bonds.**

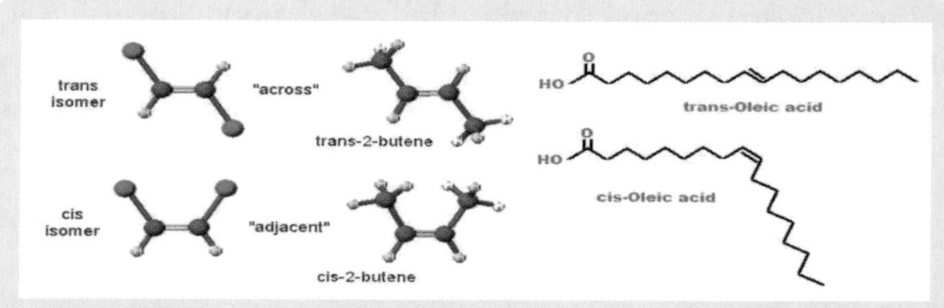


Figure 3-4. Orientation around chemical double bonds. The two carbons in a double bond each have a hydrogen atom and another atom, a carbon or, the case of FA, carbon chain. If these are on the same side of the double bond, they have the *cis*-configuration. Otherwise, *trans-*.

Almost all naturally occurring fatty acids have the *cis* configuration but it is important to understand that, by itself, it is just a designation about the millions of double bond-containing compounds in the world. **Figure 3-4** shows that UFAs have more structure than SFAs and this is why saturated fats tend to be solid (easier to pack into a solid; by analogy, it is easier to pack T-shirts into a box than to pack model Eiffel Towers or heads of Nefertiti).

## MUFAS AND THE MEDITERRANEAN DIET

The Mediterranean Diet is widely recommended for its health benefits although the data is pretty weak and it is not obvious that anybody knows what the diet is beyond the idea that you have to pour olive oil on everything. The idea probably comes from Ancel Keys, generally considered the father of lipophobia. Keys originally found a good correlation between fat consumption (actually fat availability) in six different countries and the incidence of heart disease in those countries [21]. It wasn't long, however, before the Secretary of Health in New York State and a professor at Berkeley published a paper showing that there were data from countries other than the six that Keys had studied. Had he used all of that data, the correlation would not have looked so good (described in [22-24] among others). Keys has generally been characterized as a zealot although he was probably more open-minded than some of his followers. He was, however, not easily embarrassed and undertook a study of seven countries.

## OKAY -SEVEN COUNTRIES

The Seven Countries study on dietary availability of fat had the interesting result that the two countries with the highest intake of fat were Finland, which had the highest incidence of CVD and Crete, which had the lowest [25]. It was deduced that this had to do with the type of fat, saturated in the case of Finland and unsaturated, in the case of Crete. It was later pointed out that there were large differences in CVD between different areas of Finland that had the same diet. This information was ignored by Keys who was also a pioneer in this approach to dealing with conflicting data. In any case, the finding immediately led to the recommendations to lower saturated fat, although for most people there was a lingering idea that it was good to reduce fat across the board. Health agencies were quite a bit stronger at stepping up the pressure on saturated fat but not so good at admitting the error in recommending low-fat. This is still the state of affairs. The real problem, however, is that the link between saturated fat and heart disease has been impossible to establish; direct tests failed right off and continue to fail. The story of the political triumph of an idea that was clearly contradicted by the science has been told numerous times (e.g., references [11, 22, 23, 26, 27]) and yet the phenomenon still persists. Every time you see a low-fat item in the supermarket you are looking at an artifact of one of the most bizarre stories in the history of science.

One of the rarely cited responses to the Seven Countries study was a letter written by researchers at the University of Crete and published in the journal *Public Health Nutrition* [28]. The important part of this letter:

> "In the December 2004 issue of your journal ... Geoffrey Cannon referred to ... the fact that Keys and his colleagues seemed to have ignored the possibility that Greek Orthodox Christian fasting practices could have influenced the dietary habits of male Cretans in the 1960s.... Professor Aravanis confirmed that, in the 1960s, *60% of the study participants were fasting during the 40 days of Lent*, and strictly followed all fasting periods of the church...periodic *abstention from meat, fish, dairy products, eggs and cheese*, as well as abstention from olive oil consumption on certain Wednesdays and Fridays....."
>
> "... this was not noted in the study, and *no attempt was made to differentiate between fasters and non-fasters.* In our view this was a remarkable and troublesome omission." (My *emphasis*).

The whole sorry tale has now been told many times, most recently and completely by Nina Teicholz whose exposé of the low-fat fiasco, *The Big Fat Surprise* [11] *Surprise* was published as this book was being finished, at the moment when the loyalists began scrambling to claim dedication to freedom and revolutionary ideas.

## RETURNING TO THE COMPOSITION OF DIETARY FATS

Going back to **Figure 3.1**, the composition of different dietary fats turns out to be somewhat surprising. It is true that there is a lot of oleic acid, the major monounsaturated fatty acid, in olive oil (73 %) and canola oil (58%). Less well known is that the highest amount is found in avocado oil. Probably most surprising, however, is that oleic acid makes up almost half of the fatty acids in beef tallow and lard (44% and 47 %). Beef tallow, rendered fat, was what McDonald's used to use to fry their French fries in — at the time, they got thumbs up from Julia Child — until they were pressured to switch to vegetable oil in a movement spearheaded by Michael Jacobson. Michael Jacobson, the head of the Committee for Perpetual Responsibility or something similar, might be described as humorless, up-tight and puritanical. I have been accused of inappropriate behavior in making this characterization but you can check out his interview with Stephen Colbert (http://on.cc.com/1ty5yAI; Colbert: "What is the latest thing that you're warning people not to enjoy?") Of course, when McDonald's did switch to vegetable oil the amount of *trans*-fat went up and that got Jacobson riled up again. In any case, most of the saturated fat in beef is stearic acid which was considered neutral or "heart-healthy" but the question is at least ambiguous. And, again, beef fat is only half SFA, the other half is mostly oleic acid as in the Mediterranean diet.

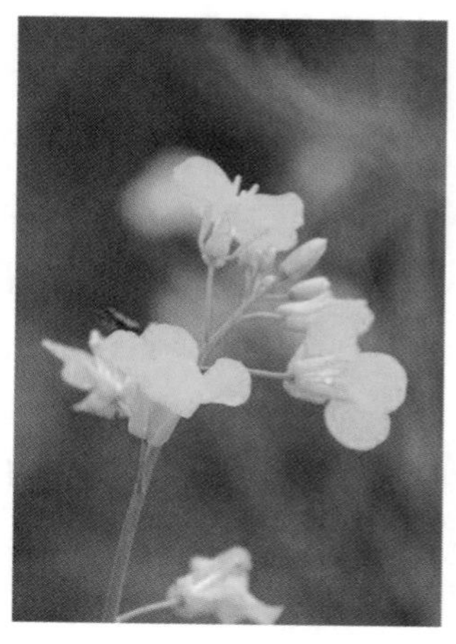

Canola oil, it turns out, is named for CANadian Oil, Low Acid, an oil isolated from rapeseed (rape, from Latin for turnip in this context) which also contains euricic acid. This fatty acid is the star of Lorenzo's oil but it not as beneficial as in the movie and is generally considered toxic and it is removed in making canola oil. My original vision of the *Quebecoise* in their native costumes picking canola fruit from the canola tree turned out not to be correct. There is no canola tree. The rapeseed plant, a member of the *Brassica* family (like broccoli) was originally processed to remove the euricic acid.

The plant has now been bred to have low euricic acid and there now really is a plant called canola and the oil is one of the major export products from Canada. Processing also produced *trans*-fatty acids but this has been removed from current versions of the product. (Wikipedia has an interesting read about canola oil: http://en.wikipedia.org/wiki/Canola).

Back to the quiz... We asked students about the "cholesterol" species that are reported in your lipid profile and that are supposed to be indictors of risk of cardiovascular disease (CVD). What is called cholesterol in this context is actually a supramolecular (more than one type of molecule) known as a **lipoprotein** which contains lipid protein. The simplified structure and the relative sizes are shown in **Figure 3-5.**

## LIPOPROTEINS. "GOOD" AND "BAD" CHOLESTEROL.

There were a few questions not shown here. Most of our students knew that low-fat diets lower low density lipoprotein cholesterol (LDL-cholesterol), the so-called "bad cholesterol." Considered bad because it is assumed to correlate well with heart disease. Not well appreciated is that the correlation is not strong. Less than half the people with a first heart attack have high cholesterol and less than half have high LDL (although "high" is subject to interpretation). The skepticism expressed in the Introduction is still appropriate here .

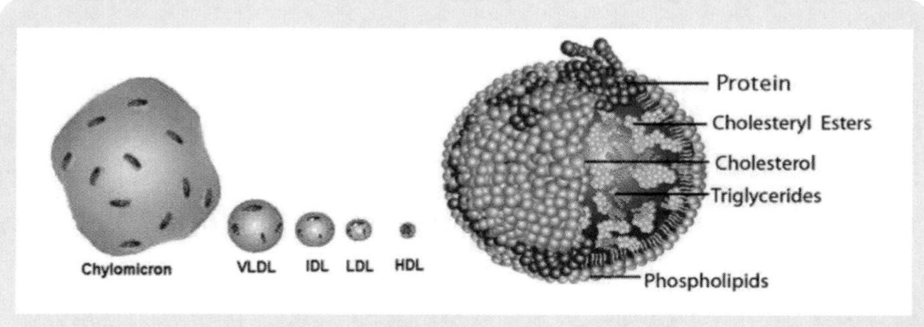


Figure 3-5. Sizes and structure of the common lipoproteins.

Cholesterol is not a cause of heart disease — we don't know what the cause is — but it is considered a risk marker, something associated with incidence of disease. There are, however, better risk markers including triglycerides and the "good cholesterol" HDL-cholesterol.

9. The diet component that is most likely to raise triglycerides (fat in the blood) is:

__X__ Carbohydrate
_____ Fat
_____ Protein

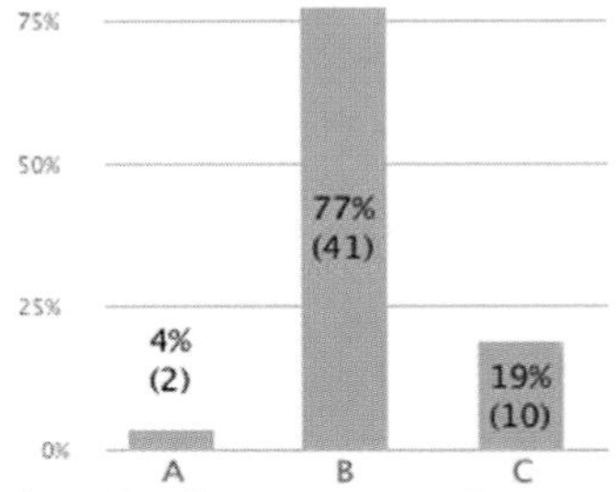

Student Performance on Question 9

The phenomenon of carbohydrate-induced hypertriglyceridemia (high blood triglyceride) has been known for at least sixty years. A major contributor is the process of *de novo* fatty acid synthesis, more usually called *de novo* lipogenesis (DNL), in which fatty acids are made from other components, mainly carbohydrate. It is significant that the fatty acid that is made in DNL is palmitic acid, the sixteen carbon saturated fatty acid. In other words, carbohydrate in the diet raises saturated fat in the blood. This was demonstrated most convincingly by experiments at the University of Connecticut [29-31] described below in Chapter 9. It turns out that saturated fatty acid in the blood may be deleterious but this is more dependent on dietary carbohydrate than dietary fat. In any case, our students completely missed the boat on this.

How much of a risk factor is high triglycerides? Well, it is impossible to tell. The American Heart Association (AHA) tends to downplay the importance of triglycerides. This is probably related to the need to avoid talking about low-carbohydrate diets, and the fact that dietary carbohydrate restriction is the most effective method of reducing high triglycerides except perhaps for total starvation. On the other hand, increases in triglycerides become a tremendous threat to the AHA in the context of sugar, or fructose in particular. Sugar is carbohydrate and whether an increase in fructose is more or less effective than glucose in elevating triglycerides or, what we really know from experiments, total carbohydrates, probably depends on how you do the study; despite what you read in the media, fructose and glucose are closely linked: as much as 60% of added fructose can be turned into glucose, so you don't even really know what you're adding. In addition, the effect of one sugar is tied to how much of the other you have. For example, fructose taken up by the liver is a signal to increase the uptake of glucose.

10. In general, what effect does a low-fat diet have on HDL-C (high-density lipoprotein cholesterol, "good cholesterol") ?

_____ Increase
__X__ Decrease
_____ No change
_____ Don't know

Student Performance on Question 10

A low-fat diet reduces cholesterol, both "good" and "bad." The bottom line on the cholesterol problem: the literature studies tend to show that a sub-type of LDL particle, the smaller LDL are generally found to be most atherogenic (highest risk for CVD). High levels of small-dense LDL are characterized as "pattern B" and this pattern is most dependent on the level of carbohydrate, not the level of fat. This critical observation has had little effect on official positions of the AHA or other agencies and anecdotally, they don't think LDL size matters but have not said exactly why not. The AHA has, however, quietly removed their proscription against total fat in 2000; you didn't know that?

LDL particle size is not generally measured in a standard lipid profile and your physician is most likely to look at total cholesterol or LDL-cholesterol to determine if you are at risk for heart disease. The recognized surrogate for pattern B is the ratio of triglycerides/HDL. The cut-off is 3.5 [32]. If your value is below that mark, there is limited risk for cardiovascular disease.

The question of whether the reduction in triglycerides or HDL, that is a consequence of a low-carbohydrate diet, has any protective effect is much harder to answer. As suggested in the introduction, it is possible that, outside of well-defined genetic abnormalities, what you eat may have no effect on your risk of heart disease. We will come back to this theme. The response to doubt separates science from religion. It is revolutionary to even consider the possibility that the diet-heart hypothesis as currently constituted is not only wrong but there is no replacement. In religion, you pray for relief from doubt. We don't want to do that.

11. The dietary change that is most likely to increase the risk of cardiovascular disease:

______unsaturated fat → saturated fat
(That is, unsaturated fat, out; saturated fat. in)
__X__unsaturated fat →carbohydrate
______carbohydrate →unsaturated fat
______carbohydrate→saturated fat
______saturated fat→carbohydrate
______saturated fat →unsaturated fat

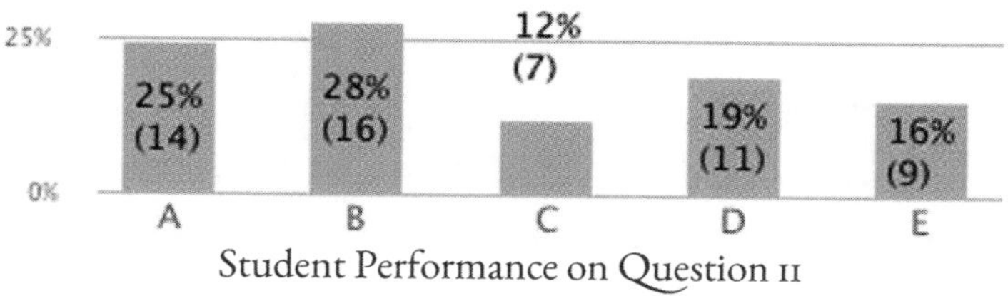

Student Performance on Question 11

This is one of the most important observations because it has been known for so long. I described in the Introduction my early research into the literature and my dismay at the results of the Nurses Health Study [4]. The study demonstrated that there was an *increase* in CVD incidence, *greater* risk, by taking fat out of your diet and putting in carbohydrate. Take out fat, any fat and replace with carbohydrate and risk goes up. This was astounding given the persistent low-fat message. It would have been reasonable for the study, done more than 15 years ago, to have been the stimulus for a change away from that low-fat message. That didn't happen. Only a few years ago, Walter Willett himself was reported in the media as embracing a low-carbohydrate diet, but little happened. It was clearly not a real passion with him and they must have gotten to him (whoever 'they' are).

## SUMMARY

Major points about lipids from the second part of the quiz:

The terms "saturated" and "unsaturated" can only be applied to fatty acids, the constituents of fats and oils. The composition of common fats and oils is different from popular conceptions, e.g., beef tallow is almost half oleic acid, the main fatty acid of olive oil.

The dietary change that has the greatest effect on cardiovascular risk factors is replacement of fat with carbohydrate. Low-fat diets reduce LDL but low-carb diets reduce the important sub-fractions, the pattern B, that are more atherogenic. Reducing carbohydrate also improves HDL. The question that is posed is whether reducing carbohydrate diminishes the actual incidence of CVD. It would be difficult to answer that question but it must be considered. What you may not have known before the quiz: our current state of knowledge does not provide evidence that what you eat will make any difference in your risk of heart disease.

The ambiguity or, more precisely, the near absolute failure of the diet-heart hypothesis contained the seeds of the first low-carb revolution. We'll look at that next and ask why another revolution is needed.

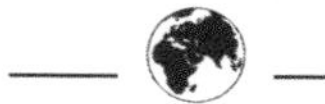

# Chapter 4

# The First Low-Carb Revolution

---

## REVOLUTIONS -POLITICAL AND SCIENTIFIC

The first low-carbohydrate revolution dates from about 2002 and as is frequently the case in politics, the revolutionaries saw themselves as a loyal opposition, and probably thought that their ideas were not particularly iconoclastic. Dr. Atkins was a physician and undoubtedly had the idea that he was only trying to help. He was obviously surprised at the vehement backlash. Unfortunately, his response to criticism was less like that of John Adams than like John's cousin, Samuel Adams, described in *Don't Know Much About History* as being better at brewing dissent than beer. However, it is doubtful that much could have been done and a real revolution can be dated to 2002 but, like political revolutions, has to be won again.

Scientific revolutions, like political revolutions, usually have to be won more than once. Gary Wills [33] described the Gettysburg Address as a statement that the Civil War was a second American Revolution. People of my generation may see the civil rights movement as a third. It's often the same for revolutions in science. We are taught that atomic theory comes from John Dalton, the Manchester school-teacher who proposed it in 1799 but atoms were not truly accepted as real things until Einstein nailed it in 1905.

The idea that dietary carbohydrate, sugars and starches, have some unique power to make people fat is pretty old. It would be hard to identify the first farmer who fattened animals for market by feeding them grain. Brillat-Savarin, the father of modern gourmet cooking, generalized the principle to fattening people and claimed that there were folks who were "carbophores" and he admitted to being one himself [34]. The mechanism: The anabolic effects of the hormone insulin, stimulated primarily by the sugar glucose, was a well established physiologic phenomenon before the first low-carbohydrate revolution. The scientific literature provides many examples of weight loss from carbohydrate restriction beyond the reduction in calories that usually went along with it. Although it has been around in one form or another for a long time, carbohydrate restriction only became revolutionary with the ascendancy of a kind of low-fat nutritional-medical monarchy with powerful influence.

The original Atkins book [20] appeared in its first edition in the seventies, just about the time of the codification of low-fat as the desirable diet. The Atkins Diet was vehemently denounced to the point of having congressional hearings. An amusing moment was the American Medical Association (AMA) asserting that one of the dangers of a low-carbohydrate diet for weight loss was that it might lead to anorexia.

As in political revolutions, the first low-carbohydrate revolution was stimulated by a kind of manifesto, a document that historians describe afterwards as being a call to action. The equivalent of Thomas Paine's *Common Sense*, which fired everybody up for the American Revolution, was Gary Taubes's 2002 article in the *New York Times* Magazine Section: *What if It's All Been a Big Fat Lie* [35] **Figure 4-1.** Later expanded into the book *Good Calories, Bad Calories* [23], Taubes documented the political ascendancy of the low-fat paradigm and the establishment of something like the Court of Low-Fat.

The AMA, the American Heart Association (AHA) and influential physicians were all received at court. The media and the government went along and that included the McGovern Committee — Tom Naughton's comedy documentary *Fat Head* [36] includes a clip of McGovern explaining that congress did not have the luxury of waiting for all the science to be in.

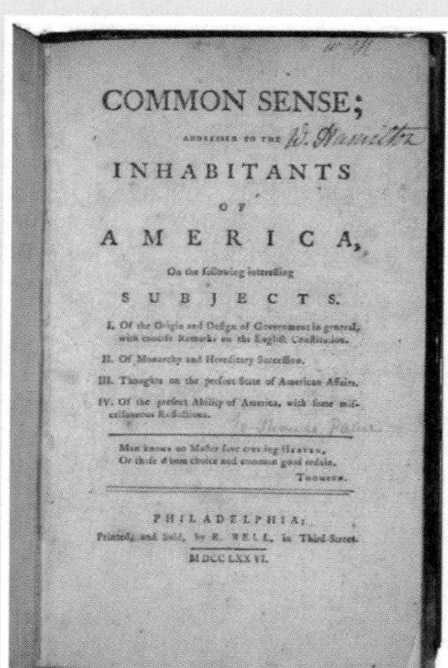

COMMON SENSE;

ADDRESSED TO THE

INHABITANTS

OF

AMERICA,

On the following interesting

SUBJECTS.

I. Of the Origin and Design of Government in general, with concise Remarks on the English Constitution.

II. Of Monarchy and Hereditary Succession.

III. Thoughts on the present State of American Affairs.

IV. Of the present Ability of America, with some miscellaneous Reflections.

Man knows no Master save creating HEAVEN,
Or those whom choice and common good ordain.
THOMSON.

PHILADELPHIA;
Printed, and Sold, by R. BELL, in Third-Street.
MDCCLXXVI.

## What if It's All Been a Big Fat Lie?

By Gary Taubes
Published: Sunday, July 7, 2002

**If the members of the American medical establishment were to have a collective find-yourself-standing-naked-in-Times-Square-type nightmare, this might be it. They spend 30 years ridiculing Robert Atkins, author of the phenomenally-best-selling "Dr. Atkins' Diet Revolution" and "Dr. Atkins' New Diet Revolution," accusing the Manhattan doctor of quackery and fraud, only to discover that the unrepentant Atkins was right all along. Or maybe it's this: they find that their very own dietary recommendations -- eat less fat and more carbohydrates -- are the cause of the rampaging epidemic of obesity in America. Or, just possibly this: they find out both of the above are true.**

FIGURE 4-1. Thomas Paine's *Common Sense* and the first page of Gary Taubes's New York Times Magazine Section piece.

The McGovern hearings set a pattern of ignoring dissenting voices. Philip Handler, Head of the National Academy of Sciences who testified that there was little science behind this rush to judgment. I recognized White as part of White, Handler and Smith, authors of one of the few comprehensive biochemistry texts at the time, that is, he was a well-known biochemist.

## THE FIRST LOW-CARBOHYDRATE REVOLUTION

There were many experimental and clinical trials that set out to prove the diet-heart hypothesis. The first, the Framingham study, still going on, was a massive study of the behavior of residents of the small town in Massachusetts. The original results showed no effect of total or saturated fat or cholesterol on cardiovascular disease (CVD). Doubly disappointing in that the study *did* find a correlation between cholesterol and CVD. The correlation is not a knock-out but there really was a correlation, now a classic in epidemiology, taught in statistics classes. The fact that diet did *not* correlate with CVD is less often discussed. In fact, the results of the Framingham study were buried for years until a statistician had them published. It should have been the death of diet-heart right there. If fat were as bad as they said, there should not be a single failure like this. Not one. In actuality, almost every one of the dozen or so large trials that have followed Framingham has failed. Science, however, was not the major force. The lipophobes, as Michael Pollan calls them [5], anointed themselves with the power to dismiss each experimental failure as loss of a minor battle in a war where victory must surely fall to them; just one more big clinical trial, just another hundred million bucks and you will see how bad fat is. Even when, in 2001, the AHA removed its proscriptions against total dietary fat, it was done without fanfare. What? You didn't know that? They're still down on saturated fat and, of course, *trans*-fat, the easy target that appeared in the food supply because of the pressure from groups like the AHA to replace butter and other sources of saturated fat. They have, however, given up on total fat.

Although preceded by other exposés, Taubes's book was the most compelling presentation of how nutritional science had been taken over by this group of lipophobes. Numerous re-tellings have followed. The recent *Big Fat Surprise*, [11] is of comparable literary quality to "*Good Calories, Bad Calories*, and is more explicit in its condemnations of the players. Ultimately, with control over even the NIH, the low-fat mafia (also a common phrase) could now resist all scientific argument and dismiss all of the experimental failures of low-fat to give us anything at all. The ascendancy of low-fat was, and still is, coupled with a special hatred for low-carbohydrate diets and especially for its main exponent, Dr. Atkins, even after his death.

The low-fat idea wasn't good to begin with, but, of the tests of the idea that failed, one after another, nothing was more embarrassing than the Women's Health Initiative (WHI) which reported in 2006: "Over a mean of 8.1 years, a dietary intervention that reduced total fat intake and increased intakes of vegetables, fruits, and grains did not significantly reduce the risk of coronary heart disease (CHD), stroke, or CVD in postmenopausal women...." A multi-center, $400 million study, the WHI had assigned 19, 541 postmenopausal women to the dietary intervention and a control group of 29,294 women, in a free-living setting. As such, its failure should have been a bombshell. It was not long before Dr. Elizabeth Nabel, director of the National Heart, Lung and Blood Institute of the NIH appeared on television to assure the nation that, instead, recommendations had not changed, that you really needed to reduce saturated fat. Nothing's changed, despite the scientific study that they had funded showing that a change *was* needed. It is serious. The refusal to accept the failure of a scientific test and the stubborn insistence on doctrine was palpably harmful. The WHI women weren't getting any better and the population at large, doing its best to adhere to low-fat, was getting fatter and more diabetic in this period. Refusal to see the WHI for what it was, represented a clear statement that the lipophobes, starting at the top at the NIH, were going to stonewall any effort to change.

## "THE SHOT HEARD 'ROUND THE WORLD"

If *What if it's All Been a Big Fat Lie* was the *Common Sense* of the first low-carbohydrate revolution, the "shot heard 'round the world" was the report by Gary Foster and coworkers [37] showing that the Atkins diet actually improved markers for cardiovascular disease, the lipophobes' main "concern" about low-carbohydrate diets.

The NEW ENGLAND JOURNAL of MEDICINE

ORIGINAL ARTICLE

A Randomized Trial of a Low-Carbohydrate Diet for Obesity

Gary D. Foster, Ph.D., Holly R. Wyatt, M.D., James O. Hill, Ph.D., Brian G. McGuckin, Ed.M., Carrie Brill, B.S., B. Selma Mohammed, M.D., Ph.D., Philippe O. Szapary, M.D., Daniel J. Rader, M.D., Joel S. Edman, D.Sc., and Samuel Klein, M.D.

ABSTRACT

RESULTS

Subjects on the low-carbohydrate diet had lost more weight than subjects on the conventional diet at 3 months (mean [±SD], −6.8±5.0 vs. −2.7±3.7 percent of body weight; P=0.001) and 6 months ... but the difference at 12 months was not significant ...

. After three months, no significant differences were found between the groups in total or low-density lipoprotein cholesterol concentrations. The increase in high-density lipoprotein cholesterol concentrations and the decrease in triglyceride concentrations were greater among subjects on the low-carbohydrate diet than among those on the conventional diet throughout most of the study. Both diets significantly decreased diastolic blood pressure and the insulin response to an oral glucose load.

CONCLUSIONS

The low-carbohydrate diet produced a greater weight loss (absolute difference, approximately 4 percent) than did the conventional diet for the first six months, but the differences were not significant at one year. The low-carbohydrate diet was associated with a greater improvement in some risk factors for coronary heart disease. Adherence was poor and attrition was high in both groups. Longer and larger studies are required to determine the long-term safety and efficacy of low-carbohydrate, high-protein, high-fat diets.

FIGURE 4-2. First page of Foster, et al. [37]

It was the specter of fat that hovered over everything. Foster's demonstration had a big impact because he spoke for the whole nutritional establishment; he later described, in public lectures, how he and his collaborators had been having lunch at a scientific meeting, bemoaning their inability to sweep the Atkins diet from their sight. They decided to get a grant to trash the diet and so they did — one suspects that their intent was clear in the grant application; not to test *whether* the Atkins diet was good or bad — try to get a grant to do that — but to show just how bad it was. They carried out a one-year study comparing a low-carbohydrate diet modeled on the Atkins diet with a low-fat diet. What they found, instead of what they wanted, was that:

> Subjects on the low-carbohydrate diet had lost more weight than subjects on the conventional diet at 3 months....

This part was not a surprise. Everybody knows somebody who has lost a lot of weight on the Atkins diet and nutritionists had more or less granted the idea that low-carbohydrate diets were good for weight loss. Although they usually insisted that it was "just a reduction in calories." (If you've tried to lose weight, though, you know that there is no "just" about it). The kicker, though, was that Foster report:

> ....After three months, no significant differences were found between the groups in *total or low-density lipoprotein cholesterol* concentrations. The increase in *high-density lipoprotein cholesterol* concentrations and the *decrease in triglyceride concentrations* were greater among subjects on the low-carbohydrate diet than among those on the conventional diet throughout most of the study. Both diets significantly decreased diastolic blood pressure and the insulin response to an oral glucose load. [37]. (My *emphasis*).

In other words, the low-carb diet was better on HDL a ("good cholesterol") and especially triglycerides. Most of all, there was no increase in LDL — low-density lipoprotein cholesterol (LDL) which is what your doctor takes as the traffic light for determining whether you need to be prescribed statins.

## MORE WORK NEEDS TO BE DONE

What was the conclusion? "Longer and larger studies are required to determine the long-term safety and efficacy of low-carbohydrate, high-protein, high-fat diets." This strange conclusion indicates the persistent difficulty in making progress. Low-fat diets do worse on most markers and can't do better than a draw on anything else but we are expected to be worried about the low-carb diet? If the low-fat diet

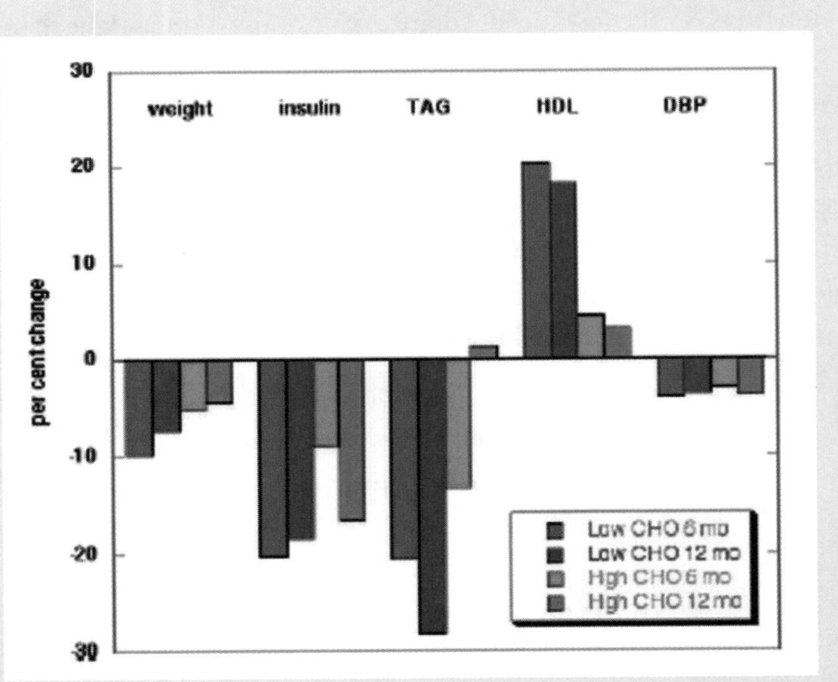


FIGURE 4-3. Comparison of low (blue) and high (red) carbohydrate diets at 6 and 12 months. Results from a multi-center trial in which 63 obese men and women were randomly assigned to either diet. Data from Foster, et al. [37]. Figure from Volek & Feinman [38], used with permission. DBP, diastolic blood pressure; HDL, high-density lipoprotein-cholesterol, so-called "good cholesterol;" TAG, triglycerides.

is worse, shouldn't we be worried about long term safety and efficacy of *that* diet? In fact, Foster's experiment was consistently described as the "diets were the same at one year" and that was supposed to be a draw. There probably are sporting events where the champion keeps the title in the case of a draw but the idea that the low-fat diet was some kind of champion with a long term record of success is absurd. The background assumption that we have some "prudent diet," some diet of "moderation," this is what is called in computers, vaporware. The "conventional diet" is exactly the one that gave us the epidemic of obesity and diabetes.

## AD LIB VS. CALORIE RESTRICTION

Beyond the obvious bias, Foster's study was compromised in its experimental design. People in the low-fat group were directed to consume an explicitly low calorie diet. They were required to eat what they were told. In the low-carb group, in distinction, participants were allowed to eat anything that they wanted as long as they kept carbs low. (Even if you believe that the diets were actually equal, which diet would you go for?) This protocol was used because Foster, *et al.* was not testing the principle of reducing insulin fluctuations as a means of controlling metabolism. The study was not testing, as in the title, "a low-carbohydrate diet for obesity," but rather "The Atkins Diet," and, perhaps in the authors' mind, what was tested was Atkins himself. The Atkins diet said that you didn't have to count calories. The experiment was testing two principles; that carbohydrate restriction meant greater satiety allowing you to regulate calories implicitly and that the Atkins diet, calorie-for-calorie will be more effective for weight loss. Testing both at once was more demanding than isolating the variables. That the low-carbohydrate diet produced the better effect may have been due to either or both the greater satiety or the reduced energy efficiency (from the standpoint of storing fat).

The dietary protocol was not the only problem. Data were analyzed according to the bizarre method known as intention-to-treat (ITT). In this method, data from the people who had dropped out of the study were included in the study by "imputing" values based on previous measurements. The difference between "imputing" and making stuff up is hard to figure out. ITT doesn't make any more sense than you think (discussed in Chapter 23) but that's how things are. Beyond the lack of reasonableness, intention-to-treat always makes the better diet look worse than it actually is. In the event, though, workers in carbohydrate restriction were sufficiently happy to see the positive outcome that they were disinclined to be too critical of the methods. At face value, the lipophobes had had their shot and they lost. They tried to maintain a façade of impartiality while still putting the burden of proof on low-carb, but basically it was a loss. So, what happened to the first low-carb revolution?

Why didn't it move forward? How did low-fat loyalists prevail in the face of such strong scientific evidence?

## WHAT STOPPED IT?

It was an opportunity. The public had a chance to see if the low-carbohydrate idea would work. Many did try it and many had good success. Popular articles were written about it. What happened? If it wasn't the thing for everybody, it seemed to work for most who tried it. Frequently, it seemed miraculous. People described it as "pounds melted away." Why didn't it move forward? First, there was poor understanding of what was involved and there was a proliferation of products designed to make it easier because it was perceived, incorrectly for most people, as a difficult strategy. This allowed the company Atkins Nutritionals® and many others to sell a lot of products many of which were not clearly helpful. They are still doing that. There was little disappointment in the low-carb community when the company declared bankruptcy. Since resurrected, Atkins

Nutritionals continues to offer substitutes for the carbohydrates that you are giving up. There was a proliferation of companies and products containing sugar alcohols — carbohydrates that are digested slowly if at all — and therefore were presumed to not contribute to blood glucose. Untested and poorly understood, sugar alcohols gave some people intestinal problems but, more important, they cast what should have been a straight-forward diet in a slightly bizarre light. But, in the end, the nutritionists and the Professors of Medicine stopped it.

## SECOND, LET'S KILL ALL THE DIETITIANS

"The first thing we do, let's kill all the lawyers"
— William Shakespeare, ***Henry VI, Part II***

What was remarkable about the whole state of affairs was that the low-fat strategy had failed in competition with a real alternative. Low-fat had failed in numerous large scale trials starting with the Framingham study but here it could not compete with a low-carb diet even with the experiment set up in their favor and with the authors' putting a positive spin on it. It was a direct challenge to nutritional orthodoxy but they did not go gentle into that good night. What torpedoed the first low-carbohydrate revolution, were the nutritionists. They had the chance to tell the public "if you do want to try a low-carbohydrate diet, this is what we recommend." Instead, they acted as if Foster's paper had never existed and they ignored those studies that followed it which further supported carbohydrate restriction.

Nutrition has never been highly thought of. The field derives from the practical job of making menus. The advances of physiology and biochemistry meant that nutrition had increasing overlap with more solid science, but the field was, and is, very slow to change. In the real world, nutritionists have attempted to put on the mantle of professionalism and are currently trying to establish the newly re-named Academy of Nutrition and Dietetics (AND) with the legal right to be the sole voice on nutrition and to legally repress anybody else. They recently exercised this power by trying to stop low-carb blogger Steve Cooksey from "offering counseling" on his blog despite appropriate disclaimers (**Figure 4-4**). Currently challenged in court on second amendment grounds, the case highlights the adversarial state of nutritional science. And for those familiar with computer logic, my witticism is to refer to our own group as OR (Objective Research) and the Cooksey affair as NAND-gate.

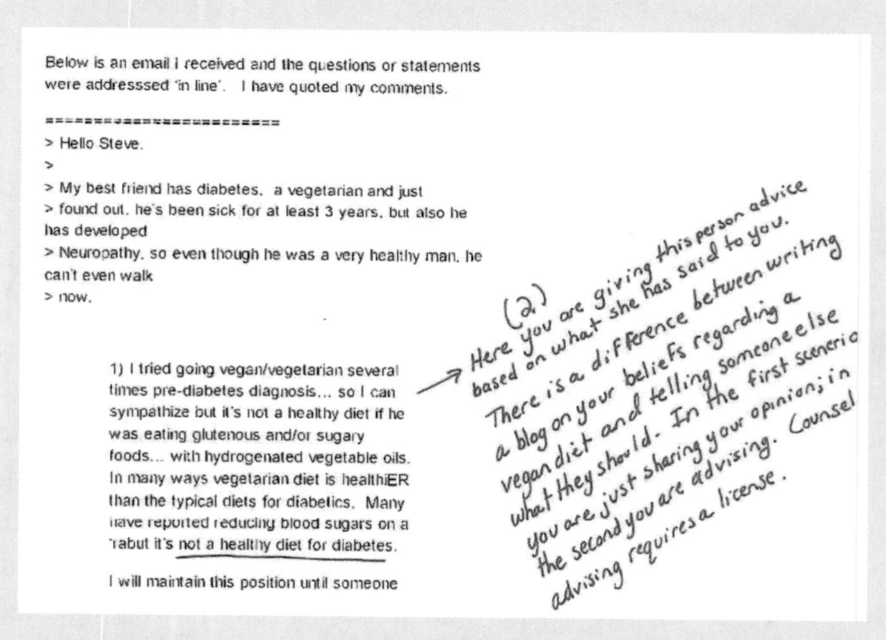
Below is an email I received and the questions or statements were addresssed 'in line'. I have quoted my comments.

========================

> Hello Steve.

>

> My best friend has diabetes. a vegetarian and just
> found out. he's been sick for at least 3 years. but also he has developed
> Neuropathy. so even though he was a very healthy man. he can't even walk
> now.

1) I tried going vegan/vegetarian several times pre-diabetes diagnosis... so I can sympathize but it's not a healthy diet if he was eating glutenous and/or sugary foods... with hydrogenated vegetable oils. In many ways vegetarian diet is healthiER than the typical diets for diabetics. Many have reported reducing blood sugars on a 'rabut it's not a healthy diet for diabetes.

I will maintain this position until someone

(2) Here you are giving this person advice based on what she has said to you. There is a difference between writing a blog on your beliefs regarding a vegan diet and telling someone else what they should. In the first scenerio you are just sharing your opinion; in the second you are advising. Counsel advising requires a license.

FIGURE 4-4. Excerpt from Steve Cooksey's blogpost and red-line by AND (Academy of Nutrition and Dietetics).

Underlying all of the resistance, however, is the idea that only long term large scale studies are important and so we are able to ignore smaller studies which, because they are better controlled, actually give you more information. And again, there was also the assumption, never said out loud, that there were long-term studies supporting a low-fat diet, a "prudent" diet, a diet of moderation that had good success and that could be the one for all of us and, even better, would fix things if you did get fat. There is no such diet and there never was. Again, vaporware. There *were* long-term studies but they had consistently failed. Not just one. Almost all failed. The Framingham Study, the Oslo Heart Study [39, 40], Western Electric Study [41] and probably two dozen others, tabulated and explained in the irreverent style that they deserve by Anthony Colpo [24] including the Women's Health Initiative [42-44]. They showed no value in reducing dietary fat or saturated fat for prevention of heart disease or anything else. And, in the biggest trial of all, the population trial, the diet of the whole American people during the obesity epidemic, it was increased carbohydrate, not fat, that was actually harmful.

To be fair to the nutritionists, the doctors did their part. Undeterred by their lack of training or experience in biochemistry or nutrition, it was *de rigeur* for junior faculty in a department of medicine to write a review trashing the Atkins diet, now taken as the generic name for all low-carbohydrate diets. Some of these critiques cited, as the major flaw, that the diets failed to conform to the USDA or other dietary guidelines. In other words, they faulted a diet that thought the USDA recommendations were bad for not conforming to those recommendations. Using the question as part of the answer is what was called "begging the question" when it meant something specific. (It was probably a dumb phrase anyway).

## FAILURE TO ACCEPT FAILURE

Stepping back and looking at the big picture, the most striking thing was the inability of low-fat diets, even those low-fat diets that did lower cholesterol, to provide a significant impact on cardiovascular outcome or, really, anything else. Very large, very expensive clinical trials of low-fat dietary strategies fail. Most failed big. And they keep doing them and our tax dollars keep paying for them. In addition, in those cases where we didn't have outcome data (how many people had a heart-attack and how many died) and instead, had to look at the risk factors, the different cholesterol forms, HDL, LDL and their sub-fractions, it turned out that reducing fat was at best ambiguous and it was frequently dietary carbohydrate that had the major effect. As carbohydrates were increased, most of the risk markers got worse. The markers and their association with outcome were not sufficient to attribute cause but that had not stopped interpretation when it was low-fat that reduced risk factors.

As we go beyond the original idea of total blood cholesterol as a major risk factor — less than half of the people who have a first heart attack have high cholesterol — as we look at the different forms of the lipoprotein particles (this is what is really measured in the clinical tests of blood cholesterol), carbohydrate restriction becomes the "default diet," the remaining alternative, the one to try first for general health. At the same time, though, while low-carbohydrate diets look better for CVD risk factors, we have the same problem that we have with fat; there is little in the way of evidence that lowering carbohydrate could actually prevent CVD. Given its success in treatment of the collection of health markers referred to as metabolic syndrome (again, our main arguing point), it would be surprising if reducing carbohydrate did not help in prevention but at this point, what we know is very little. We are left with the real possibility that, not only is there nothing at all to the diet-heart hypothesis, that is, not only is dietary fat not involved, but there is the possibility that, outside of well-defined genetic conditions like familial hypercholesterolemia, diet is just not a major player in cardiovascular disease. Very surprising given our current view of things and likely to change as we learn more but you have to go with the data.

## Summary

The first low-carbohydrate revolution, around 2002, was precipitated by Gary Taubes's deconstruction of the diet-heart paradigm, probably more accurately described as calling attention to the self-deconstruction by continued failure of experimental tests. In combination with the multi-center study headed by Gary Foster, the door was open for examination of just what scientific support there was for low-fat ideas and whether the iconoclastic diets based on carbohydrate restriction might not be better. The nutritional establishment, however, refused to accept the results and more or less continues to stone-wall carbohydrate restriction. It will require a second revolution. To understand what the issues really are requires some familiarity with nutritional biochemistry. The macronutrients are the main focus. That's next.

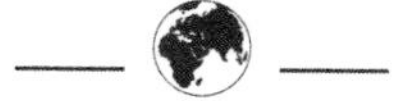

# Chapter 5

# Basic Nutrition: Macronutrients

---

Carbohydrate, fats and protein. These are the **macronutrients** because of the quantities in which they are consumed. *Micronutrients* include vitamins and minerals, obviously to be taken in small amounts. It has become common to refer to foods as "nutrient-rich" or "nutrient-dense," or not, according to whether somebody thinks that they have high amounts of *micro*nutrients. This annoying imprecision is taken by some people — I'm certainly one of them — as an indication of how unscientific, that is, how lacking in attention to detail, the field of nutrition is.

During the period from 1970 to 2000, roughly the time in which observers began to notice an "obesity epidemic," there was an excess of consumption of calories, almost all of which was due to carbohydrates. Protein is usually the most stable part of the diet. In the absence of financial considerations, the generally higher satiety of protein probably makes intake self-limiting although there may be unique metabolic regulation of nitrogen sources. During this period, the total amount of protein in the American diet did not change. **Figure 2-2** shows, that fat, if anything, went down.

## BASICS OF CARBOHYDRATE CHEMISTRY

Chemically, the class of compounds called carbohydrates includes the **simple sugars (monosaccharides)** like glucose and fructose, and combinations of the simple sugars, disaccharides like sucrose (one glucose, one fructose) and polymers (polysaccharides) like starch and glycogen, as well as derivatives of the sugars, for example, the so-called "sugar alcohols."

"Alcohol," that is, ethanol, is not a carbohydrate despite what you may hear on YouTube. Whatever the extent to which sugar can make you as loopy as alcohol, chemically, ethanol is not a carbohydrate. A horse is not a dog. One of the reasons that we make pre-meds study organic chemistry is that the precision in naming organic compounds is presumed to carry over into pharmacology. It is likely that manufacturers started spelling klonopin (antidepressant) with a 'k' because they didn't want physicians to accidentally prescribe clonidine (antihypertensive).

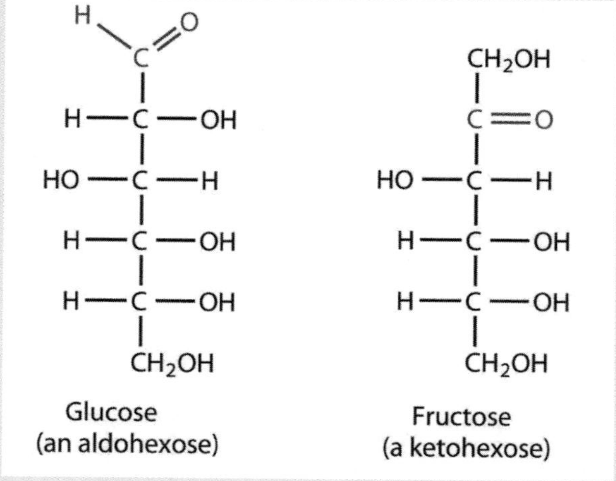

FIGURE 5-1 Structure of simple sugars.

The formal chemical description of sugars is that they are polyhydroxy aldehydes and ketones: **Figure 5-1** shows the chemical structures of glucose and fructose. To simplify where they fit in, in biochemistry, the common sugars and related polymers, can be represented cartoon-style as in **Figure 5-2**.

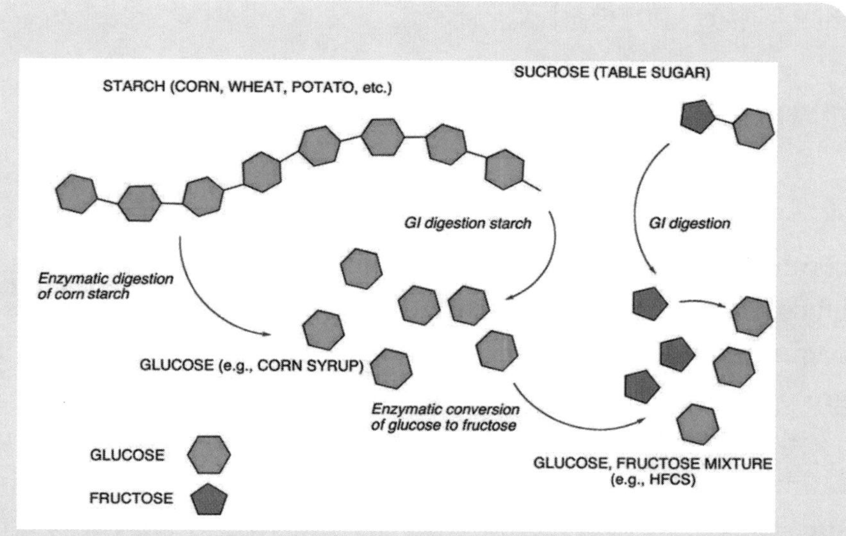


FIGURE 5-2. Structure and transformations of the common carbohydrates. Starch is a polymer of glucose. In digestion, the glucose units are released and absorbed as such. Sucrose is a dimer of fructose and glucose and digestion produces the two monosaccharides.

The most common sugar is glucose and it almost always cyclizes (folds up) in the form of a hexagon, at least in aqueous (water-based) solutions. Fructose can also form a six-membered ring but is more likely to cyclize in a pentagonal shape, as in the cartoon representation in the figure.

**Figure 5-2** reveals that starch is a polymer of glucose (polysaccharide), and that the breakdown to simple sugars is brought about in digestion. If you never did the experiment in grade school, you can try chewing a piece of bread for several minutes. The sweetness that develops is an indicator of the digestive enzymes in saliva which are catalyzing the conversion of the starch in the bread into sugar (glucose). Most starch has a somewhat more complicated structure than that shown in the figure: While some starch molecules, called **amylose**, do have a linear structure, other types, **amylopectin**, have many branch points.

## GLYCOGEN — GLUCOSE SAVINGS ACCOUNT

Glycogen is a polymer of glucose, very highly branched, and it is the storage and supply depot for body glucose flux. Liver, the main command center of metabolism and muscle, the main consumer of glucose, are the sites of glycogen metabolism. Liver has the highest concentration but there is overall much more in muscle where most glycogen is stored.

Branching means that there are a lot of ends so that glucose units can be chopped off as needed. Glycogen is a very dynamic storage site. The extensive branching and 3-D structure means that glycogen occupies a lot of space (**Figure 5-3**). Children with one of the inborn errors of metabolism known as glycogen storage diseases will have visibly distended abdomens due to the increased *size* of the liver (hepatomegaly) needed to accommodate the glycogen stores which can no longer be broken down.

We think of glycogen as desirable because of the association with endurance in sporting events. This is the basis for carbohydrate loading the day before a marathon but, even in the area of athletics, things are not clear cut — marathons are mostly run on fat, even if you are not adapted to a low-carbohydrate diet. A sprinter may depend more on glycogen. And marathon runners train, that is, they use and store carbohydrate. For the rest of us, analogous to fat, glycogen is a storage site for calories so any benefit from carbohydrate loading depends on what you've been doing. Storing calories that you don't use is not a good thing.

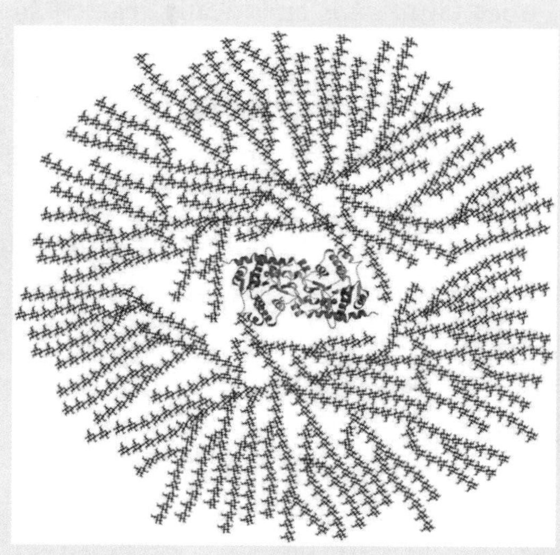

FIGURE. 5-3. Structure of glycogen. Each repeating unit is a glucose molecule. There are rarely more than nine units before the structure branches. The colored object in the center is the protein glycogenin on which the glycogen structure is assembled.

On a low-carbohydrate diet, glycogen storage tends to be reduced, typically, around 60 % on a very low-carbohydrate intake (<100 g)/day. However, metabolism does not run on mass action, (the chemical principle that the amount of a compound will drive its chemical reactivity) but rather on hormones and enzymes. So under conditions of low dietary intake, glycogen will be replenished by the glucose produced from gluconeogenesis and storage will be maintained. It is important to understand that gluconeogenesis and glycogen metabolism are really one process: Glucose synthesized from protein may be stored as glycogen and then only later appear in the blood. An important feature of a carbohydrate-restricted diet, however, is the switch to a metabolic state that runs on fat rather than carbohydrate.

Glucose is at the center of metabolism. Looking ahead, the main theme in human biochemistry is that there are two major fuels — glucose and acetyl-CoA (derived largely from fat, pronounced ass-a-teel-co-ay). Two fuels and two goals; provide energy and maintain blood glucose at a constant level. Too little blood glucose (hypoglycemia) is not good because some tissues, particularly the brain and central nervous system require glucose but too much (hyperglycemia) is also not good. Glucose is chemically reactive and interacts with body proteins. Glycation (reaction with a sugar) may inhibit the protein or it may be cleared from the cell or circulation. You need glucose but, again, you don't have to ingest any. You can make it from protein and other sugars.

A major motif that reappears in this book is that carbohydrate and protein can be turned to fat but, while glucose can be made from protein, with a few exceptions, you can't make glucose from fat. Looking at the two fuels, glucose can provide acetyl-CoA, but acetyl-CoA cannot be converted to glucose.

*Glucose can be made from protein, but, with a few exceptions, you can't make glucose from fat.*

## LIPID CHEMISTRY: GOOD FATS, BAD FATS

Most of the fatty acids have common names — many were discovered before we had systematic chemistry and before we had the professional panels to set the rules. Some of the names tell you how they were discovered — palmitic acid is found in palm oil, oleic in olives and you can guess that caproic and caprыllic acids smell like goats.

There are a lot of disclaimers about "good fats, bad fats" but in one way or another, the government and private agencies, and individual researchers are still recommending that you reduce fat. The recommendation for reduced fat may be accompanied by an explanation that the type of fat is more important than the total amount but when you get down to it, the recommendation, usually runs along the lines of the following contradictory statements: "Fat is not bad. Only saturated fat is bad. Eat low-fat foods." The big targets are saturated fat and, of course, *trans*-fat. The juxtaposition of saturated fat and *trans*-fat is an indicator that it is the politics, not the science, that is at work here.

The American Heart Association (AHA) website provides a truly maniacal cartoon video on the hideous Sat and Trans brothers (**Figure 5-4**):

> "They're a charming pair, Sat and Trans. But that doesn't mean they make good friends. Read on to learn how they clog arteries and break hearts --and how to limit your time with them by avoiding the foods they're in."

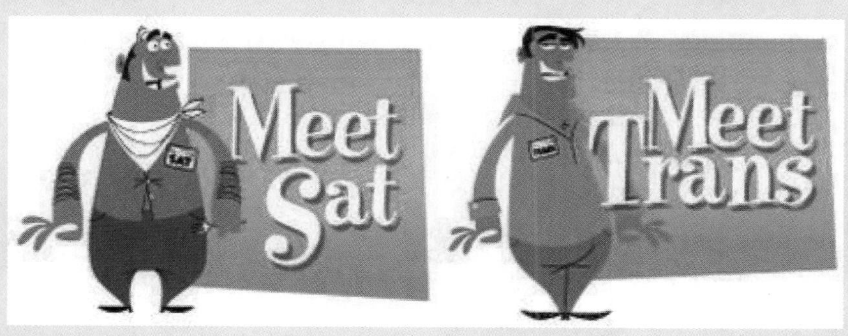


**Figure 5-4.** The evil Sat and Trans brothers from the American Heart Association Website (http://bit.ly/OhiHNC).

What's missing from the website is the story behind *trans*-fat. The crusade against dietary saturated fat, in which the AHA and other health agencies fought so vigorously, led to a search for alternatives to butter and lard. It is important to understand that this mission was led by physicians, not by physiologists, not by biochemists. The movement was accused of trying to carry out a grand experiment with the American people as guinea pigs but there's no stopping zealots. Butter was seen as the quintessential high saturated fat food and it was clear that no progress could be made without deposing it and installing a substitute.

Wide availability of vegetable oils provided a potential alternative to butter, lard and other sources of saturated fat. Vegetable oils, however, are liquids and, at least for baking, have to be converted to a more useable form (like margarine or Crisco). You can do this with the process of hydrogenation; unsaturated oils are "unsaturated" with respect to how much hydrogen is attached to the carbon atoms. Hydrogenation turns some of the unsaturated fatty acids to saturated fatty acids, in effect converting the oil to a solid form. Unsaturated fatty acid molecules have more rigid structure (**Figure 5-5**) and are harder to pack into a solid which is why unsaturated fats tend to be liquid. Converting some of the unsaturated fatty acids into saturated ones made the material more solid and easier to work with. A side-reaction in the manufacture of hydrogenated oil, however, is the conversion of some of the oil to the *trans*-form. The names refer to structure.

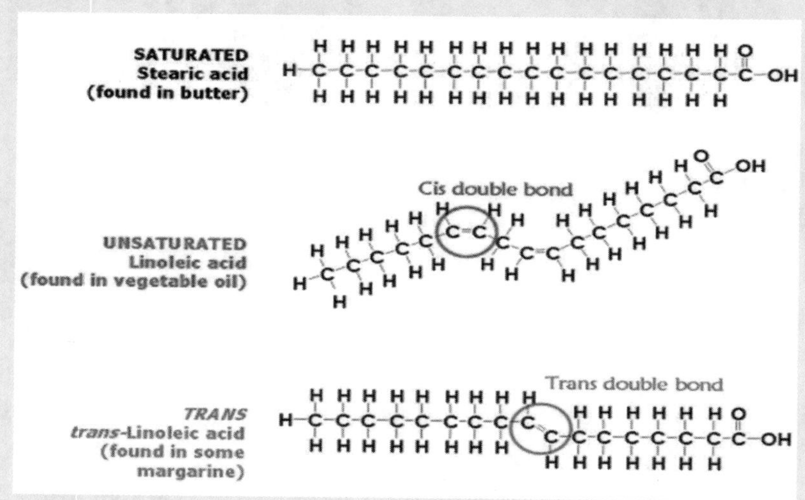


FIGURE 5-5. Structure of fatty acids showing that double bond have two different possible geometric forms: *cis* (large parts of the molecule on the same side of the double bond, or *trans* (opposite sides of the double bonds. There is free rotation around single bonds so they have no such geometrical differences.

As shown in **Figure 5–5**, double (unsaturated) bonds can be *cis* or *trans*; most naturally occurring fatty acids are *cis* so *trans*-fatty acids are not normally processed to a great extent. (Note: *trans*-fats are unsaturated; *cis*-or *trans*-can only refer to unsaturated bonds).

Some biochemists— notably Mary Enig —tried to stop the introduction of products containing *trans*-fatty acids but most chemists did not know much about *trans*-fatty acids and with little support, the low-saturated-fat forces prevailed. At least for a while. When it turned out that *trans*-fat was the form that correlated best with cardiovascular disease, this was a ready-made scapegoat and, presumably because it is an artificial product, it became the target of health agencies. These groups did not mention that *trans*-fat in the food supply arose from their own campaign against saturated fat. In the end, *trans*-fat is a very small part of the diet, its risk is probably greatly exaggerated and there is universal acceptance of the need to remove it, but there is nothing inherently good about it and nobody wants to defend it.

In distinction to *trans*-fat, saturated fat has always been part of the normal human diet and is a normal part of metabolism. Saturated fatty acids are synthesized in your body, a process that is stimulated by a *high carbohydrate* diet. This has been known for years. The process is called *de novo* lipogenesis and is in the biochemistry textbooks, and while it is acknowledged that high dietary carbohydrates led to *de novo* synthesis of saturated fatty acids, the idea is immediately forgotten when official dietary recommendations are being written. So where did we get the idea that fat and saturated fat, in particular, is unhealthy? Again, the story has been told many times, most succinctly in *The Rise and Fall of Modern Medicine* [90], most engagingly in *Good Calories Bad Calories* [23] and *The Big Fat Surprise* [11] but the death knell for the low-fat idea was, or should have been, the meta-analyses from several groups [6-8]. A collection of studies, some going back 25 years was not able to find any risk in dietary saturated fat.

## THE GLUCOSE-INSULIN AXIS

Carbohydrates are food. They are part of the human diet. They are not poison but they can be a problem. We don't know the amount, if any, that's best for any particular person; there is no biological requirement for any carbohydrate as there is for protein or, to a lesser extent, for some fat. Nor do we know whether the type really matters. And glycemic index, or "good carbs, bad carbs" are still weak ideas. But we do know a lot. It's simple: "*High* in carbohydrates" is bad advice for people who are overweight or especially for people who have diabetes or metabolic syndrome. For many of them, reducing carbohydrate can constitute a cure. And while we don't know for sure, it is likely that "*high* in carbohydrates" plays a role in how we *get* fat and diabetic in the first place. And we know that insofar as it's true, it's because we have the underlying basic science; carbohydrates, directly or indirectly, through the hormone **insulin**, control the response to other foods. **Anabolic hormones** stimulate building up of body protein and storage of body material (anabolic steroid hormones are most common in stories in the media because of their effect on muscle protein). Hormonal systems are very complex but surprisingly, in metabolism, insulin has an overpowering effect. Insulin is predominant in the storage of nutrients. It encourages storage of fat. It encourages storage of carbohydrate as **glycogen** and increases the synthesis of body proteins. Hormones communicate with living cells through the docking proteins known as receptors and they trigger the metabolic machinery within the cell.

Carbohydrates are the major stimulus for secretion of insulin. Persistent high insulin fluxes will bias the body towards storage, in particular, storage of fat. So *dietary* fat is important but it plays a more passive role than is generally said. The rate at which fat gets stored depends on the hormones that are present. A "high-fat diet" with high carbohydrate is very different from a diet with the same amount of fat but lower carbohydrate; the carbohydrates may make the effect of the fat deleterious instead of beneficial. That's the bottom line.

We teach first year medical students that the flow of fat from the diet into stored fat or into the lipid markers used to characterize cardiovascular risk is like the flow of water through a faucet. Carbohydrates control the faucet. If carbohydrates are low, flow stops and the fat is oxidized. In the presence of high carbohydrate, insulin increases the rate of storage. This is overly simplified, of course, but it is not greatly oversimplified. The main idea, that it is a control problem not a too-much-stuff problem, is on target.

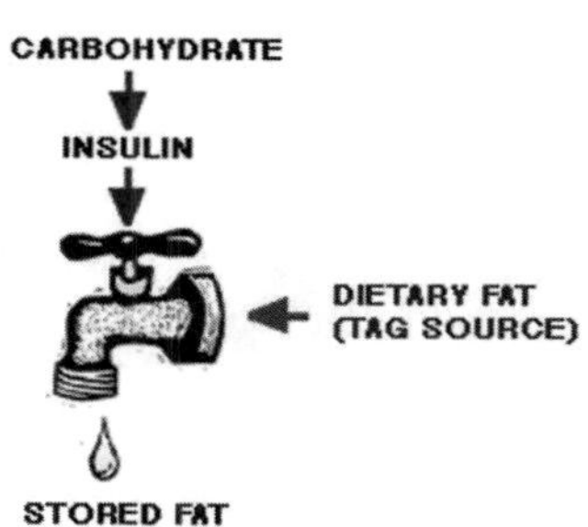


Fat metabolism is only part of the picture. Insulin is a global hormone and regulates carbohydrate and protein metabolism. Everybody knows this but not everybody wants to face it. If you confront naysayers, they tell you that the problem is very complex. So, how does it play out in the real world?

It should be easy to get the answer. Here's an experiment that is pretty clear, or at least, should have been pretty clear. Brehm, *et al.* [45] assigned 50 healthy, slightly obese women to an *ad libitum* low-carbohydrate diet or an energy-restricted, low-fat diet for four months. The results (**Figure 5-6**) tells you that the low-carb people lost significantly more weight.

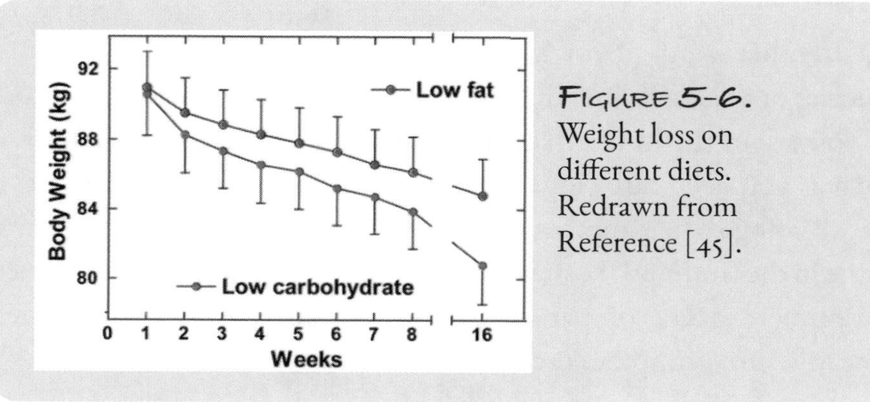


Figure 5-6. Weight loss on different diets. Redrawn from Reference [45].

## DIET COMPARISONS AND THE NUTRITIONAL LITERATURE

Reference [45], however, has good news and bad news. Bad news first. The actual spread of individual values is way bigger than what is shown in the figure. It depends on statistical details but, put simply, there are different ways of showing variation in the data and the one in the figure — if you are already familiar with the terms, the standard error of the mean (SEM) — always makes your data look better than it is. The actual spread is about four times the size of the error bars. So the bad news is that outcome on the two diets are not highly predictable and from the presentation of the data you can't tell who did what. The good news is that the big winners must have been the people in the low-carb group. So, in this kind of experiment you don't know your odds but you do know which has the possibility of the bigger payoff.

Really good news; read the Methods section and you find that this experiment followed the protocol for Foster's paper described above:

> "... One group of dieters was instructed to follow an ad libitum diet ...The other group of dieters was instructed to follow an energy-restricted, moderately low-fat diet with a recommended macronutrient distribution of 55% carbohydrate, 15% protein, and 30% fat."

In other words, if you are in the low-fat group, you have to count calories or at least follow the low-calorie meal plan that they give you. If you are in the low-carb group, you can do whatever you want as long as you keep carbs low. If the results are even the same, most of us are going to be happier doing the low-carb diet. This is how it was done in the landmark Foster paper and the pattern has been continued for numerous diet comparisons; the low-fat group must limit calories. The low-carb group can eat *ad lib* as long as carbs are low.

You don't always read the Methods section of a paper unless you are actually planning to repeat the experiment yourself or if there is something unusual that is specifically due to the details of how the experiment was carried. If there is something important in the methodology, it should be described in the body of the paper. I admit that when this was published in 2005, I didn't realize that a low-calorie diet was pitted against an *ad lib* low-carb diet and, in fact, that it was a pattern for diet comparisons of this type. The rationale, of course, was that since the Atkins diet did not restrict calories, participants in the low-carb arm would only be instructed to reduce carbohydrate intake. This may be reasonable from a clinical point of view but it does make "the diet," rather than carbohydrate, that is, something easier to control, the independent variable.

Brehm's experiment is far from the best but it is representative of the type of experiment, the low-carb diet does better but there is big spread in the values.

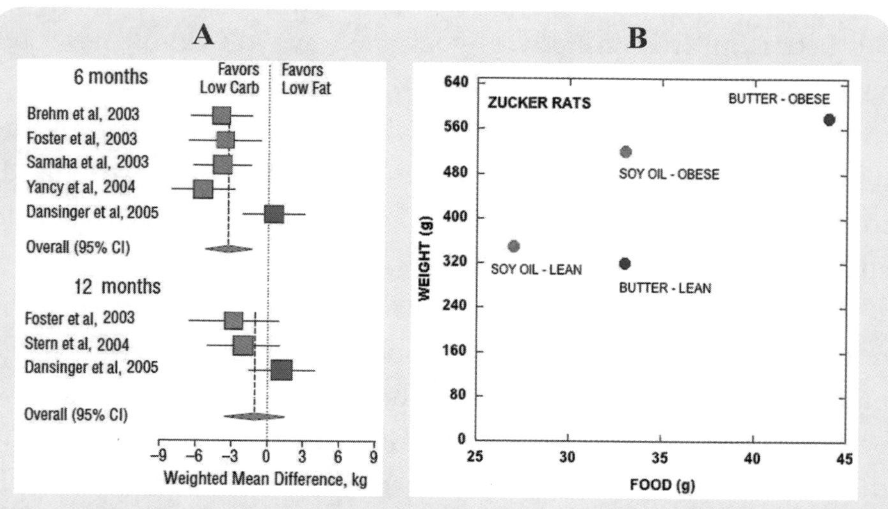


Figure 5-7 A. Meta-analysis of comparisons of weight loss on low-fat and low-carbohydrate diets. Data from reference [46]
B. Responses to different lipids in Zucker rats.

In 2006 a meta-analysis, that is, a re-examination of previous studies, was performed by Nordmann *et al.* Meta-analysis is a weak, possibly useless method. The idea is to average previous studies but most of us think that averaging errors makes things worse, not better. On the other hand, a meta-analysis usually does give you a chance to see the results from several different studies. **Figure 5-7 A** shows the conclusion, that low-carbohydrate diets lead to better weight loss. In interpreting the graph, it is important to understand that when the error bars (horizontal lines in this figure) cross the line at 1.0, it means that there is no effect, either way. Most of the studies found the low-carbohydrate diet to be more effective at six months but, again, no difference at one year. The reason things got worse after six months is that the experimenters let them get worse — they didn't know how to keep everybody on track. When it's your diet, you won't let that happen.

Several other studies have been done since and with the same conclusion. They present the same picture; the shorter ones turn out better but it almost always goes one way, you almost never see a study showing that low-fat is better. Nutritionists tend to consider that a draw means low-fat wins, and when low-carbohydrate wins the results are simply ignored or, as in Foster's study, "more work needs to be done." That's why we have the recommendations that we do and why we have the nutritional mess.

There is always the objection that studies that depend on diet records, as most of these do, are prone to error and that the people in the study are mis-reporting what they eat. Errors in reporting have been documented but they are not completely inaccurate — usually they are about 80 % accurate. All experiments have error, however. It is only a question of how you deal with the error. For inaccuracy in dietary reporting to account for the difference between diets it would be necessary for subjects in the low-fat group to under-report what they ate and for the low-carbohydrate people to *over*-report what they ate, or both. These are certainly possible but, again, from a practical standpoint it might be good to be on a diet where you think you ate more than you actually did.

In nutrition, animal studies have obvious limitations — it is considered a departure from normality when we "eat like a bird," or "like a pig" — but experimentally, such studies have an advantage because the subjects eat what you tell them to eat. The experimenter can control food intake; **Figure 5-6 B** shows that weight gain in a species of rats depends on how much they eat, of course. But there is also a difference in whether their source of oil is butter or soy oil; butter is less fattening for rats in general but the obese ones really go for it. You can't generalize the specific result to humans but it shows that there is nothing strange about weight gain being dependent on the exact composition of the diet. Finally, biochemistry tells us that there is no receptor for calories, that is, no way for cells to sense how many calories are coming in, only how much of each type of macronutrient. The available chemical energy will ultimately show up but there is no reason to think that there will be a direct relation between calories and weight gain or loss. Calories do count but not in a simple way.

## FAT — THE FAILURE TO ACCEPT FAILURE

The decline in the percentage of dietary fat in the past thirty years was described in the last chapter. The reduction in *percentage* is partly due to the increased intake of total calories but, at least for men, the absolute amount of total and saturated fat has also gone down. The fact that a decrease in dietary fat has been accompanied by overeating and noticeable increases in diabetes and metabolic syndrome stands as an inescapable indictment of the low-fat doctrine. And, while survival has increased due to treatment, the incidence of heart disease has not changed substantially, at least in the United States. In other countries where it has, it is more likely due to reduction in smoking. It is widely said that association does not predict causality — does not *necessarily* predict causality is more accurate — but a *lack* of association is strong evidence for a *lack* of causality.

## ANIMAL MODELS

To be fair to the low-fat doctrine, it is easy to be misled. Animal studies are critical in biological science and it seems that mice, especially the mice bred for laboratory work, will get fat on high fat diets even without any carbohydrate [47-49]. How is that possible? People don't usually get fat on high fat diets, or at least, don't over-consume fat to such a high degree on high fat diets, unless the diet is also high in carbohydrate. Mice aren't men but they are a generally good metabolic model for many things so this is a drastic difference. Carbohydrate is key in human metabolism. Not necessarily so in rodent metabolism where a high fat diet can bring on obesity, diabetes and cardiovascular disease even in the absence of carbohydrate. We don't yet have a theory to encompass the differences. If our understanding of the catalytic role of insulin is correct, then it may well be that mice (who normally live on high carbohydrate diets) may maintain a functionally high level of insulin all the time, so the bias toward an anabolic state that occurs with high carbohydrates in humans is always 'on' in mice.

Whatever the explanation, it may be hard to recognize that the model system that we have used so extensively might have most impact because it is *different* from the way people respond. In this case, animal models might offer a clue to what people do *because* humans do not behave like the animals.

The real problem is that we have not faced the practical, experimental tests in humans. We have large expensive clinical trials with a consistent and reliable outcome; there is no effect of dietary fat on obesity, cardiovascular disease or just about anything else. The unwillingness to face these failures makes this a remarkable phenomenon in the history of medicine — that it persists in a period of sophisticated science and technology makes it nearly unbelievable.

"Unbelievable" is the key word. That a science is incomplete or has flaws is what one expects but that the whole of the establishment opinion on diet-heart is totally meaningless is hard to understand. How could they keep doing the same experiment over and over without success? How could that be? How could they get away with it? Why would they *want* to get away with it? New trials continue to show nothing. Well, not nothing. They clearly show that low-fat is ineffective for weight loss or just about everything else.

In science, excluding a theory is always stronger than showing consistency. In this case, if the fat-cholesterol-heart story were as they say, as salient and inescapable a risk as they make it out to be, then none of these big studies should fail. Not one. In fact, almost all fail. An occasional one shows an effect. There has been an increasing admission that high carbohydrate is not a good thing. The admission usually comes with a qualifier; "especially refined sugar" or "refined starch", but no study has directly compared "refined" and "unrefined" — high-GI and low-GI are not measures of refinement and they are, in any case weak predictors. The drastic increase in total carbohydrate that has accompanied the obesity epidemic is its most salient feature. You may choose to ignore it if you don't like it, but it is there.

So, does this mean we can add more fat? Is fat still bad? It's probably fair to say that most people think that, in some way, fat it still bad. It will turn out that the role of fat in the body is itself controlled, directly or indirectly through hormones, by carbohydrates. Deleterious effects of lipid metabolism are under the control of carbohydrates. Perhaps, most surprising, the biochemistry shows that it is the fat (more precisely the fatty acids) in your *blood* that are the problem but they are more likely to come from dietary carbohydrate than from dietary fat.

## ARE CARBOHYDRATES FATTENING

"I don't understand. I went to this conference and they had a buffet every night and I really pigged out on roast beef and lobster but I didn't gain any weight."

— Author's brother.

Nobody ever says that after going on a cruise where they pigged out on pasta and didn't gain any weight. In the faucet analogy, in the area of weight gain and loss, fat can be packaged into fat cells. Insulin opens the faucet for fat storage but it shuts down the faucet for fat oxidation. At this point, though, you might ask whether all this matters. Doesn't it all even out in the end? Isn't it just calories in, calories out, or, as they always say in the news releases "a calorie is a calorie?" And, don't the laws of thermodynamics tell us that?

It is hard to tell the extent to which you can lose more weight calorie-for-calorie by changing the composition of the diet. One clue, though, is that when an experiment shows that one macronutrient is more inefficient than another (wastes calories as heat), it is usually the low-carbohydrate arm that is less fattening. Critics say that the results are due to inaccurate reporting of food intake and that it is just about calories. Low-carb diets, they say, simply reduce total energy intake. As in the Brehm study, food frequency records can have substantial error and, again, if that is why the low-carb group always wins in these face-offs, low-carb participants would have to be over-reporting what they ate or low-fat comparisons groups would have to be under-reporting what they ate, or both. Again, there might be a real benefit of being on a diet where you think you ate more than you did. And if you thought that reducing calories was "just," you wouldn't be reading this book.

And thermodynamics does not predict that "a calorie is a calorie." Most people who quote the "laws of thermodynamics"— they usually mean just the first law — have never studied thermodynamics and simply don't know what it is about. The essential feature of thermodynamics rests, not with the first law which is about energy conservation, but rather with the second law which says that all (real) processes are inefficient. Energy is dissipated. The variable efficiency (the extent to which energy is wasted as heat) of fat, protein and carbohydrate is well known but, in the medical literature, ignored at will. Often, however, total calories may turn out to be the controlling variable but insofar as it is independent of macronutrient composition, it is because of the homeostatic (stabilizing) mechanisms of biological systems, not because of thermodynamics. Thermodynamics is my special interest and we'll come back to it in Chapter 14. Promise. First, look further at some of the underlying chemistry.

## "The Atkins Diet is a High Calorie Starvation Diet"

The quotation is from George Cahill, one of the pioneers in the study of metabolism and the response to starvation. The idea is that the reduction in blood glucose and insulin, and the increase in glucagon that accompanies reductions in carbohydrate intake, resembles the changes that are associated with total reduction in calories. In starvation, insulin goes down and glucagon goes up and fat oxidation increases, and at some point ketone bodies are generated.

In 1992, Klein & Wolfe [50] carried out a defining experiment. They had subjects go without food for three days and then, after a period of rest, they went through another three days of starvation. This time, however, the people in the experiment received intravenous injection of a lipid emulsion that was designed to meet their resting energy requirements. Klein & Wolfe measured several physiologic parameters in both experiments and as shown in Table 5-1, there was not a great difference between the two tests despite the very large difference in energy intake. The levels of free fatty acids (FFA) were the same and, in both cases, ketone bodies were reasonably high. The presence of fat if anything reduced the rates of fat oxidation. The conclusion from the study was that "these results demonstrate that restriction of dietary carbohydrate, not the general absence of energy intake itself, is responsible for initiation of the metabolic response to short-term fasting." The statement is undoubtedly something of an exaggeration, but the experiment brings out one of the major themes in diet and metabolism: Carbohydrate is a controlling element while dietary fat plays a relatively passive role. This is not to say that circulating fat, body fat or fatty acids do not play a role in metabolism but assuming that dietary fat equates to body lipids is wrong, way wrong. This is a major theme in this book: "You are what you eat" is not a good principle.

**Table 1: Similarity of starvation and carbohydrate restriction**

| | FFA (µmol/l) | fat oxidation (µmol/kg/min) | Glucose (mg/dl) | β-hydroxybutyrate (mM) |
|---|---|---|---|---|
| **Fast 84 h** | 0.92 | 1.94 | 68 | 2.56 |
| **Fast + Lipid** | 1.02 | 1.67 | 66 | 2.54 |

## WHEN YOU WAKE UP IN THE MORNING...

There are two goals in human metabolism. You have to provide energy and you have to maintain blood glucose at a relatively constant level. In the **fed state**, which nutritionists call the **post-prandial state**, the eight hours or so after a meal, diet can provide a greater or lesser amount of the material needed to meet these two needs. The period at which ingested food no longer provides material for metabolism directly is referred to as **fasting, or post-absorptive state**. When you wake up in the morning (**Figure 5-8**), after an overnight fast, insulin is low and glucagon is high, fat is broken down (lipolysis) to fatty acids and glycerol — lipolysis is inhibited by insulin and stimulated by glucagon. The fatty acids are oxidized for energy. Blood glucose is maintained by the processing of liver glycogen. Muscle also stores glycogen which can be broken down. This glucose is used by the muscle itself and is not exported. Again, we think of muscle as a consumer of glucose and the liver as a supplier, or more generally, as a command center for metabolism.

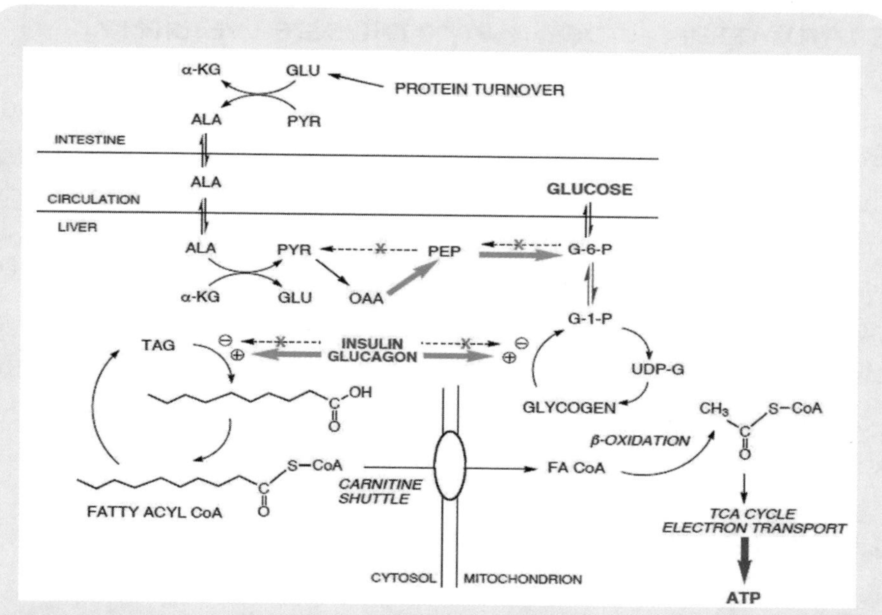


FIGURE 5-8. After an overnight fast or low-carbohydrate diet, insulin is low and glucagon is high, fat is broken down (lipolysis) to fatty acids and glycerol. Gluconeogenesis (GNG) from protein is another source of glucose.

## GLUCONEOGENESIS

Frequently described as a kind of last ditch source of glucose or energy when no food is coming in and glycogen is depleted but, in fact, gluconeogenesis (GNG) goes on all the time. When you wake up in the morning, more than half of the free glucose in the blood or produced from previously stored glycogen comes from GNG. Although there is no form of protein formally defined as a storage site as there is for stored fat or glycogen, muscle can be thought of as providing an internal source of protein, a source that must be replenished from the diet, a dynamic store of amino acids for metabolism. (More information in reference [51]).

## STARVATION -GOOD WAY TO LOSE WEIGHT?

In the fasting state, then, adipocytes (fat cells) supply fatty acids from the breakdown of fat. Most tissues, including the heart, oxidize the fatty acids for energy. Some tissues, primarily brain and central nervous system require glucose and that is provided by the combination of glycogen breakdown and replenishment from gluconeogenesis. The two goals of metabolism are taken care of. Is starvation a good way to lose weight? Of course it is not. The requirement for amino acids from protein for the maintenance of blood glucose is the problem. In the absence of dietary protein, your body will turn to its own sources.

## ARE CARBOHYDRATES FATTENING?

*Harper's Illustrated Biochemistry* is one of the standard texts in medical and graduate schools. Now in its 29th edition, it is a multi-authored comprehensive view of the field. I am grateful to Adele Hite of University of North Carolina for pointing out that in the *8th edition* (1961), when it was called *Review of Physiological Chemistry* and Harper himself was the sole author, the close connection between carbohydrate and fat was evident. The Chapter on Metabolism of Carbohydrates begins as follows.

> In the average diet carbohydrate compromises more than half of the total caloric intake. However, only a limited amount of this dietary carbohydrate can be stored as such. It is now known that

> the un-stored portion of the ingested carbohydrate is converted to fat by the metabolic processes of lipogenesis [52].

In other words, the third sentence of the carbohydrate section of a biochemistry text emphasized the closeness of carbohydrate and fat. In the twentieth edition (1985), the Chapter, now written by Peter Mayes, begins similarly and continues,

> It is possible that in humans the frequency of taking meals and the extent to which carbohydrates are converted to fat could have a bearing on disease states such as atherosclerosis, obesity and diabetes mellitus [53].

In the current edition, the process of conversion of carbohydrate to fat now has a chapter of its own. The process is known as de novo lipogenesis (DNL), new synthesis of fat, or more precisely de novo fatty acid synthesis since the immediate product is a fatty acid, the saturated fatty acid, palmitic acid (C16:0). DNL appears to be the explanation of the counter-intuitive result, demonstrated in several studies that dietary carbohydrate diet leads to increases in saturated fatty acids in the blood. Chapter 9 describes an experiment from Jeff Volek at the University of Connecticut where such an increase in saturated fatty acids was greater in the blood of people on a high carbohydrate diet compared to those on a low-carbohydrate diet even though the latter had three times the amount of dietary saturated fat.

## WHAT ABOUT PROTEIN?

In some classes that I teach, I ask the students for the definition of life. I get different answers but I usually say "no, a one word definition." I try not to drag it out too long or to overact, but the answer that I am looking for is "protein." Everything that goes on in life is controlled by proteins either as the actual component or as the source for other things. Because of its multiple roles in biology and the far more complicated chemistry, I will present here only broad outlines in the context of an answer to an email.

I received the following question:

> If one is on a very-low-carbohydrate/high-fat diet, what happens to excess protein that is not needed for muscle repair and growth, and gluconeogenesis? I see two alternatives:
>
> 1. It's excreted
>
> 2. More glucose is created.
>
> #2 seems so unreasonable to me...would your metabolism actually make more than the little bit it needs? I'm open to a #3 that I might be too unimaginative to think of. I'm interested in the theory, this isn't a request for diet advice. I like to understand things at the cellular level.

The answer is that it depends on what else is going on, but protein, *per se*, is not excreted (in the absence of some disease). Protein is a polymer. Unlike glycogen which is a homopolymer of identical glucose units, the individual units, amino acids, are picked from about twenty different choices. In digestion, protein is broken down to individual amino acids and are absorbed and re-assembled into body protein. The sequence of amino acids defines the biologic function and this sequence is encoded in the genetic material. The genetic code is largely the code of amino acid sequences.

After digestion and absorption, some of the amino acids that are not used for protein synthesis may be trashed. The nitrogen is converted to ammonia which is converted to the compound urea and excreted. The remaining carbon skeleton can be used for energy either directly in the TCA cycle or converted to ketone bodies, especially on a very low-carbohydrate diet. Some amino acids can be converted to glucose. Much more than a little bit is needed. The carbon skeleton from amino acids, directly or indirectly can be converted to fat. So, a practical answer is that, "excess" protein is re-cycled, used for energy or for synthesis of glucose.

Protein, as such, is not normally excreted. Proteinuria is an indication of some abnormality, kidney malfunction or other disease-related nephropathy. Amino acids are excreted at some low level. High excretion of particular amino acids is usually an indication of some metabolic disturbance or inborn error of metabolism. It is important to understand that everything that goes on in the body is mediated by proteins which turn over all the time and whereas muscle "repair and growth" is important, it is not the only thing. Body proteins, unlike glycogen or other homopolymers, have specific amino acids sequences so require a particular make-up. Some amino-acids are interconverted and some (essential amino acids) are required from diet.

Current tendencies are to try to encourage vegetarianism or, at least, reduce meat consumption. Whatever the moral or practical arguments are, the scientific case is highly questionable. The proliferation of studies trying to demonstrate an associations between meat consumption and one disease or another are largely bogus and a couple of these studies are deconstructed in Chapters 18 and 19.

## What We Eat

Protein is a stable part of the diet. Total consumption of protein has not changed during the obesity epidemic. Sources of protein have changed. Consumption of red meat has gone down and chicken consumption has gone up (**Figures 5-9** and **5-10**). Other things have increased to a greater extent. **Figure 5-10** is from a paper by George Bray [54].

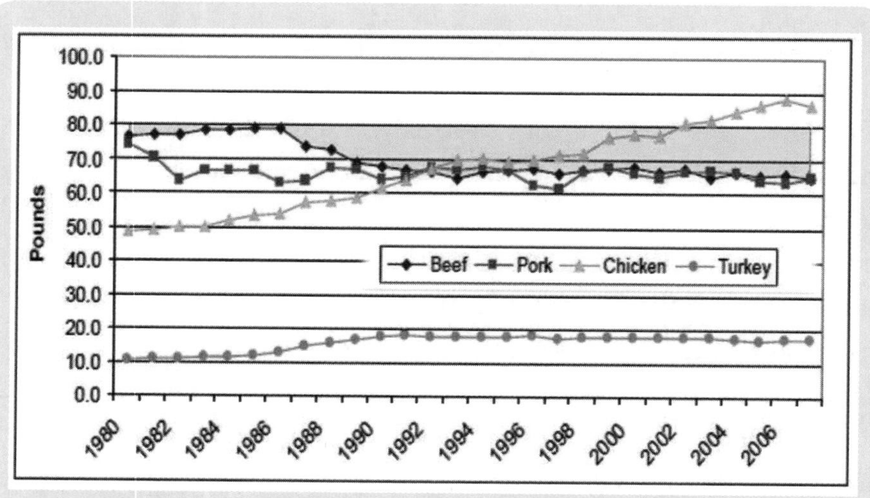


FIGURE 5-9. Meat Consumption in the indicated period.

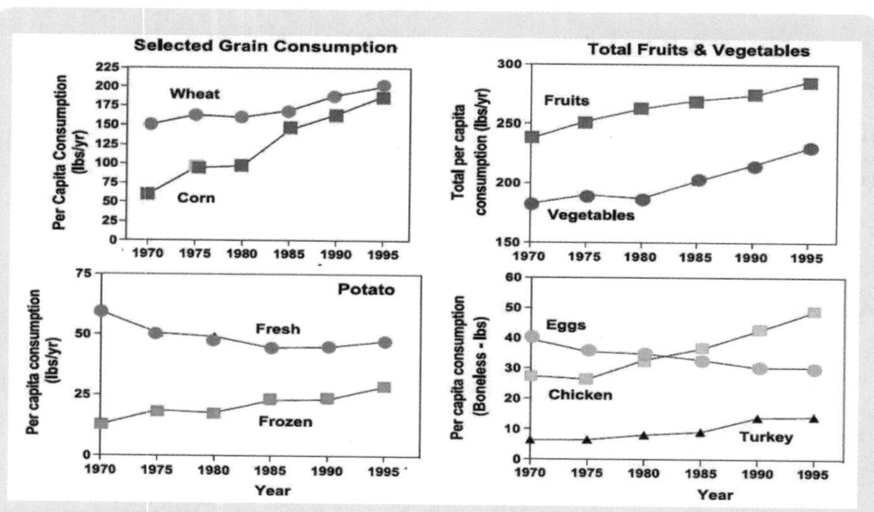


FIGURE 5-10. Food Consumption in the indicated period. Figure redrawn from Bray, et al. [54].

The original caption attached to **Figure 5-10** included the rather odd comment that "none of the foods in this figure show changes that would help to pinpoint this epidemic." Something about the increase in wheat and corn would seem to be relevant.

**Figure 5-10** also suggests that, contrary to almost everybody's recommendations, we are not going to make great headway simply by increasing "healthy" fruits and vegetables.

## SUMMARY

Carbohydrate, fats and protein are the macronutrients. They provide the major building blocks for body material and are their transformation, primarily via oxidation is the source of energy. They are not just fuels and raw materials. Macronutrients are involved in regulating their own utilization. Carbohydrates, in particular, directly or indirectly, through the hormone insulin, control the response to other macronutrients in foods. Primarily anabolic, insulin controls storage of nutrients (favors storage of fat, stimulates glycogen) storage and increases the synthesis of body proteins.

Deleterious effects of lipid metabolism are under the control of carbohydrates. Glucose can come from dietary input or can be produced by other cell processes and in both cases, can be used directly for energy or stored as glycogen, primarily in muscle or liver. Liver glycogen can supply glucose for other tissues. Muscle stores glycogen only for its own use. Gluconeogenesis and glycogen metabolism are really one continuous process; glucose synthesized from protein may be stored as glycogen and then only later appear in the blood.

The pivotal idea in metabolism is that while fat can be made from glucose, with few exceptions, glucose cannot be made from fat.

During the period of the obesity epidemic excess consumption of calories was almost entirely due to carbohydrates. Protein in the American diet did not change and fat, if anything, went down.

There have been major revolutions in the history of nutrition. A short historical digression in the next chapter may bring some things about glucose and glycogen into focus.

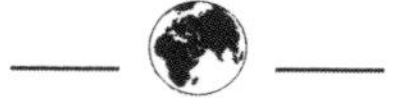

# Chapter 6

# Another Revolution: Glycogen And Gluconeogenesis

The nineteenth century was a period of political, intellectual and scientific revolution. Politics makes more noise but there may be greater long term impact from turnarounds in intellectual and scientific fields. The summer of 1848 in Paris was the site of yet another French Revolution. People had taken to the streets. They were building barricades just as in *Les Mis*. There was dissatisfaction over rights of assembly and the autocratic government but rising food prices were probably more important. Whatever it was about, there was much turmoil leading the faculty at the *Collège de France* to complain that it had all "slackened the zeal for research among all of the chemists, and all of their time...is absorbed by politics." The intellectual revolution at the *Collège*, however, was in Claude Bernard's laboratory.

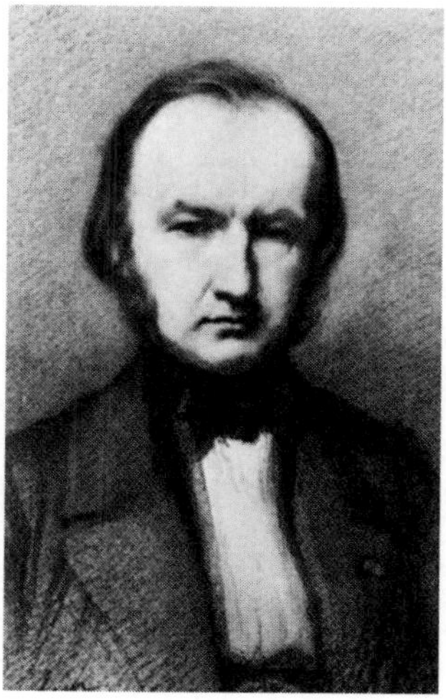

Figure 6-1. Claude Bernard, 1858

Bernard, generally considered the father of modern physiology had been studying digestion in dogs. He found sugar in a dog that he had been dissecting, a dog that had not been fed any sugar. It was revolutionary because it was generally assumed at the time that any sugar in an animal had to have come from the diet and it was expected that, in the end, the sugar would be destroyed by oxidation; animals eat sugar — or any food — for energy and the energy comes from oxidation of the food just as if you were burning food in a furnace. Lavoisier had shown that more than 100 years before. Sugar *was* a food. How did it wind up undigested in the animal? Bernard's first reaction was that there might be something wrong with the reagent that he had used to detect the sugar. But the reagent was okay, the dog really was making its own sugar. In fact, he soon found that if he fed a dog only meat, there was as much sugar in that animal as there was in another dog that had been fed on a "sugary soup." Strange as it seemed, the dog must be making its own sugar. It must be making sugar from something else.

## GLYCOGEN AND GLUCONEOGENESIS

> "Although Bernard's experimental findings were occasionally at fault and at times influenced by preconceptions ... his strength appears to lie in his ability to discard a theory once its experimental basis had been undermined. Even though he was apt not to state frankly that he had been wrong, he nevertheless did change his ideas."
>
> — F. G. Young [55]

It took some doing to show that the sugar was actually being produced in the dog's liver but, by 1857, Claude Bernard had isolated the *matière glycogene*, that is, **glycogen**. We know now that glycogen is a storage form of carbohydrate, a polymer of glucose. It is actually made from glucose, although the glucose that goes into the glycogen may come from something else.

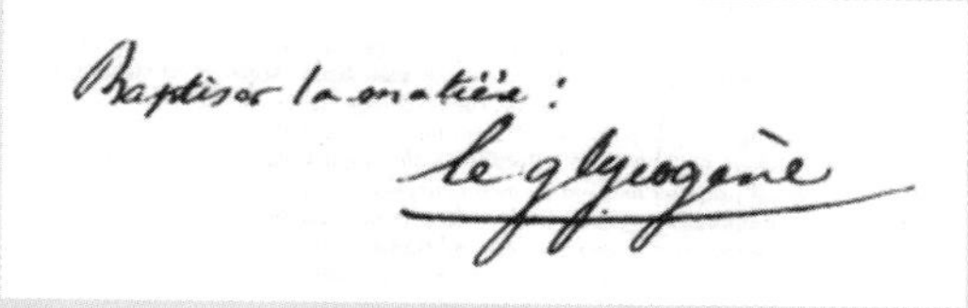

FIGURE 6-2 The first mention of the word glycogen as recorded by Claude Bernard in 1857

Glycogen is, a highly branched, highly structured polymer as in **Figure 5-3** and it is the key player in maintaining blood glucose at a constant level. Glucose is a major energy source and when cells take up glucose, the liver breaks down glycogen to re-establish a constant level. Bernard emphasized this role of glycogen as a supplier, providing glucose to the circulation, but he was not quite right on how it got there. He knew that glycogen didn't come from fat and further experiments showed that feeding protein seemed to be even better than feeding sugar (he used fibrin, the blood coagulation protein). The picture that evolved was that protein was the source of glycogen which, in turn, could produce glucose. This was not exactly right — if carbohydrate intake is high, ingested sugar is converted to glycogen — but Bernard had not only discovered glycogen but had also seen the need for the process which converted other things to glucose, the process now understood as **gluconeogenesis**. This would not be fully understood for another hundred years.

Our current understanding focuses on glycogen synthesis and breakdown as a control point in metabolism. Sugar in the diet or in the circulation can be stored in glycogen and can be made available when needed. But, it is not only dietary glucose that shows up in glycogen. Bernard was right that sugar could be made in the liver from protein, that is, amino acids from proteins. (It is sometimes said, even in textbooks, that gluconeogenesis is a "last ditch" source of glucose but, in fact, the process goes on all the time). The glucose synthesized in gluconeogenesis may be exported to the blood or, alternatively, may be used to replenish previously used glycogen and the new glucose molecules may only appear in the blood at a later time.

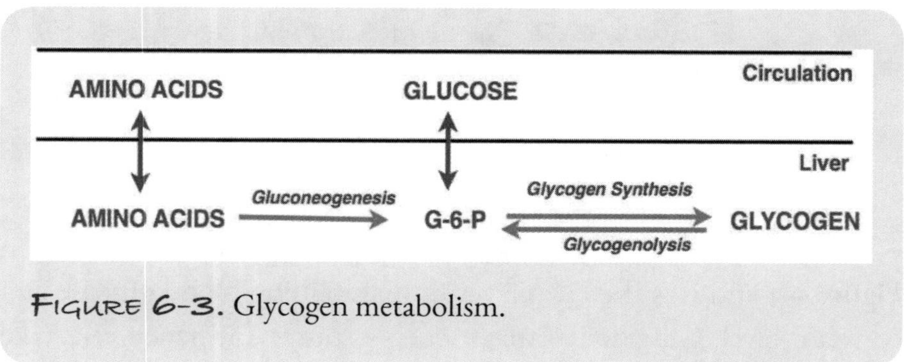


FIGURE 6-3. Glycogen metabolism.

Bernard was right that glucose came from glycogen but he did not understand that glycogen could also be *made* from ingested sugar. The key mistake is that Bernard did not understand that glucose is present in the blood all the time and it is maintained at a constant level (**Figure 6-3**). He didn't get it because he had actually made an experimental error. A lucky one, it turns out.

## SOMETIMES WE LUCK OUT

The reason for believing that glycogen was not made from glucose came from his measurements of the inputs to and outputs from the liver. Bernard determined the amount of sugar in the portal vein which brings blood from the digestive tract to the liver — it's not a true vein (red in **Figure 6-4**.) He measured, as well, the amount of glucose leaving the liver in the hepatic veins (blue). His original observations showed that there was little or no glucose in the inputs from the portal vein, that is, it seemed that no sugar was coming into the liver. But he could identify sugar in the hepatic veins *leaving* the liver. In other words, he could see glucose exiting the liver but no glucose coming in. This pretty much made his case that the liver was a sugar-producing organ and that glycogen was being made from something else.

Some of Bernard's scientific rivals said that he was wrong; they said that they themselves had, in fact, been able to detect sugar coming into the liver in the portal vein. They were right, of course — we know that there is sugar throughout the circulation and that glycogen is assembled from blood glucose.

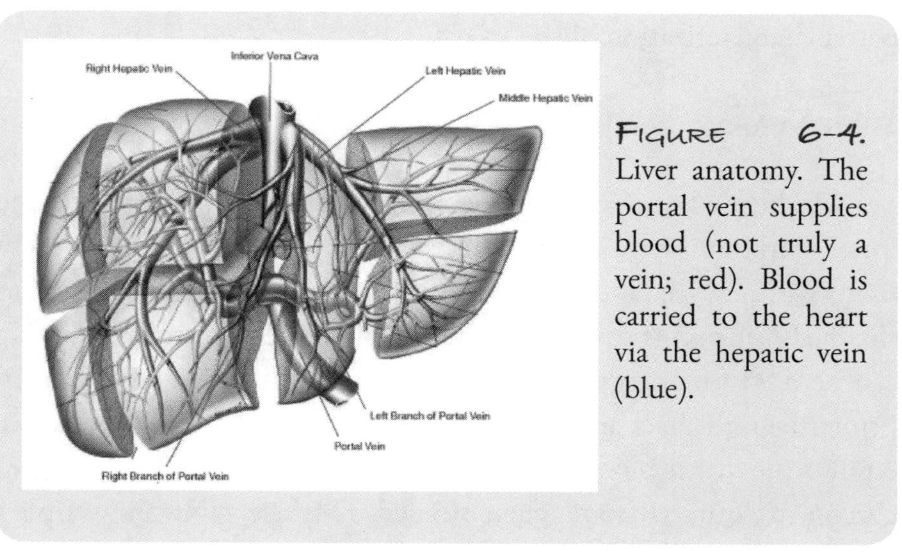


Figure 6-4. Liver anatomy. The portal vein supplies blood (not truly a vein; red). Blood is carried to the heart via the hepatic vein (blue).

What went wrong? Bernard had made the mistake of letting some of his preparations sit around too long and the sugar in the portal vein that was the input to the liver was being metabolized. His basic idea was right — usually, more sugar is leaving the liver than is coming in (the liver does produce glucose) but the differences are not that great and, given the methods that he had at the time, he probably would have missed it. It was this error that allowed him to piece together a picture of a more complicated part of metabolism. He got it slightly wrong and had to modify his ideas later but he identified glycogen *and* generated the idea of gluconeogenesis. Sometimes we luck out.

Today, we emphasize the need to keep blood glucose constant; we understand that almost all cells in the body can use glucose as an energy source so too little is not good. It turns out that too much is also not good because glucose has some chemical reactivity and will react with proteins in the blood and in the tissues to form what are called **advanced glycation end-products** or **AGEs**. The modified proteins may lose function as a consequence. In the popular press and on social media, the effects of high glucose have evolved into the idea of glucose as a toxin which is surely exaggerated or at least awaits better characterization of the AGEs.

## SUMMARY

We already knew in the nineteenth century that metabolism, the inner workings of the body, controlled how sources of energy were used. We knew that blood glucose came from the liver as well as from the diet. Glucose is supplied in the diet from sugars and starches. It can be used for energy immediately or it can be stored as glycogen, primarily in the liver and muscles. Glycogen in the liver is in dynamic equilibrium with blood glucose and, in this way, the liver supplies glucose to other tissues when needed. (Muscle glycogen supplies glucose only to the muscle itself; muscle is a consumer of glucose). A third source of blood glucose is gluconeogenesis (GNG) which, as the name implies, makes glucose anew from existing metabolites. The primary source of carbon in GNG is amino acids from protein.

Looking ahead, under conditions where there is no food or low dietary carbohydrate, there will be a continuing drain on body protein. In the latter case it can be supplied by dietary protein but ketone bodies provide an alternative source of energy to reduce the dependence on protein. Ketone body synthesis and utilization interact, as one would expect, with glycogen metabolism.

To put this in context, the next chapter will provide an overview of energy metabolism illustrating the principle that, in metabolism, there are two goals and two fuels.

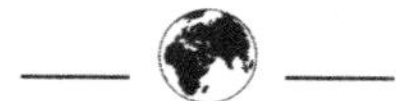

# Chapter 7

# An Introduction To Metabolism: Two Goals -Two Fuels

Metabolism — the conversion of food to energy and cell materials — is as complicated as you would expect but it is possible to get an idea of the big picture. The approach here is the systems or "black box" strategy — getting some information just by looking at the inputs and outputs to a system even if we don't know the details of what's going on inside. As we find the details we can nest black boxes inside each other. It is a way of organizing limited information. The method is favored by engineers who are the people most unhappy with the idea that they don't know anything at all.

## THE BLACK BOX OF LIFE

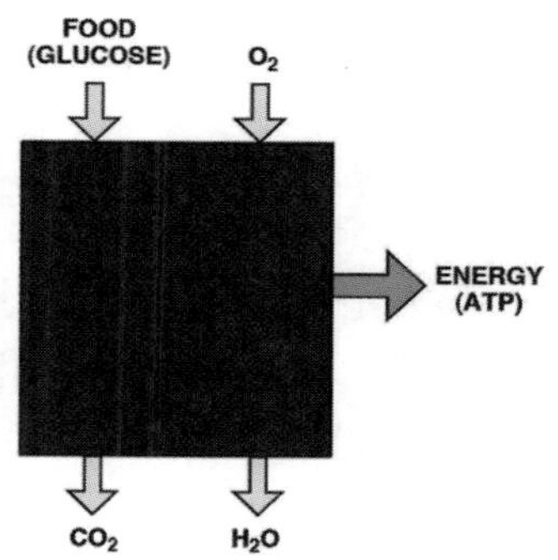


You knew, before you started this, what we do in metabolism; we take in food and oxygen. We put out $CO_2$ and water. Somehow this gives us the energy for life and provides the material to build body components.

Looking at the inputs and outputs, you don't have to know too much chemistry to figure out that inside the black box, living systems use oxidation, like burning fuels for heat or to run a machine. Technically speaking, this is an oxidation-reduction reaction (**redox**, for short). Oxidation, in this context, means combination with oxygen or loss of hydrogen atoms; reduction means loss of oxygen or gain of hydrogen; we say that the carbon atoms in the food get oxidized and the oxygen gets reduced (to water). Like the common oxidation reactions you know (combustion in a furnace or in an automobile engine), this produces energy which can be used to do work. Some work is mechanical work — moving muscles — but most of the energy is used for chemical work; making body material and keeping biological structures intact and generally keeping things running.

## CHEMICAL ENERGY

Energy in physics is not too different from common usage. It means the ability to do work. Complicated as systems can get, basically we are talking about lifting a weight on a pulley. In chemistry, energy is identified with the progress of a reaction. If a chemical reaction goes by itself (not necessarily quickly) without addition of work, we know that, in the end, we can use it to lift a weight. If you have studied any chemistry, you remember the equilibrium constant which tells you how much product you have at the end of the reaction. If the constant is favorable, if you have a lot of product, the reaction is said to be exergonic, down-hill and spontaneous. You can get energy from it.

## METABOLISM: TWO GOALS

Two major goals in human energy metabolism: first, provide energy for life processes and second, maintain more or less constant levels of blood glucose. Too little glucose is not good because it is a major fuel but too much is also not good because glucose is chemically reactive and can take out body proteins in side reactions as described in the previous chapter.

**Energy in biochemistry** is described in terms of a particular chemical reaction. When you study biochemistry, you get to examine what the compounds do precisely but then you use them as the abbreviations.

**Important note:** In biochemistry, the names of acids are interchangeable with the salt name of the acid — if you know a little chemistry, it is because at pH 7, carboxylic acid or phosphoric acid, are completely converted to the charged form (phosphate). So, pyruvic acid is the same as pyruvate; lactic acid is the same as lactate; phosphoric acid is the same as phosphate, etc.

Phosphate is abbreviated Pi. The "i" stands for "inorganic." It is a slightly archaic term but still used and Pi is sometimes read as "inorganic phosphate." So, the big energy system in biology is:

$$ADP + P_i \leftrightarrows ATP + H_2O \quad (1)$$

Energy storage in living systems is taken as the synthesis of ATP from ADP (the other reactants are assumed). Utilizing energy is accompanied by the conversion of ATP back to the low energy form ADP. The reverse reaction in equation (1) is called hydrolysis (adding water) of ATP. The reaction is favored in the reverse direction. You need energy to make ATP from ADP. In metabolism, the "energy" in food is used to make ATP. The energy in the ATP is used to do chemical work, make proteins, cell material. The ATP is converted to ADP.

Textbooks frequently refer to ATP as a "high energy molecule" but it is not exactly the compound itself but rather the reaction (synthesis and hydrolysis) that is high energy. For the moment, we can think of ATP as the "coin of energy exchange in metabolism" and, roughly, the ATP:ADP ratio as the energy state of the system.

## METABOLISM: TWO FUELS

In fulfilling the two goals, two kinds of fuels are used: glucose itself and the **two carbon compound, acetyl-Coenzyme A.** (abbreviated **acetyl-CoA** or acetyl-SCoA the S, meant to show that the compound contains sulfur, is not pronounced). Coenzyme A is a complicated molecule, but, like many such molecules, like ATP and ADP, it is always referred to in this way so it is not important to know the detailed structure.). Definitions:

> **Coenzymes** are small molecules that take part in the metabolic changes in living systems. They can be involved in energy metabolism (like ATP/ADP) or other reactions. The oxidation-reduction coenzymes are the NAD molecules (always abbreviated but stands for nicotinamide adenine dinucleotide if you are bothered by free-floating abbreviations). Two forms: Oxidized, NAD+ and reduced, NADH.

Most ATP in the cell comes from the oxidation of acetyl-CoA but glucose can be converted to acetyl-CoA. Acetyl-CoA also comes from fat and, to a smaller extent, from protein. Glucose, itself, can also be formed from protein but glucose *cannot* be formed from acetyl-CoA. The significance of the last statement is that; **fat can be formed from glucose** but, with a few minor exceptions, **glucose cannot be formed from fat**. Historically, the challenge for biochemistry was to explain how the energy from an oxidation-reduction reaction could be used to carry out the synthesis of ATP which has a different mechanism (phosphate transfer). The process is called oxidative phosphorylation and was only figured out about fifty years ago and was only worked out relatively recently.

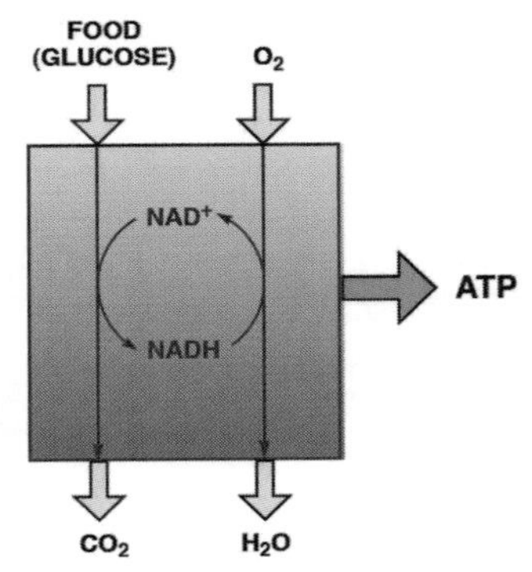

Again, two goals; provide energy as ATP and maintain a pretty much constant level of blood glucose for those cells that require it; the brain in particular, can't use fat, that is, fatty acids, as a fuel.

Breaking into the black box, oxidation of food by oxygen is separated into two different processes. The food never sees the oxygen but instead there is an intermediary player. The intermediate agent, the redox coenzyme, NAD+ does the oxidation of food and the NADH (the product, the reduced form) is re-oxidized by molecular oxygen. Why do we do it this way? In general, biochemical reactions proceed in small steps to allow for control and for capturing energy. Even if we could do it all in one big blast, like an automobile engine — living tissues do not do well with explosive, high temperature reactions — we would have little control over it and we would not be able to capture the energy in a usable chemical form.

## Glycolysis

Glucose is at the center of metabolism. Glycolysis, the collection of early steps in its processing is common to almost all organisms. Glycolysis (sugar splitting) ultimately provides two molecules of the three-carbon compound known as pyruvic acid (pyruvate). In most cells, the pyruvate from glycolysis is oxidized to acetyl-CoA which is the input for aerobic (oxygen-based) metabolism and the main source of energy for most mammalian cells. One of the functions glycolysis is to provide acetyl-CoA. Some cells, however can run on glycolysis alone. Such cells are said to have a glycolytic metabolism and can convert pyruvate to a number of different compounds, most commonly lactic acid.

## GLYCOLYTIC METABOLISM

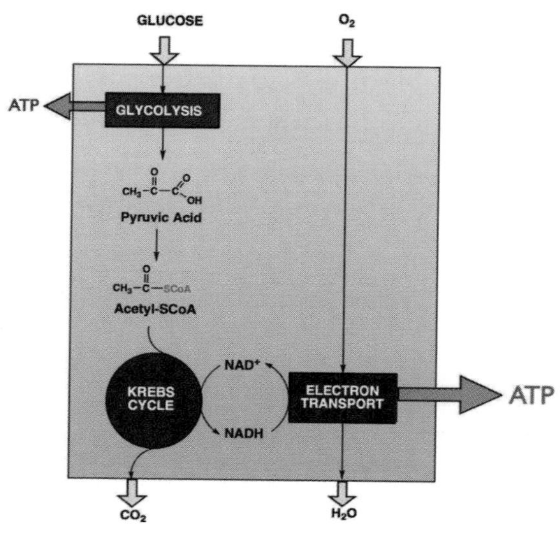


Many microorganisms are glycolytic. Much of our understanding of glycolysis comes from the study of bacteria and the process of fermentation. The final product can be very different for different organisms. Alcoholic fermentation involves the conversion of pyruvate to a two carbon compound acetaldehyde which, in turn, is converted to ethanol. (When you ingest alcohol your liver runs this reaction backwards, converting alcohol to acetaldehyde and then to acetyl-CoA which is further oxidized.) Other kinds of glycolytic bacteria, like those in yoghurt, convert pyruvate to lactic acid (lactate) accounting for the acidity of yoghurt. Mammalian cells can also carry out this transformation. Brain, central nervous system, red blood cells and rapidly exercising muscle are the most common of the glycolytic tissues producing lactate. It used to be said that the lactate produced by exercising muscle was the cause of delayed-onset muscle soreness (sometimes written DOMS, pronounced as the letters) but this is not true. The cause of DOMS is not known but the lactic acid is metabolized, that is, provides fuel for other muscle cells, and is long gone by the time soreness sets in.

## Oxidative Metabolism

Acetyl-CoA is the main substrate for the oxidative process that produces $CO_2$ released from the black box of life. The process is frequently called the Krebs cycle after Sir Hans Krebs who was the major researcher in assembling the observations on where particular carbon atoms went when different foods were fed to a tissue or organism, into a coherent mechanism. Oxidation of such a small molecule by itself would have to take place in a small number of steps and would not allow the kind of control that it is necessary to keep a biological system responsive to different conditions, so the two carbons of actetyl-CoA are attached to a carrier to form a 6-carbon molecule, called citric acid, or citrate. For this reason the cycle is also frequently referred to as the citric acid cycle. In the way of knowing the names, citric acid is a tricarboxylic acid, or TCA for short, so the process is also referred to as the TCA cycle. All three names are used. Krebs called it the TCA cycle and we will use that most of the time.

## Where Does the Energy Come From?

The TCA cycle is complicated but a rough description is that the substrate, acetyl-CoA is bound to a carrier to form a compound, citric acid, that is oxidized step-wise, primarily by the redox coenzyme NAD+. The product of the reaction is $CO_2$ and the reduced form of the coenzyme, NADH. NADH is the ultimate reducing agent (transfers H) that turns oxygen to water as in the black box picture. This process, the electron transport chain is, as the name tells you, a sequence of reactions that, in effect, transfer electrons. The net effect is the reduction of molecular oxygen to water. Somehow this converts ADP to ATP. This is the mechanism for capturing the energy of burning food in the potential to convert ATP back to ADP, that is, store chemical energy. The process, still mysterious when I was in graduate school, is now understood. The idea behind it, the

Chemiosmotic Theory — really no longer a theory — is due largely to a single man, Peter Mitchell. The overall process would be a major digression from where we are now, so *Chemiosmotic* and *Peter Mitchell* are the things to Google. Because it involves oxygen, obtaining energy from The TCA cycle-electron transport chain is referred to as oxidative metabolism, distinct from glycolytic metabolism which may precede it. Glycolysis provides acetyl-CoA for the TCA cycle.

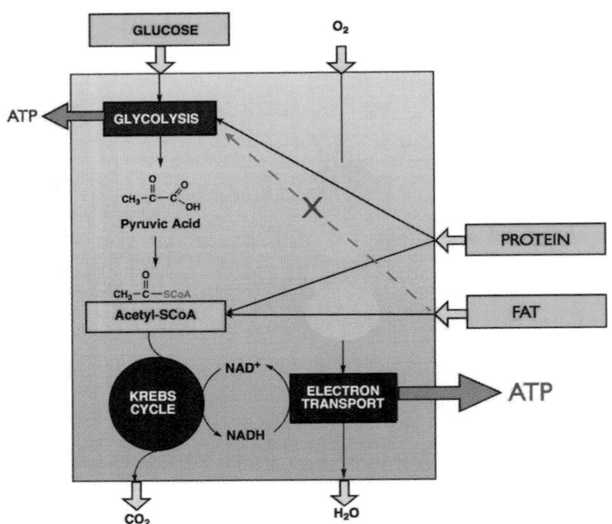


## SOURCES OF ACETYL-COA

Glycolysis is not the only source of acetyl-CoA for the oxidative metabolism of glucose. The major source, for many cells, is fatty acids from fat. The process of converting fatty acids is called β-oxidation. The long chain fatty acids are chopped two-at-a-time from the carboxyl end. It's called "β-" because the break is at the second carbon in the fatty acid chain.

## KETONE BODIES

First, the bottom line: The ketone bodies have evolved as an alternative energy source under conditions of starvation or carbohydrate restriction. Synthesis and utilization of ketone bodies provide a way of dealing with the biochemical principle stated so many times in previous chapters: You can make fat from glucose but you cannot make glucose from fat. This means that all of the energy stored in the form of fat will not help you in providing glucose for the brain and CNS. In the absence of dietary carbohydrate or total calories, protein will be the main source of carbons for gluconeogenesis and the risk is that you will break down body protein to meet this second goal of metabolism.

Created in the liver from acetyl-CoA, the ketone bodies, β-hydroxybutyrate and acetoacetate, are four carbon compounds. They constitute a way for acetyl-CoA units (from fat) to be transported from the liver to other tissues where they are turned back into acetyl-CoA and used for energy. The selective advantage is that it takes the pressure off protein having to provide glucose under extreme conditions.

The brain and central nervous system (CNS) cannot use fatty acids for fuel. These and some other tissues are dependent on glucose, at least under normal well-fed conditions. In starvation, or on a low-carbohydrate diet, the problem is how to supply energy to these tissues. Because you cannot make glucose from fat (the fuel that you have stored to provide for lean years), amino acids from protein must supply glucose *via* gluconeogenesis. In starvation, that protein must come from muscle and other body proteins. It is the demand for glucose rather than total energy that is the problem under extreme conditions.

The ketone bodies are derived from fatty acids, but ketone bodies, unlike fatty acids themselves, *can* be used by brain and CNS because they supply **acetyl-CoA** directly. The evolutionary advantage of ketone bodies is that they provide a way to avoid the breakdown of body muscle stores. Ketosis is generally described as "protein-sparing." Under conditions of starvation or low-carbohydrate input, protein must be broken down to provide glucose for the brain unless another source of energy can be found. The ketone bodies are that source of energy so as they become available, less protein is required for gluconeogenesis; protein is spared. In the beginning stages of ketosis, muscle tends to get most of the ketone bodies for fuel. As things proceed, most ketone bodies are diverted to the brain. The ketone bodies can reduce the need for glucose by more than half.

A low-carbohydrate diet will supply the protein in the diet but the protective mechanism that has evolved to spare protein in starvation is still operative and very low-carbohydrate diets will show some of the same adaptive mechanisms as starvation. George Cahill, who did the pioneering work in ketone bodies and starvation, described the Atkins Diet as a "high calorie starvation diet."

When does ketosis kick in? There is no requirement for dietary glucose, but what is the requirement for glucose in the body — from gluconeogenesis or whatever — as a fuel?

The number that you see in the literature for the body's need for glucose is 130 grams/day. This number has a strange history. In a classic study by George Cahill on the response to starvation [56], it was found that this much glucose was consumed by the brain under normal conditions, that is, before the starvation phase of the experiment was started. After several days of starvation, however, it was found to be substantially less, in the range of 50 g/d but this was obviously not from the diet since it was measured under starvation conditions. Somehow, nutritionists picked up on the baseline 130 g/d which is the value before the starvation period and even morphed this into a dietary requirement. Cahill told my colleague Gene Fine that by the time he realized this had happened it was too late to stop it. So the mistake is propagated in the literature, compounded by the more or less subtle suggestion that, not only do you need 130 g of glucose (not always true), but that you need to get the 130 g from the diet (never true).

In summary, brain and CNS require about 50 g/d of glucose and, under conditions of low glucose, other fuels, the ketone bodies, may become more important. Who is directing all this? How does the fat cell know when to provide fatty acids to the liver? How does the liver know to make ketone bodies? How does the body keep from making too many ketone bodies? In fact, what controls whether glucose is burned for energy or stored as fat? That is the real problem in metabolism. A metabolic map, like any map, only tells you about possible routes. It doesn't tell you where the traffic lights are. And a metabolic map may or may not tell you where the traffic cops are. The most important of the traffic regulators, not surprisingly at this point, is insulin.

## THE ROLE OF INSULIN

Insulin is an anabolic (building up) hormone. Of the numerous regulators of metabolism, insulin turns out to be the most important. **Figure** 7-2, a duplicate of the figure in the Introduction shows some of the targets of insulin; primary is blocking the breakdown of fat to fatty acids. Indirectly insulin favors fat storage. Glucose storage, as glycogen, is also favored. Uptake into muscle is also stimulated by recruitment of the glucose transporters, the GLUT4 receptors. GLUT4 is described as an "insulin-dependent receptor" and clearance through this receptor used to be considered the main effect of glucose but current thinking is that it is secondary. Overall, though, insulin clears glucose and stores it. The hormone also catalyzes fat storage and builds new proteins. It is generally anabolic. Physiologically, it is a sign of good times.

Looking ahead, in diabetes, where there may be an absence of insulin (type 1 diabetes) or poor response to circulating insulin (type 2), the effects on lipid metabolism may be more important than the effects on carbohydrate even though the primary problem is an inability to deal adequately with ingested glucose (in sugar or starch). The most immediate and salient feature of diabetes, however, is the hyperglycemia (high blood glucose). This is due, as in the figure, to a failure to prevent hepatic production from the breakdown of glycogen and the synthesis of new glucose via gluconeogenesis. Addition of dietary glucose on top of this will obviously make things worse.

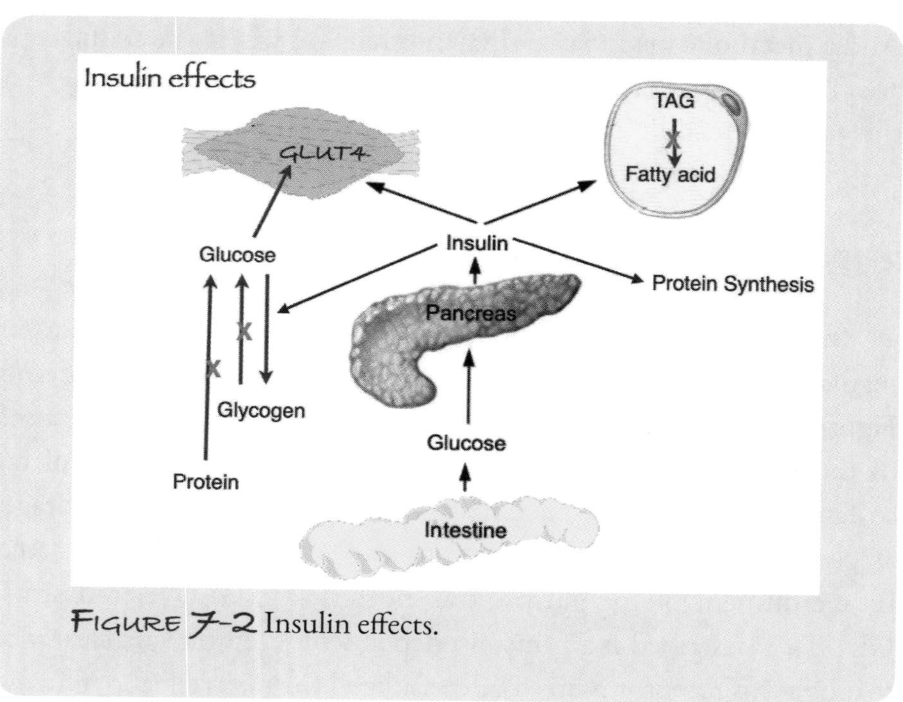


FIGURE 7-2 Insulin effects.

## KETONES, KETOACIDOSIS AND INSULIN

Ketone bodies are acids and, as such, the circulation must be protected against acidosis. Ketosis can become very high in type 1 diabetes and ketoacidosis is one of the major threats of untreated type 1. How is ketoacidosis prevented in normal people and why does it occur in diabetes? The major idea is that, like most processes in metabolism, ketone body synthesis and utilization is controlled by feed-back loops. Here's the process:

1. When glucose is low, insulin is low and glucagon is high (starvation, low-carbohydrate diet). This leads to *dis*inhibition of lipolysis in the fat cell, the process of fat breakdown which is normally repressed by insulin. The net effect is that fatty acid is increased and exported in the blood. Fatty acids in the blood, again, are referred to as free fatty acids (FFA) or non-esterified fatty acids (NEFA).

2. The fatty acids are oxidized in the liver. Fatty acids are degraded by β-oxidation which chops off two carbon acetyl CoA molecules step-wise.

3. Acetyl-CoA is the substrate for energy metabolism in liver and other cells, but...

4. As acetyl-CoA increases it is converted to the four-carbon ketone-bodies, β-hydroxybutyrate and acetoacetate and transported to other tissues where they regenerate acetyl-CoA. As before, ketone bodies are a way of transporting acetyl-CoA.

5. Ketone bodies regulate their own production in several ways. One way is to reduce the FFA that goes to the liver. Two major feedback inhibitors:

6. Back at the adipocyte (fat cell), the level of ketonemia (ketone bodies in the blood) is sensed by receptors. When the concentration is high, the ketone bodies turn off their own synthesis, that is, they inhibit lipolysis.

7. In addition to this direct effect, ketone bodies stimulate secretion of insulin from the pancreas. The effect is to feed back to inhibit lipolysis. So, lower fatty acids, lower acetyl-CoA in the liver, lower ketone bodies.

8. If glucose is still low, lipolysis is increased, fatty acids "go back up."

9. Which happens first? It all happens at once. Again, it is not a pin-ball machine. It all goes on at once. The whole system may not move because it is locked into the steady state of interlocking effects of glucose, insulin, the ketone bodies, fatty acids and everything else. The level of insulin biases the whole system in one direction or the other, but everything controls the final state.

A person with type 1 diabetes, lacking insulin, cannot exert feedback control and is in danger of ketoacidosis — since the ketone bodies are acids high levels will increase acidity.

A good analogy is an electronic amplifier. The input from your sound system, for example, can be amplified greatly — the amplifier is said to have very high open loop gain. Such a large signal, however, will amplify the distortion and small changes will cause large noise in the output. This is dealt with by connecting the amplifier so that some of the output is fed back into the amplifier in the opposite sense of the incoming signal, so-called negative feedback. The gain (amplification) is greatly reduced but the fidelity is increased. The effect is similar in metabolism where you don't want big fluctuations. In type 1 diabetes, the fatty acid signal cannot be adequately controlled, analogous to hooking your system up to an electric guitar which may provide a signal that can't be controlled and is said to drive your amplifier into saturation and you will have an increase in distortion.

## Summary of Fuel Sources and Synthesis

1. There are, roughly speaking, two kinds of fuels: glucose and acetyl-CoA.

2. Acetyl-CoA can come from carbohydrates and other nutrients, fat (that is, fatty acids) and protein (amino acids). Glucose is not required for acetyl-CoA synthesis. Under conditions of low-carbohydrate or low total food, fatty acids become the major source of acetyl-CoA.

3. Not all tissues use every fuel source. Brain, CNS and red blood cells, for example, cannot use fatty acids. Red blood cells only use glucose and, to a first approximation, brain and CNS are also dependent on glucose for metabolism but acetyl-CoA can also be a fuel. For these cells, however, it cannot be obtained from fatty acid.

4. Under conditions of starvation or carbohydrate restriction, ketone bodies, can become a source of acetyl-CoA. Made in the liver and transported to other tissues, ketone bodies can provide an alternative energy. Red blood cells are still dependent on glucose but the brain's total demand for glucose is reduced by the availability of the alternate fuel, the ketone bodies.

5. Ketoacidosis is prevented by negative feedback. Ketone bodies inhibit fatty acid production and also promote release of insulin which, in turn, inhibits lipolysis.

6. There is no dietary requirement for carbohydrate. Amino acids can also supply glucose through the process of gluconeogenesis.

7. Fat as a source of acetyl-CoA. It also works the other way; acetyl-CoA can be converted to fat.

8. Whereas glucose can be converted to fat, with a few exceptions, fat cannot be converted to glucose. This will be a key idea behind the therapeutic use of dietary carbohydrate restriction.

9. Glucose can also be stored as the polymer glycogen.

10. Bottom line is the limitation of "you are what you eat." Metabolism means the interconversion of foods.

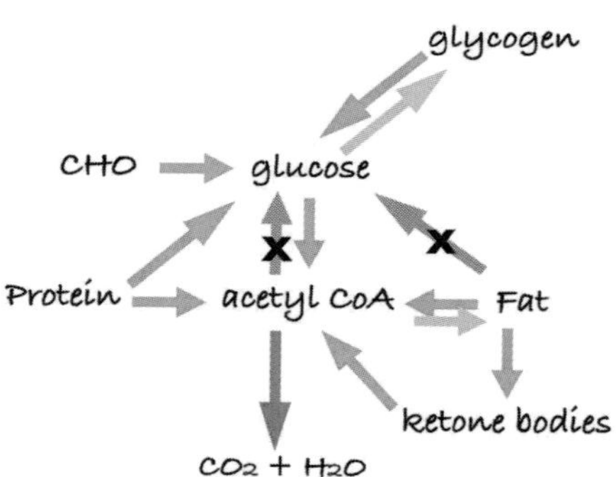


## NEXT

What kind of carbohydrate? The major effect of dietary carbohydrate stems from the effect of glucose on the insulin pathway. However, a significant part of carbohydrate intake is fructose in the form of sugar or high fructose corn syrup (HFCS) — Figure 5-2 . Fructose is a potential source of glucose and glycogen and, as played out in the popular and scientific press, a great threat to life. The threat is obviously exaggerated and the next chapter will try to put it in perspective.

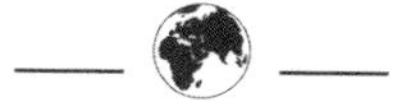

# Chapter 8

# Sugar, Fructose And Fructophobia

If you have an interest in nutrition, or maybe even if you don't, you are likely familiar with the media blitz on sugar. There are now numerous scientific articles with titles like "Consuming fructose-sweetened, not glucose-sweetened, beverages increases visceral adiposity and lipids and decreases insulin sensitivity in overweight/obese humans [57]." The sudden and pervasive appearance of high fructose corn syrup (HFCS) has made fructose a particular object of fear and loathing, notwithstanding the fact that HFCS has about the same proportions of fructose and glucose (55:45) as sucrose (table sugar; 50:50). The strange bedfellows in this political movement include Michael Bloomberg, the former mayor of New York and Robert Lustig, a pediatric endocrinologist. On the face of it, neither has the credentials to make the case for the science — physicians do not have any special training in biochemistry or nutrition although not all of them know this — and the popular discussion is at a low intellectual level. Hizzona' saw that banning large bottles of soda would solve the problem and Lustig told us that sugar was like alcohol or cocaine. Can we make sense of all this?

(Note: as this book was in its final stages, Michael Bloomberg recognized that maybe guns were a threat at least comparable to 16 oz.

sodas and now that gun control is his current interest, all is forgiven).

**Table 1 – Sugar Content of Selected Common Plant Foods (g/100g)**

| Food Item | Total Carbohydrate | Total Sugars | Free Fructose | Free Glucose | Sucrose | Fructose / Glucose Ratio | Sucrose as a % of Total Sugars |
|---|---|---|---|---|---|---|---|
| *Fruit* | | | | | | | |
| Apple | 13.8 | 10.4 | 5.9 | 2.4 | 2.1 | 2.0 | 19.9 |
| Apricot | 11.1 | 9.2 | 0.9 | 2.4 | 5.9 | 0.7 | 63.5 |
| Banana | 22.8 | 12.2 | 4.9 | 5.0 | 2.4 | 1.0 | 20.0 |
| Dates | 75.0 | 63.4 | 19.6 | 19.9 | 23.8 | 1.0 | 37.6 |
| Grapes | 18.1 | 15.5 | 8.1 | 7.2 | 0.2 | 1.1 | 1.0 |
| Peach | 9.5 | 8.4 | 1.5 | 2.0 | 4.8 | 0.9 | 56.7 |
| Pear | 15.5 | 9.8 | 6.2 | 2.8 | 0.8 | 2.1 | 8.0 |

We have always known that if you sit around all day eating candy, you will get fat. Conversely, removal of sugar, which is a carbohydrate, from your diet will contribute to the total benefits, including weight loss, of a low-carbohydrate diet. Whether or not sugar, that is, sucrose, or its component fructose (sucrose is half glucose and half fructose) have unique roles in obesity and other effects of carbohydrate is not known, although you could not tell from the assurances of the fructophobes.

The problem with the numerous scientific papers showing the dangers of fructose is that, when you actually read these articles, they are all carried out against a background of 55 % total carbohydrate. If you are going to remove carbohydrate, you might want to know whether it should be fructose or glucose, that is, whether sugar is better or worse than starch. What these studies show you instead is how bad it is to add fructose on top of existing nutrients, or to replace glucose with fructose, which are not the same thing. It is not reasonable to think that we will solve things by keeping high carbohydrate and switching from orange juice to the whole grain bread that always seems slightly indigestible (at least to some of us).

The problem here is that we don't really have the answer. For people with diabetes or metabolic syndrome or even those who are overweight, the data are clear. Total carbohydrate restriction is the most effective therapy, more effective than other diets and more effective than most drugs. And diet is safer than most drugs. But, we don't know the extent to which removing fructose is a player in these therapeutic effects. And we can't guess. You don't need credentials to do science but what professionals know is that you can't simply make guesses. Sometimes, you need the data. Biochemists are rare in nutrition because we simply don't know enough. I continue to admit that I am just about the only biochemist dumb enough to get involved here.

## IN DEFENSE OF SUGAR (AND FRUCTOSE)

Writing a "defense" of sugar seems very odd. In some way, it's a remake of the defenses of saturated fat that I have written in the past. In those cases, I stressed the need for some perspective. Saturated fat. People have been making and eating cheese for as long as they knew how. What am I defending? Eggs Benedict? *Béarnaise* sauce? *Soppressata* sausage? These have been part of our culture for generations. Were we really supposed to believe that some recent earth-shattering scientific discovery meant it was really poison? It didn't seem to make sense, and in fact, when you looked at the science, it was very poor, sometimes embarrassingly poor. (We all get tarnished by bad science.) And we don't have the sense that expert dietary advice has really improved our health.

It's the same thing here. Sugar is a food and, while nobody denies that many in the population are plagued by excessive availability and over-consumption, it is still a feature of *la cuisine, haute* and otherwise. Chocolate mousse is as much a part of our culture as Wagner. Some of us have to have mousse in very small doses but, for many, that is also true of Wagner.

## THE THREAT OF FRUCTOPHOBIA

Rob Lustig is a nice guy. Everybody says this before criticizing his increasingly unrestrained ideas on sugar. He is almost as ubiquitous as HFCS itself; his YouTube and *60 Minutes* performances, among others, have raised him to the standard of scientific spokesperson against fructose.

Lustig's YouTube begins with the question "What do the Atkins diet and Japanese food have in common?" The answer is supposed to be the absence of sugar but, of course, that is not true and that was the starting point for my blogpost, a modified version of which follows:

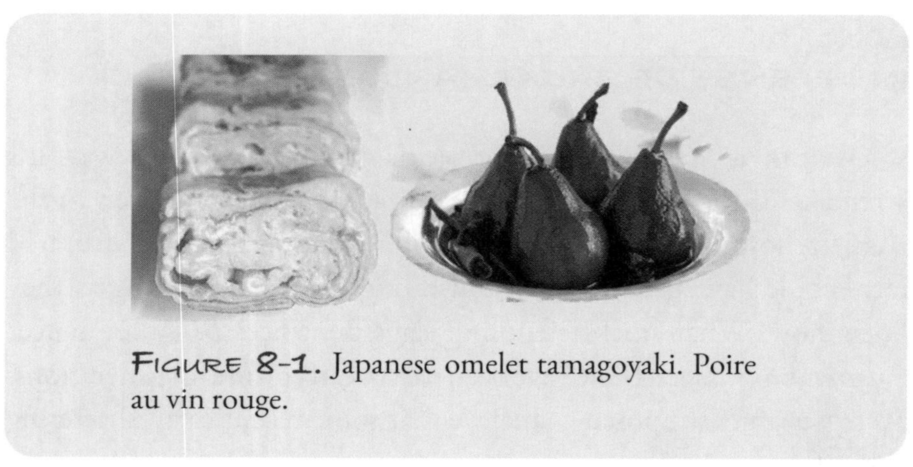

FIGURE 8-1. Japanese omelet tamagoyaki. Poire au vin rouge.

Sugar is an easy target. These days, if you say "sugar," people think of Pop-Tarts® or Twinkies®, rather than pears in red wine (Ingredients: 3 cups red wine, 1 cup sugar...) or *tamagoyaki*, the sweet omelet that is a staple in Bento Boxes. Pop-Tarts® and Twinkies® are especially good targets because, in addition to sugar (or HFCS), they also have what is now called solid fat. I don't think that I'm really being ironic when I say that the USDA thinks that "saturated" is too big a word for the average American. The American Heart Association and other health agencies are still down on solid fat while initiating a program against sugar. Here's a question, though: If you look on the ingredients list for Twinkies®, what is the first ingredient, the one in largest amount? Answer at the end of this Chapter.

## THE THREAT

Most people agree, whether or not they think that carbohydrates are inherently fattening, that by focusing on fat, the nutritional establishment gave people license to over-consume carbohydrates and that this contributed to the obesity epidemic. The new threat is that by focusing now on fructose, the AHA and USDA and other organizations are giving implicit license to over-consume starch — almost guaranteed since these agencies are still down on fat and protein. The additional threat is that by creating an environment of fructophobia, the only research on fructose that will be funded are those studies at high levels of carbohydrate where, because the two sugars interact metabolically and sometimes synergistically, deleterious effects of fructose are likely to be found. The results will be generalized to all conditions. As in lipophobia, there will be no null hypothesis.

The barrier to introducing some common sense into the discussion is that we really don't have the answers. We don't have enough data. The idea that fructose is a unique agent in increasing triglycerides (fat in the blood) is not true. High carbohydrate diets lead to high triglycerides and there are conditions where sugar has a worse effect than starch but the differences are small compared to the overall effect of any kind of carbohydrate. The greatest threat of fructophobia is that we won't find out what the real effect of fructose is. Figure 8-2 does show a difference between fructose and glucose but the differences are small and the large error bars mean that there is little predictive value. Most of all, the two regimes to be compared are both high in carbohydrate and because the absolute level of the triglycerides are high in both cases, it is likely that the biggest difference would be seen if either of the outcomes were compared to the results of a low-carbohydrate diet. This is the single most important question to ask in the sugar problem; for a person on the so-called standard American diet with high carbohydrate, is it better to replace carbohydrate, any carbohydrate, with fat, any fat (except *trans-*) or to replace fructose with glucose? Ignoring subtleties. To a first approximation. Replace carbohydrate with fat, or replace sugar with starch. Which is better?

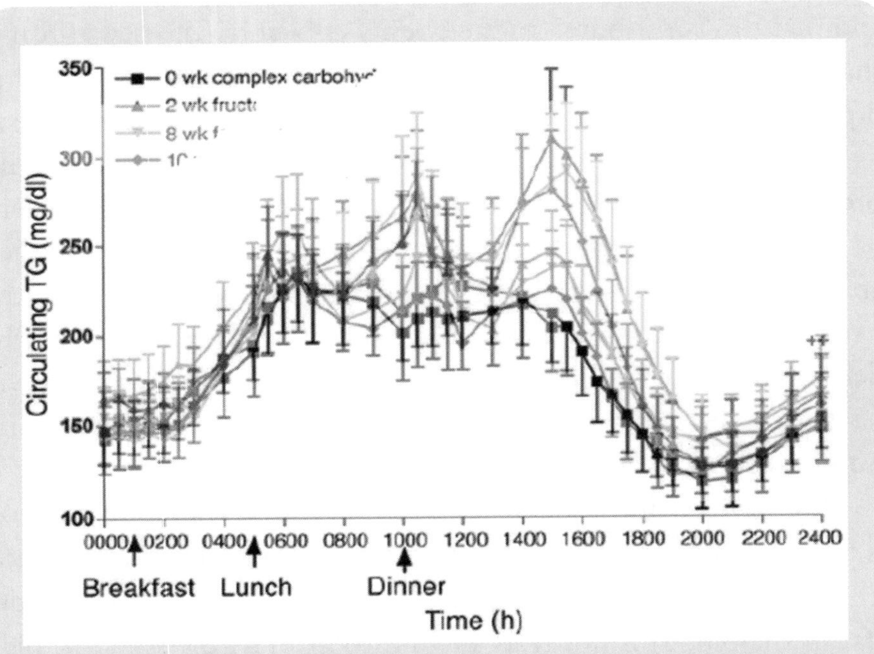


FIGURE 8-2. Effect on plasma triglycerides of fructose compared to glucose. 24-hour circulating triacylglycerol before (black) or after 2, 8 and 10 weeks of consuming glucose-sweetened (blue) or fructose-sweetened beverages (red) providing 25% of energy. Superposition of two figures, redrawn from Stanhope, et al. [57]

We do know something, however. We do know that ethanol is not processed like fructose despite how often it is said on the internet. Not at all. The pathways are completely different although they converge, like almost all substrates that are used for energy at the entry to the TCA cycle. It's just not true that there is a similarity. And people say that glycogen is not formed from fructose and Lustig shows a metabolic pathway from which glycogen is absent. Fructose, however, does give rise to glycogen. Under most conditions, fructose is a preferred substrate for glycogen synthesis. For some period in the history of chemistry, fructose was primarily considered a "glycogenic substrate." Of course, fructose must first be converted to glucose. Claude Bernard knew that fructose could give rise to glycogen but he couldn't understand why he wasn't able to find any fructose within the glycogen itself. I pointed out in my blogpost, "Wait a Minute, Lustig. The Threat of Fructophobia. And the Opportunity." now incorporated into our review [79 ], that conversion of fructose to glycogen is especially true when you consider the effect of exercise and that Gatorade® may actually be a good thing if you are in a football game rather than watching one. A major misunderstanding in fructophobic thinking, however, is the assumption that metabolism is static. Rather, metabolism has evolved to deal with changing conditions of diet and environment. A metabolic chart, like any map, only tells you where you can go, not whether you go there. In any case, the most important factor in trying to assess the role of fructose is the lack of straightforward experiments. What we want to know is, as above, what happens when you remove sugar and replace it with starch —compared to what happens when you remove any carbohydrate and replace it with fat. Oddly, we don't know. It is likely that we would find that exchanging one sugar for another has a small metabolic effect compared to exchanging sugar for fat.

*"...nobody has ever been admitted to a hospital for an overdose of fructose."*

It is possible that sugar and ethanol have behavioral effects in common, but this is not due to similarities in metabolism. And the behavioral effects are not even settled within the psychology community; alcoholism is far different from "sugar addiction," if there is such a thing. While there is no definite agreement, 'addictive' has formal definitions in behavioral psychology and polishing off the whole bag of chocolate chip cookies may not technically qualify as addictive behavior.

In the end, nobody has ever been admitted to a hospital for an overdose of fructose. People may say that your diabetes was caused by fructose but you can't be admitted to a hospital on somebody's opinion of what you did wrong. There is no diagnosis "fructose poisoning." If you are admitted to the hospital for type 2 diabetes, that is the diagnosis.

## THE THREAT OF POLICY

All of this might be okay; the numerous scientific papers that find something wrong with fructose probably have little impact on people's behavior, but, possibly for that reason, the fructophobes have gone to the next step. Convinced of the correctness of their position, they have taken the case to politicians who are always eager to tax and regulate. There is an obvious sense of *déja-vu* as another group of experts tries to use the American population as guinea pigs for a massive population experiment, along the lines of the low-fat fiasco under which we still suffer (not to mention the example of Prohibition). It is not just that we got unintended consequences (think margarine and *trans*-fats) but rather that, as numerous people have pointed out, the science was never there for low-fat to begin with (brilliantly explained in Tom Naughton's *Fat Head*). In other words, leaving aside the question of when we should turn science into policy, is the science any good?

## FRUCTOSE IN PERSPECTIVE

So where are we on fructose? It is important to understand that fructose is not a toxin. There is no such thing as "fructose-poisoning." Contrary to popular myth, the "Twinkie Defense," did not argue that the defendant was possessed by some kind of sugar rush. The defense claimed that he was propelled to homicide by his depressed state and that this deranged mental condition was indicated by his consuming junk food. (He had previously been a health-nut). Strange defense in that most of us think of depressives as going for suicide rather than homicide, but in any case, sugar did not make him do it.

Some restraint is necessary. Alcohol-associated liver disease is a well-characterized life-threatening condition, and, in fact, many people do die from it. The idea that fructose can have the same effect has no basis in science and is deeply offensive to people who have had personal experience with alcohol-related illness and death.

Fructose is a normal nutrient and metabolite. It is a carbohydrate and it is metabolized in the metabolic pathways of carbohydrate processing. If nothing else, your body makes a certain amount of fructose. Fructose, not music (the food of love), is the preferred fuel of sperm cells. Fructose formed in the eye can be a risk but its cause is generally very high glucose. The polyol reaction involves sequential conversion of glucose to sorbitol and then to fructose. One truly bizarre twist in the campaign against fructose is the study by Lanaspa and coworkers [58] that attempted to show the deleterious effects of glucose were due to its conversion to fructose *via* the polyol reaction. The paper is technical but many people reading the paper published in *Nature* don't think that the conclusion really follows from the data. If the idea is not actually excluded, it sounds much like an expression of the need to say that somehow or other everything bad is caused by fructose.

Our review, "Fructose in perspective" was published in 2013 in *Nutrition & Metabolism* (available without subscription at http://bit.ly/1i5svGR). Our conclusion:

> "We all agree that reducing sugar intake as a way of reducing calories or limiting carbohydrates, is a good thing, especially for children, but it is important to remember that fructose and sucrose are carbohydrates. We know well the benefits of reducing total carbohydrate. How much of such benefits can be attributed to removing sugar is unknown. The major point is that these sugars are rapidly incorporated into normal carbohydrate metabolism. In some sense, any unique effects of sucrose that are observed are due to fructose acting as a kind of super-glucose."

That was the general take in Feinman and Fine [79]. It is frequently said, however, that our metabolism is not designed to handle the high input of fructose that was absent in our evolution and that is present in what is frequently called our toxic environment. Although fructose may not have been widely available in Paleolithic times, that doesn't mean that high consumption was not common. It is likely that, for our ancestors, finding the rare berry bush was like finding a coupon for Häagen-Dazs. Moderation was not the key word. This was probably true of all carbohydrates, accounting for the likely low satiety of the wild corn that accidentally got popped in the forest fire.

While few would argue that the wide-availability or high consumption is without risk, it is important to hew to the science. There is a big difference between saying that continued ingestion of high sugar (or high carbs, or high anything) is not good and saying that we do not have the metabolic machinery to deal with high intake, or that it is a foreign substance.

Again, the threat is thinking that fructose is sufficiently different from glucose that substituting glucose for fructose is guaranteed to be better. It's not. Our review was a technical analysis of the literature summarized in a rather complicated figure showing what is known of the two sugars. It may not be easily accessible to everybody but Figure 8-3 is an annotated version of that figure explaining some of the key points.

Fructose and glucose follow separate paths ... initially, but both six-carbon sugars are broken down to three carbon fragments, the triose-phosphates. The intermediates in the effects of high carbohydrate ingestion — high plasma triglycerides and low HDL ("good cholesterol"). The conundrum for anybody who wants to attribute special properties to fructose is how an atom in a triose-phosphate knows whether it came from fructose or glucose. Of course, it doesn't, and the outstanding feature of fructose metabolism is that it is part of glucose metabolism.

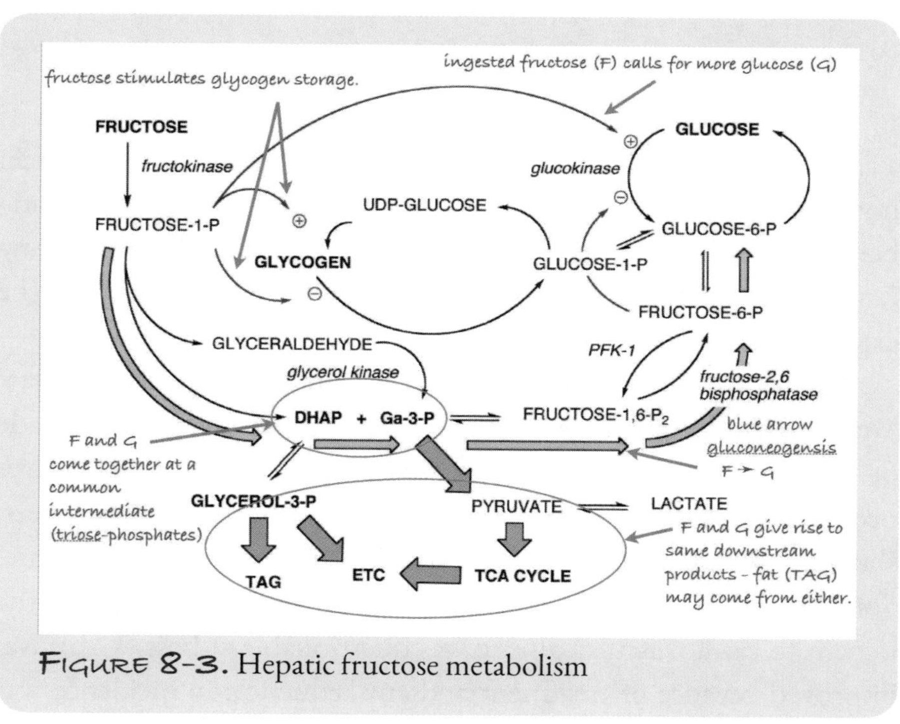


Figure 8-3. Hepatic fructose metabolism

The sequence of blue arrows in Figure 8-3 shows the path by which fructose can be turned into glucose and, under the appropriate conditions, into glycogen. As much as 60 % of ingested fructose can be converted to glucose via gluconeogenesis. So, is there really no difference between fructose and glucose? It turns out that the differences are small and due to kinetic (rate) effects rather than overall pattern of processing. Fructose is rapidly processed. Technically, fructokinase has a low Km. That means that it doesn't take much fructose to get its metabolism going at a high rate. The carbons from fructose appear in the triose-phosphates very quickly so that, if one wanted to make a grand statement, it might be that fructose is a kind of "super-glucose."

*"As much as 60 %, of ingested fructose can be converted to glucose via gluconeogenesis."*

It is not academic. We need to know whether sugar acts mostly as a carbohydrate. Again, if we remove sugar and replace it with starch, how will the effects compare to the results from the many trials showing benefits of removing carbohydrate across the board and replacing it with fat? In fact, nobody has directly made the comparison. The experiment has never been done.

Do we have the same rush to judgment that we had with fat? We said that dietary fat would give you heart disease and a cascade of changes in medical practice flowed from that. But it had never been shown that fat gives you heart disease. And it still hasn't been shown. A whole society went all out to replace fat with carbohydrate. Somehow this led to an increase in obesity and diabetes and the benefit to cardiovascular disease was questionable at best — survival improved because of treatment and any reduction in incidence was more likely due to reduction in smoking. The conclusion of our review on fructose is: "Dietary carbohydrate restriction remains the best strategy for obesity, diabetes and metabolic syndrome. The specific contribution of removal of fructose or sucrose to this effect remains unknown." Unknown is the key word.

## SWEETENER CONSUMPTION

What about sweetener consumption? Did it really go up so dramatically? Surprisingly, not as much as one might have thought. According to the USDA, about 15 %. One question is whether this increase is disproportionately due to fructose. The figures below show that, in fact, the ratio of fructose to glucose has remained constant over the last 40 years. While sugar or HFCS is the main sweetener, pure glucose is sometimes used in the food industry and has remained at a constant 20 % explaining the deviation from 1:1 which would be expected. There is, however, more glucose than fructose in the food supply. One might argue that despite the constant ratio, the absolute increase in fructose has a more pernicious effect than the increased glucose but, of course, you would have to prove that. The figures suggest, however, that you will have to be careful in determining whether the effect of increased sweetener is due to fructose or to glucose, or whether it is the effect of one on the other, or the effect of insulin and other hormones on both.

## SCAPEGOATS

As a good example of the hyperbole attending discussion of fructose, consider an article in *Mother Jones* by Gary Taubes and Cristin Kearns Couzens called "Big Sugar's Sweet Little Lies." [59] The article is a well-researched and quite fascinating story of how the sugar industry has been pushing its products, but the analogy is made between sugar producers and the tobacco industry's attempts to bury any information that might cut into profits. I suspect one does not have to look hard for industries that try to sell their product by underhanded means but the ethical problems relate to the product, not its promotion. Sugar does not functionally resemble tobacco in any way. Whether the reduction in cigarette consumption was a response to financial pressure rather than education is testable; in the first case, reduction in smoking should be greater in lower income economic groups and should be opposite in the second case which is observed, for example, in Gallup polls. (http://bit.ly/1kWzhiE).

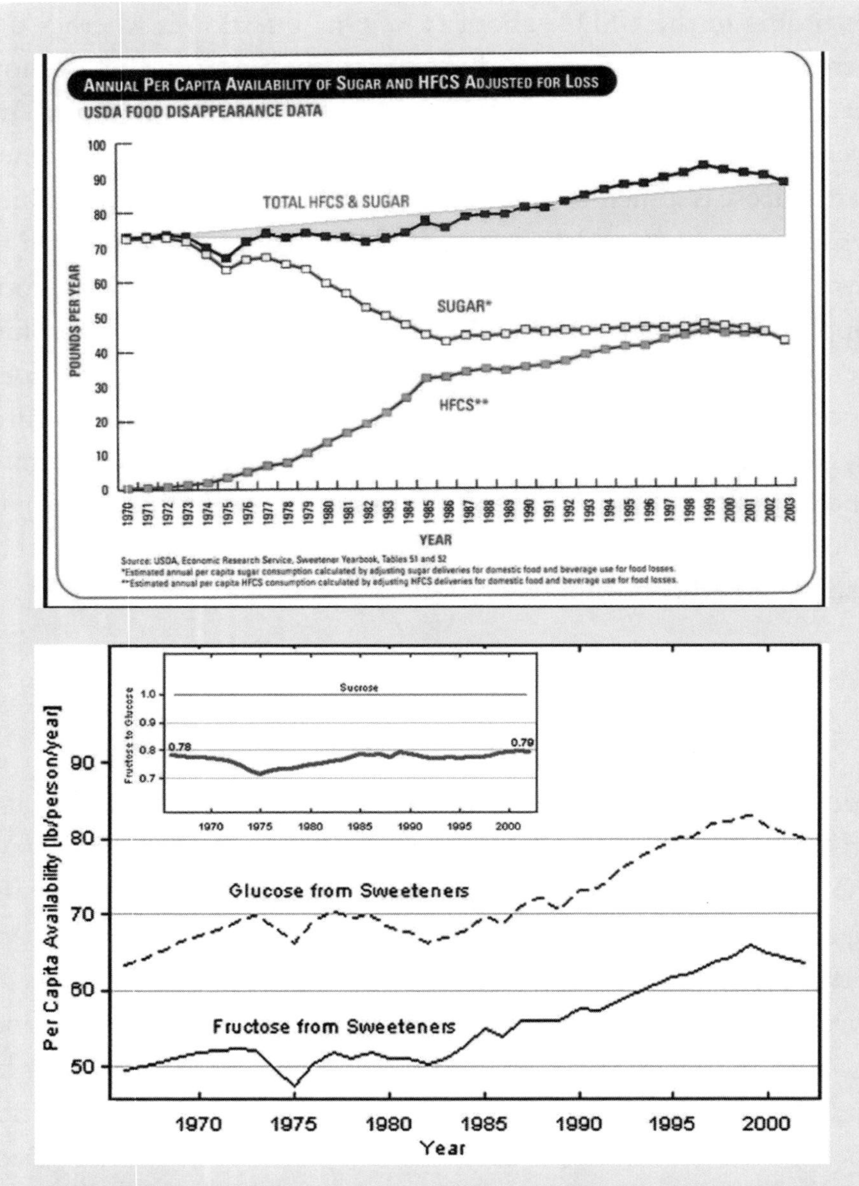


FIGURE 8-4. Sweetener consumption. Source: USDA

The graphics from *Mother Jones* are reproduced in **Figure 8-5** which is supposed to illustrate "a significant rise in Americans' consumption of 'caloric sweeteners,'.... This increase was accompanied, in turn, by a surge in the chronic diseases increasingly linked to sugar." The sentence is tricky, really illogical. It says that "the increase" in sugar is linked to diseases "linked to sugar." You can't use "linked" twice. The link of chronic disease to sugar is exactly what's in question. The graphics in the article are also a little odd.

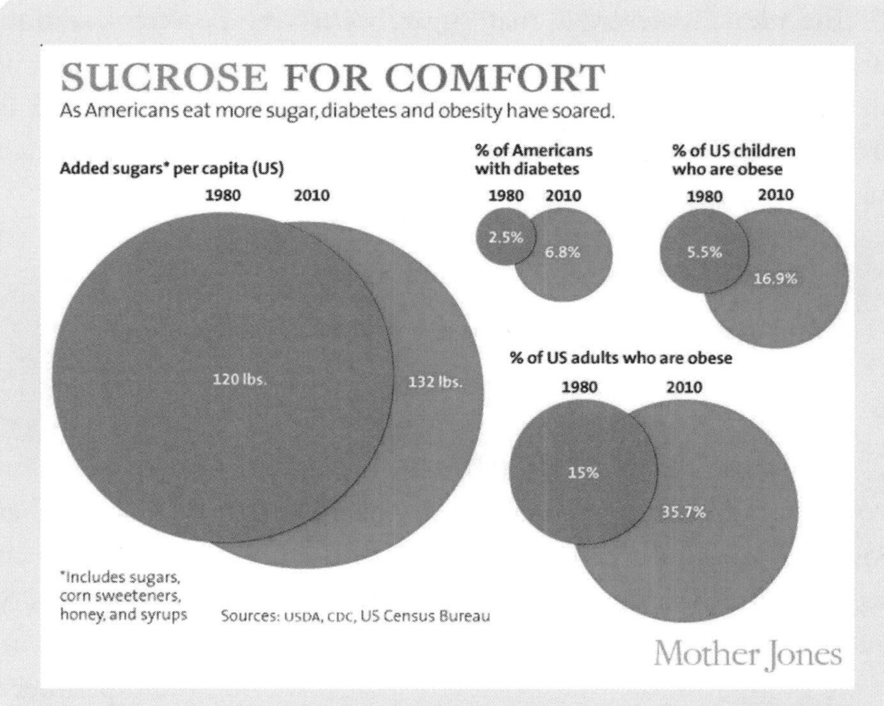


Figure 8-5. Graphic from the article "Big Sugar's Sweet Little Lies." in by Gary Taubes and Cristin Kearns Couzens [59].

The sugar graphic is huge and over-powers the figure. Since it has different units, there was no particular reason to make the sugar graphic so large but *Mother Jones* is not *Annalen der Physik*. In fact, the increase in the past 30 years is quite small. Using the numbers in the figure:

% Increase in sugar = 120/132 = 9 %

Other data shows that the increase was 15 % so we can even go with that number. For comparison, in a comparable time period, the increase in the US for total carbohydrate was, for men, 23.4 % and, for women, 38.4 %.

The idea, however, is that sugar has a very powerful, almost catalytic effect. A little increase in sugar is supposed to be causal in making big changes. So, what happened in the thirty years that is presumed to have been a consequence of the 9 % increase in added sugars? Again, from the figure:

% Increase in % diabetes = 4.3/6.8 = 63 %.

% Increase % US children obese = 11.4/16.9 = 67%

% Increase % US adults obese = 20.7/35.7 = 58%

Is fructose that powerful? If it is, the recommended reduction would certainly be a good thing. How likely is that? And, if it is that powerful, could it even be adequately reduced. A 9% increase, even a 15% increase in sugar consumption, caused a major increase in obesity and diabetes; the absolute changes are small but represent the entire population. To show that fructose is that powerful, the experiment would be easy to do — compare removal of fructose with removal of glucose and the results should be evident. Again, that experiment hasn't been done. Why not? We have good experiments showing that if you take out carbohydrates and put in fat, you get significant benefit. Clear benefit; not a judgment call, not statistics. And it's carbohydrates across the board. If fructose is the most effective of the carbohydrates, it should not be hard to show that it was the player in these comparisons. That the experiment hasn't been done is suspicious. Or, at least, surprising.

High fructose corn syrups comprise different mixtures of fructose and glucose, but by far the most common is 55:45, more or less the same ratio as sucrose. Numerous papers have tried to show that they are different in their effects on humans or animals but it is clear that they are not. Interestingly, they do have different tastes and there are certain advantages to HFCS in that the fructose has a different effect than sucrose. While fructose, glucose and sucrose all taste sweet, they have different kinetic (time) effects. Fructose comes on strong and then disappears quickly allowing the overtones of other tastes, as in fruits, to appear while the longer acting sucrose may mask more subtle flavors. However much you think that fructose has been misused in industry, it is a part of cooking and should be understood for what it can do.

## SUMMARY

Sugar, that is sucrose, and HFCS, or their components, glucose and fructose, are carbohydrates. They must have participated in whatever effects the dramatic increase in carbohydrate had on the epidemic of obesity and diabetes. Whether and to what extent it is fructose as a carbohydrate as opposed to fructose as a unique agent, even toxin, that is responsible for its deleterious effects is the question to be answered. The numerous studies on the dangers of fructose, however, are almost always carried out at high total carbohydrate making it hard to address the problem accurately. While reduction in fructose is recommended, what happens when you actually do this is rarely studied and there is the suggestion of another rush to judgment analogous to lipophobia. A sober perspective on fructose may be difficult but a review of what we really know reinforces the close relation between fructose and glucose. Metabolism of the two sugars comes together at the level of the three carbon fragments, the triose-phosphates. Thus, either can give rise to the downstream products, triglycerides and lipoproteins. Fructose can be converted to glucose and to glycogen. The conclusion still seems to be that carbohydrate restriction is therapeutic while unique effects of removing sugar are still to be demonstrated. Both the media and a major part of the nutritional establishment appear to be unwilling to wait for that proof and the ascendancy of fructophobia seems to be real.

One of the threats of fructophobia is that we have not really given up on lipophobia. Saturated fat is still seen as a threat. But is it? And if it is, is it saturated fat in your blood or on your plate? That's next.

Kellogg's®
Pop-Tarts®
*Frosted Strawberry*

**Nutrition Facts**
Serving Size 1 Pastry (52g)

**Amount Per Serving**
**Calories** 200 Calories from Fat 45

| | **% Daily Value*** |
|---|---|
| **Total Fat** 5g | **8%** |
| Saturated Fat 1.5g | **8%** |
| *Trans* Fat 0g | |
| Polyunsaturated Fat 2g | |
| Monounsaturated Fat 1g | |
| **Cholesterol** 0mg | **0%** |
| **Sodium** 170mg | **7%** |
| **Total Carbohydrate** 38g | **13%** |
| Dietary Fiber less than 1g | **3%** |
| Sugars 17g | |
| **Protein** 2g | |

Vitamin A 10% • Vitamin C 0% • Calcium 0% • Iron 10%
Thiamin 10% • Riboflavin 10% • Niacin 10% • Vitamin $B_6$ 10%
Folic Acid 10%

* Percent Daily Values are based on a 2,000 calorie diet. Your daily values may be higher or lower depending on your calorie needs:

| | Calories | 2,000 | 2,500 |
|---|---|---|---|
| Total Fat | Less than | 65g | 80g |
| Saturated Fat | Less than | 20g | 25g |
| Cholesterol | Less than | 300mg | 300mg |
| Sodium | Less than | 2,400mg | 2,400mg |
| Total Carbohydrate | | 300g | 375g |
| Dietary Fiber | | 25g | 30g |

Calories per gram: Fat 9 • Carbohydrate 4 • Protein 4

**INGREDIENTS:** ENRICHED FLOUR (WHEAT FLOUR, NIACIN, REDUCED IRON, THIAMIN MONONITRATE [VITAMIN $B_1$], RIBOFLAVIN [VITAMIN $B_2$], FOLIC ACID), CORN SYRUP, HIGH FRUCTOSE CORN SYRUP, DEXTROSE, SOYBEAN AND PALM OIL (WITH TBHQ FOR FRESHNESS), SUGAR, CONTAINS TWO PERCENT OR LESS OF CRACKER MEAL, WHEAT STARCH, SALT, DRIED STRAWBERRIES, DRIED PEARS, DRIED APPLES, CORNSTARCH, LEAVENING (BAKING SODA, SODIUM ACID PYROPHOSPHATE, MONOCALCIUM PHOSPHATE), MILLED CORN, CITRIC ACID, GELATIN, CARAMEL COLOR, SOY LECITHIN, PARTIALLY HYDROGENATED SOYBEAN AND/OR COTTONSEED OIL†, MODIFIED CORN STARCH, XANTHAN GUM, MODIFIED WHEAT STARCH, COLOR ADDED, VITAMIN A PALMITATE, RED #40, NIACINAMIDE, REDUCED IRON, PYRIDOXINE HYDROCHLORIDE (VITAMIN $B_6$), YELLOW #6, RIBOFLAVIN (VITAMIN $B_2$), TRICALCIUM PHOSPHATE, THIAMIN HYDROCHLORIDE (VITAMIN $B_1$), TURMERIC COLOR, FOLIC ACID, BLUE #1.
† LESS THAN 0.5g *TRANS* FAT PER SERVING.

**CONTAINS WHEAT AND SOY INGREDIENTS.**

NLI#06583

## ANSWER TO FRUCTOSE PUZZLER

The major ingredient in Pop-tarts is enriched flour. When I posted this on my blog, one person said that although flour is the first ingredient, if you add up the high fructose corn syrup, dextrose and other things that contribute sugar, the sum of those will be larger. It is suggested that this is to hide the sugar content rather than the separate physical and food properties. An interesting idea but easily testable. The label says that there are 38 g of total carbohydrate but only 17 g of sugar.

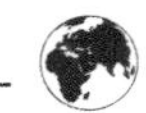

# Chapter 9

# Saturated Fat - On Your Plate Or In Your Blood?

---

Acceptance of carbohydrate restriction is still very slow. Even as the nutritional establishment shifts its focus to fructose, it has yet to admit the failure of the war on saturated fat. This leaves us with two barriers to bringing carbohydrate-restriction into focus. There may be three or four — we can't forget meat as a presumed source danger, possibly as a source of saturated fat. When the experiments on the risk of sugar fail, the careful misleading writing and statistics will inevitably explain that it hasn't failed but it will have failed. And, there is always fiber waiting in the wings but when you look at the original data on fiber it is very weak. In the end, though, there is too much information out there. The trials in which saturated fat improves health when substituted for carbohydrate must come to the fore. The average consumer, however, will have trouble piecing it together and will have a tough time benefitting from the second low-carb revolution. Some consumers do recognize that whatever is wrong with fructose might need to be generalized to all carbohydrates.

An important principle, rarely tested directly but surely critical: "A high fat diet in the presence of carbohydrate is different than a high fat diet in the presence of low-carbohydrate." Failure to understand this principle and therefore failure to adequately test for the effect of control exerted by carbohydrate, accounts for numerous reports in the medical and popular literature describing the effect of a "high-fat diet" or even "a single high fat meal." The source of the high fat, however, may be a slice of carrot cake, a Big Mac® or something else that is also very high in carbohydrate.

On saturated fat, the studies from Jeff Volek's laboratory at the University of Connecticut provide the most telling evidence. There is a tendency to look for truth in a multitude of studies especially in nutrition where it is hard to control all the variables. But the number of experiments is less important than the scientific design of the individual trials and whether it is easy to interpret the results. A study on 40 volunteers with metabolic syndrome from Volek's lab provides a classic case, carefully controlled and unambiguous.

A particularly striking result from the study was the demonstration that when the blood of volunteers was assayed for saturated fatty acids, those people who had been on a low-carbohydrate diet had lower levels than those on an isocaloric low-fat diet. This, despite the fact that the low-carbohydrate diet had three times the amount of saturated fat as the low-fat diet. How is this possible? Well, that's what metabolism does. What happened to the saturated fat in the low-carbohydrate diet? The saturated fat was oxidized while (the real impact of the study) the low-fat arm was making new saturated fatty acid. Volek's former student Cassandra Forsythe extended the idea by showing how, even under eucaloric conditions (no weight loss) dietary fat has relatively small impact on plasma fat [29].

A barrier to understanding the role of saturated fat, is the emphasis on "diets" where it is impossible to even get agreement on definitions and where an accidental or individual response may produce a strategy that works for somebody; the grapefruit diet is the generic ad hoc diet. We will do better speaking, instead, of basic principles. The key principle is that carbohydrate, directly or indirectly, through insulin and other hormones, controls what happens to ingested (or stored) fatty acids. Carbohydrate is catalytic, that is, exerts its effect on other nutrients. The fat in the Big Mac will not constitute any risk if you chuck the bun. You are what you do with what you eat.

The question is critical. The scientific evidence shows that dietary saturated fat, in general, has no effect on cardiovascular disease, obesity or probably anything else, but *plasma* saturated fatty acids do. In particular, plasma saturated fatty acids can be a cellular signal. If you study dietary saturated fatty acids under conditions where carbohydrate is high or, more important, if your study effects in rodents where plasma fat better correlates with dietary fat, then you will confuse plasma fat with dietary fat. An important study from Lin, *et al* identified potential cellular elements that control gene transcription whose products bear on lipid metabolism [60] although, again, in rodents, where dietary fat correlates with plasma fat (**Figure 9-1**).

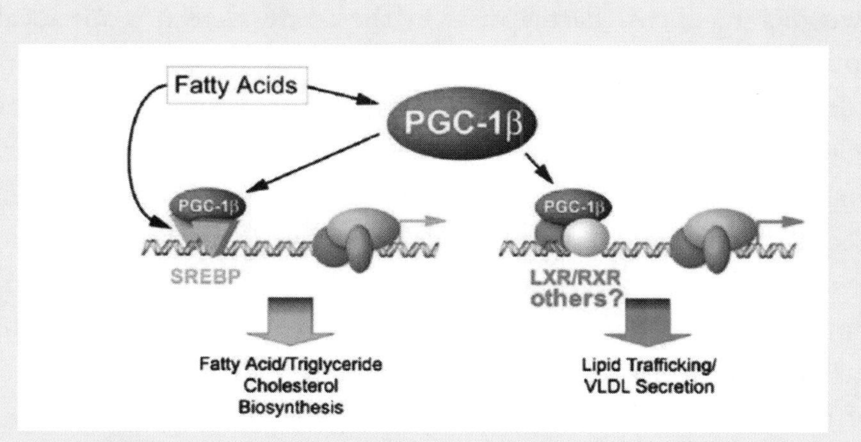


Figure 9-1. The Role of Plasma Fatty Acids in Cell Signaling. PGC-1β, SREBP are intracellular signals that control cell responses.

It is important to know about plasma saturated fatty acids. First, recall that, strictly speaking, there are only saturated fatty acids (SFAs). What is called saturated fats simply means those fats that have a high percentage of SFAs — things that we identify as "saturated fats," like butter, are usually only 50 % saturated fatty acids. Coconut oil is probably the only fat that is almost entirely saturated fatty acids but, because they are medium chain length, they are usually considered a special case.

In Volek's experiment, 40 overweight subjects were randomly assigned to one of two diets [30, 31, 61]. A very low-carbohydrate ketogenic diet, (VLCKD) provided a macronutrient distribution of about 12% carbohydrate and 59% fat (28% protein). The low-fat diet (LFD) composition was %CHO:fat:protein = 56:24:20. The group was unusual in that they were all overweight and would be characterized as having metabolic syndrome; all demonstrated the features of atherogenic dyslipidemia, a subset of metabolic syndrome markers that describes a poor lipid profile (high triacylglycerol (TAG), low HDL-C, high small-dense LDL (so-called pattern B)).

Volek's work is striking for the differences in weight loss between two diet regimens. Participants in the study were not specifically counseled to reduce calories but both groups spontaneously reduced caloric intake. People in diet studies tend to automatically reduce calories. The response in weight loss between the two groups, due to the macronutrient composition of the plans, was dramatically different. People on the very low-carbohydrate ketogenic diet (VLCKD) lost twice as much weight on average as the low-fat controls despite the similar caloric intake. And, although there was substantial individual variation (**Figure 9-2.**), 9 of 20 subjects in the VLCKD group lost 10% of their starting body weight, more weight than that lost by any of the subjects in the LFD group. In fact, nobody following the LFD lost as much weight as the **average** for the low-carbohydrate group. The major differences between the VLCKD and LF appeared in the changes in whole body fat mass (5.7 kg vs 3.7 kg).

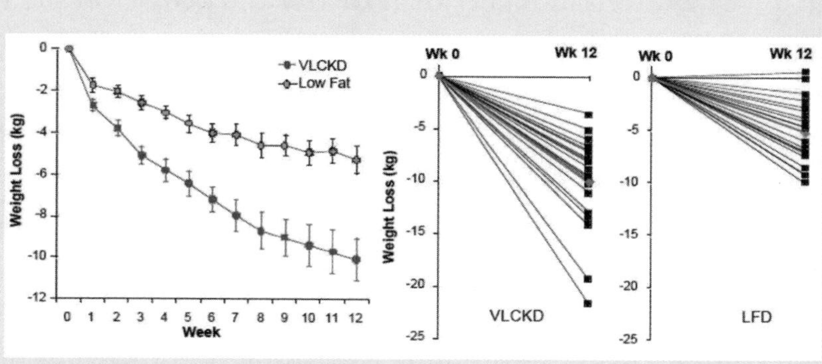


FIGURE 9-2. Weight Loss in the study of 40 overweight subjects with metabolic syndrome. Data from Volek, et al. [30, 31, 61].

It is generally considered that deposition of fat in the abdominal region is more undesirable than subcutaneous fat. This fraction was found to be reduced more in subjects on the VLCKD than in subjects following the LFD (-828 g vs -506 g). Volek's study thus provides one of the more dramatic effects of carbohydrate restriction on weight loss. Similar results had preceded it, though, and these have been frequently criticized for increasing the amount of saturated fat (whether or not any particular study actually increased saturated fat). Although the original "concern" was that this would lead to increased plasma cholesterol, eventually saturated fat became a generalized villain and, insofar as any science was involved, the effects of plasma saturated fat were assumed to be due to dietary saturated fat. The surprising outcome of Volek's study was that there was, in fact, inverse correlation between dietary and plasma SFA. Surprising because the effect was so clear cut (no statistics needed) and because an underlying mechanism could explain the results.

## ON YOUR PLATE OR IN YOUR BLOOD?

The dietary intake of saturated fat for the people on the VLCKD was 36 g/ day, threefold higher than that of the people on the LFD (12 g/day). When the relative proportions of circulating SFAs in the triglyceride and cholesterol ester fractions were determined, however, they were actually lower in the low-carb group. Seventeen of 20 subjects on the VLCKD showed a decrease in total saturates (the others had low values at baseline). In distinction, only half of the subjects consuming the LFD showed a decrease in SFA. When the absolute fasting TAG levels are taken into account (low-carbohydrate diets reliably reduce TAG), the absolute concentration of total saturates in plasma TAG was reduced by 57% in the low-carbohydrate arm compared to 24% reduction in the low-fat arm, again, despite the fact that LFD group had reduced their dietary saturated fat intake. One of the saturated fatty acids of greatest interest was palmitic acid or, in chemical short-hand, 16:0 (16 means that there are 16 carbons and 0 means there are no double bonds, that is, no unsaturation).

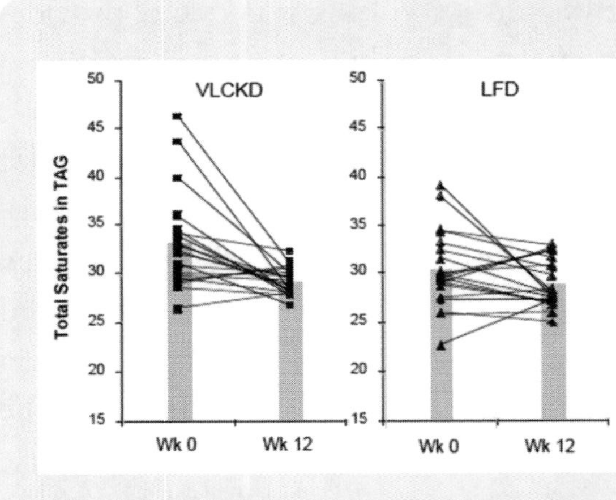


FIGURE 9-3. Total saturated fatty acids in the plasma triglyceride fraction in the study of 40 overweight subjects with metabolic syndrome. Data from Volek, et al. [30, 31, 61]

How could this happen? The low-fat group reduced their SFA intake by one-third, yet had more SFA in their blood than the low-carbohydrate group who had actually increased intake. Metabolism is about change. Chemistry is about transformation.

## DE NOVO LIPOGENESIS

We made the generalization that there were roughly two kinds of fuel, glucose and acetyl-CoA (the two carbon derivative of acetic acid that went into aerobic metabolism). The big principle was that you could make acetyl-CoA from glucose, but (with some exceptions) you couldn't make glucose from acetyl-CoA, or more generally, you can make fat from glucose but you can't make glucose from fat. How *do* you make fat from glucose? Part of the picture is making new fatty acids, the process known as *de novo* lipogenesis (DNL) or more accurately *de novo* fatty acid synthesis. The mechanism for making new fatty acids is, in a rough sort of way, the reverse of breaking them down. You successively patch together two carbon acetyl-CoA units until you reach the chain length of 16 carbons, palmitic acid. This fatty acid can be further processed. Palmitic acid can be elongated to stearic acid (18:0) or de-saturated to the unsaturated fatty acid, *palmitoleic acid* (16:1-n7, 16 carbons, one unsaturation at carbon 7).

The critical part is getting the process going. The first step is formation of a three carbon compound, malonyl-CoA. The process is under the control of insulin. Malonyl-CoA enters into the synthetic process and simultaneously prevents transport of fatty acid into the mitochondrion where it would be oxidized. If you are making new fatty acid, you don't want to burn it. New fatty acid is a reasonable explanation for the increased SFA in the low-fat group; the higher carbohydrate diet has higher insulin levels on average, encouraging diversion of calories into fatty acid synthesis and repressing oxidation. How could this be tested?

It turns out that the unsaturated fatty acid, palmitoleic acid (16:1-n7) is not common in the diet and is therefore a good indicator of synthesis. The same enzyme that catalyzes conversion of palmitic acid also catalyzes conversion of stearic acid (18:0) to the unsaturated fatty acid oleic acid (18:1n-7) as in olive oil. The enzyme is named for the second reaction, stearoyl-CoA desaturase-1 (SCD-1), (luckily the only one that is important). SCD-1 is membrane-bound, that is, it is not swimming around the cell looking for fatty acids but is, rather, closely tied to DNL (waiting at the end of the assembly line so to speak), and preferentially de-saturates newly formed fatty acids, palmitic acid to palmitoleic acid and stearic to oleic.

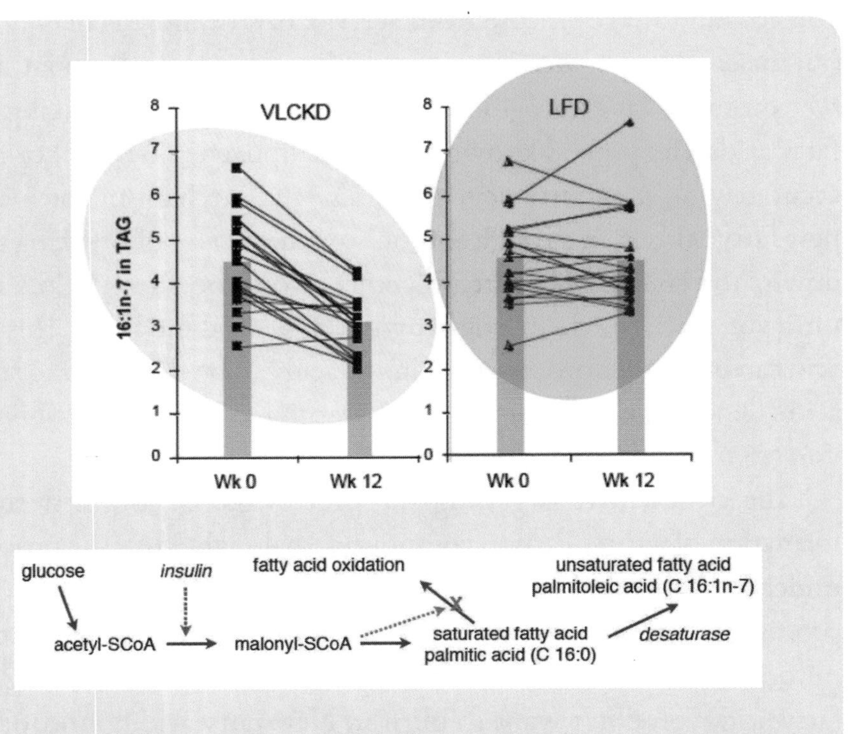


FIGURE 9-4. Changes in palmitoleic acid (16:1-n7) in the plasma triglyceride fraction and mechanisms for control of de novo lipogenesis: malonyl-CoA initiates palmitic acid synthesis and inhibits uptake of the product into the mitochondria. Data from Volek, *et al.* [30, 31, 61].

The data from Volek's experiment show a 31% decrease in palmitoleic acid (16:1n-7) in the blood of subjects on the low-carb arm with little overall change in the average response in the low-fat group.

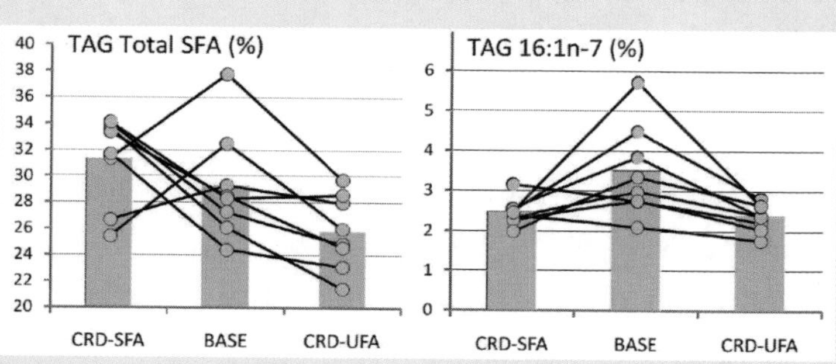


Figure 9-5. Levels of total saturated fatty acids and of palmitoleic acid (16:1-n7) in plasma triglyceride fraction. Data from Forsythe, et al. [29]

## Saturated Fat: In Your Blood or On Your Plate?

Cassandra Forsythe, Volek's student at the time, extended this work to the case of weight maintenance. It is common to say that physiologic effects of low-carb diets are due to the effect of weight loss rather than the inherent response to reduction in carbohydrate and it is good to remove this objection. In the experiment, men were assigned to one of two different weight-maintaining diets, both low in carbohydrate, for 6 weeks. One of the diets was designed to be high in SFA (dairy fat and eggs), and the other was designed to be higher in unsaturated fat from both polyunsaturated (PUFA) and monounsaturated (MUFA) fatty acids (high in fish, nuts, omega-3 enriched eggs, and olive oil). The relative percentages of SFA:MUFA:PUFA were, for the SFA-carbohydrate-restricted diet, 31: 21:5, and for the UFA diet, 17:25:15. The results as stated in Forsythe [29]:

> "The most striking finding was the **lack of association between dietary SFA intake and plasma SFA concentrations**. Compared

> to baseline, a doubling of saturated fat intake on the CRD-SFA (carbohydrate-restricted diet with high saturated fatty acid) did not increase plasma SFA in any of the lipid fractions, and when saturated fat was only moderately increased on the CRD-UFA, the proportion of SFA in plasma TAG was reduced from 31.06% to 27.48 mol%. Since plasma TAG was also reduced, the total SFA concentration in plasma TAG was decreased by 47% after the CRD-UFA, similar to the 57% decrease we observed in overweight men and women after 12 week of a hypocaloric CRD."

The bottom line, again, it is dietary carbohydrate rather than dietary SFA that controls plasma SFA. Thus, while it is widely held that the type of fat is more important than the amount, this is not a universal principle and is not important if carbohydrates are low. But, what about the amount? A widely cited paper by Raatz, *et al.* [62] suggested, as indicated by the title, that "Total fat intake modifies plasma fatty acid composition in humans," but the data in the paper shows that the differences between high fat and low-fat were, in fact, minimal. How can you do that? How can you say one thing when your data shows something else? One doesn't know what was on the authors' minds and maybe they interpreted things differently but the sense is that the literature maintains an attitude somewhat like the approach of lawyers. If the jury buys it, it doesn't matter whether or not it's true. In scientific publishing, the jury are the reviewers and the editors. If they are already convinced of the conclusion, if there is no *voir dire*, you will surely win the case.

The bottom line is that distribution of types of fatty acid in plasma is more dependent on the level of carbohydrate then the level or type of fat. Volek and Forsythe give you a good reason to focus on the carbohydrate content of your diet. What about the type of carbohydrate? In other words, is glycemic index important? Is fructose as bad as they say? Consistent with the small perturbation caused by fructose compared to glucose shown in the previous chapter, we have a good general principle: no change in the type of carbohydrate will ever have the same kind of effect as replacing carbohydrate across the board with fat.

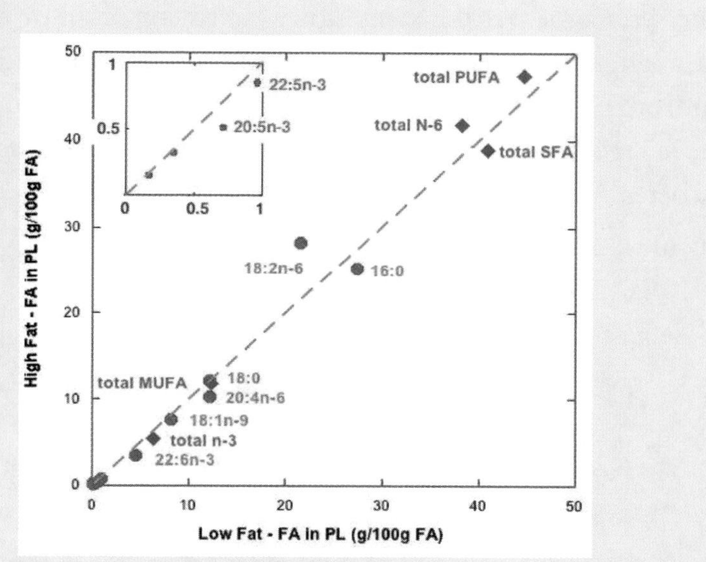


Figure 9-6. Comparison between types of fat in phospholipid fraction (PL) depending on whether the diet was high or low in total fat. Dotted line indicates identity (same amount in PL from each diet) . Data from Raatz, et al.[62].

## Summary

Sometimes a single classic experiment makes things clear. Volek's experiment demonstrates that saturated fat in your blood is controlled by carbohydrate in your diet and some of it comes directly from *de novo* lipogenesis. Saturated fat in the blood is better controlled by regulating carbohydrate intake than lipids. Volek's results also reinforce the observations that no regimen is better for weight loss. More important, the study covered a very wide range of physiologic markers and all of the participants fit the criteria for metabolic syndrome. It would not be too much to say that this is a clear experimental verification of the proposal in Chapter 12 that response to a low-carbohydrate diet is a good operational definition of the syndrome. At the same time, treatment of all of the markers with a single intervention provides support for the designation as a syndrome. The multiple physiologic markers in metabolic syndrome make it a risk for many disease states. The most unambiguous of these is diabetes. That's next.

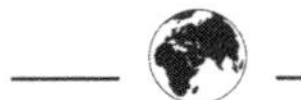

# Chapter 10

# Diabetes

At the end of our clinic day, we go home thinking, "The clinical improvements are so large and obvious, why don't other doctors understand?" Carbohydrate-restriction is easily grasped by patients: because carbohydrates in the diet raise the blood glucose, and as diabetes is defined by high blood glucose, it makes sense to lower the carbohydrate in the diet. By reducing the carbohydrate in the diet, we have been able to taper patients off as much as 150 units of insulin per day in 8 days, with marked improvement in glycemic control-even normalization of glycemic parameters.
— Eric Westman [63]

## "WHO GIVES CARBOHYDRATES TO DIABETICS?"

The scene is lunch in the cafeteria at SUNY Downstate Medical Center. I am going on about how strange it is that carbohydrate is recommended for people with diabetes, a disease whose most salient symptom is high blood glucose. Overhearing my story, several clinicians at the table ask incredulously, almost in unison, "who gives carbohydrates to diabetics?" "Who? The American Diabetes Association (ADA). They recommend 55-60% carbs (or whatever their values were at the time)." Their response? I believe the cliché is deafening silence. It's true. The ADA recommends high carbohydrate diets to be compensated for with medication. Sugar is okay as long as you "cover with insulin." That's really what they say "sucrose-containing foods can be substituted for other carbohydrates in the meal plan or, if added to the meal plan, covered with insulin or other glucose lowering medications." At least until 2013. They have finally quietly dropped this bizarre and ultimately harmful recommendation but it stands as a document of willingness to recommend a dietary treatment that will make things worse so that more drugs can be taken.

The folks at the table were not endocrinologists and they were of my generation. They grew up thinking that you don't give carbohydrates to people with diabetes. After all, it will increase their blood sugar, something that you are trying to prevent when you have the disease. Because of the specialization in the field of medicine, they were unaware of how recommendations had evolved at official agencies or even that it is currently politically incorrect to refer to patients as "diabetics" (unless you yourself are a person with diabetes). They believed in the old common sense idea that because diabetes was a disease of carbohydrate intolerance, cutting out carbohydrate was the first line of attack. And they probably knew that it worked. Why wouldn't it work?

## DIABETES -TYPE 1 AND TYPE 2

Diabetes is a disease (or several diseases) of carbohydrate intolerance due either to the inability of the pancreas to produce insulin in response to carbohydrate (type 1) or to poor cellular response to the insulin that is produced (insulin resistance) accompanied by deterioration of the insulin-producing cells of the pancreas (type 2). The most salient symptom (and a major contributor to the pathology) is high blood sugar which, not surprisingly, is most effectively treated by reducing dietary carbohydrates. The common clinical measurements are 1) fasting blood glucose (sometimes written FBG), usually given in units of mg/dl and normal is considered to be around 100, 2) an oral glucose tolerance test (sometimes OGTT), the response in the blood to a dose of glucose, and 3) the percent of hemoglobin A1c (HbA1c), a modified form of hemoglobin (has reacted with blood glucose) that is a measure of the cumulative effect of the high blood sugar. Normal levels are about 5%. People with diabetes can have values of 20%. In type 1, patients are required to inject insulin. People with type 2, if they cannot lower their blood sugar with "diet" — the diet that their doctor recommends is unlikely to adequately do so — they will also require insulin or other drugs for glucose reduction of which there are many. The insulin level of 150 U/day cited in the introductory quotation is a very high dose.

## Why Diabetes?

Diabetes stands at the forefront of the nutrition problem because it's so clearly linked to carbohydrate metabolism and what carbohydrate restriction can do for you. Diabetes is, in a real sense, the extreme version of the nutritional problem in obesity and possibly heart disease. The Atkins diet, most commonly used as a therapy for overweight or obesity, has become more or less synonymous with low-carbohydrate diets along the lines of Kleenex® or Styrofoam®. Atkins or other low-carbohydrate diets, however, are not just about weight loss. They are not even primarily about weight loss, although there are many more people who are overweight than there are people with diabetes. Lots of diets work for weight loss (especially if you are young, or male or reasonably active or, best, all three) and calorie restriction may or may not be part of the reason that a low-carbohydrate diet makes you lose weight. But to bring diabetes under control, we know that you have to reduce carbohydrate whether or not calories go down, whether or not you lose weight.

The intuitive idea that people with diabetes should not consume much sugar or starch is a good principle. Everybody knows this. Nothing in the science contradicts this. However effective a diet is for treatment, nobody really knows what is required for prevention since it is a kind of hidden disease, and, type 2 in particular, can have a very slow onset. As a dietary treatment, however, a low-carbohydrate diet is better than drugs for most people. And diabetes is a terrible disease, the major cause of acquired blindness and the major cause of amputations after accidents.

## WHERE DOES IT COME FROM?

Chapter 6 described Claude Bernard's revolutionary discovery of the supply of blood glucose by glycogen and gluconeogenesis and his astonishment at finding sugar in a dog that hadn't consumed any sugar. Historians suspect that, writing about it later, he may have exaggerated how much the original observations really took him by surprise. He wasn't the first and undoubtedly will not be the last scientist to revise the history of his discoveries for dramatic effect. It is a great story to have the answer fall from heaven especially if you can describe the intervention of your prepared mind, as Pasteur put it.

It is likely that Claude Bernard had suspected for a long time that animals could make their own sugar. He guessed that it could be made from fat — which was not true — or from protein — which was right. One clue that must have led him in this direction was his observation that people with diabetes had more glucose in their blood than could be accounted for by dietary intake alone. He must have suspected that those people with diabetes were making their own sugar. In fact, gluconeogenesis goes on all the time in normal people as well as in people with diabetes. GNG is not, as the textbooks sometimes imply, a last resource during starvation, after glycogen is depleted.

GNG is always present. As described in Chapter 5, when you wake up in the morning half of your blood glucose may come from GNG.

What is different for people with diabetes is that they have lost the ability to turn it off at the right time. This is due to the reduction or absence of insulin as in type 1 or the poor response to the insulin that occurs in type 2. In normal people, the presence of glucose coming in from the diet causes insulin secretion. Insulin inhibits gluconeogenesis and glycogen breakdown (**Figure 10-1**).

Many people think that the high blood sugar seen in diabetes is due to a failure in clearance because the cells cannot take up the glucose in the blood for fuel. Even the textbooks say it. Glucose enters cells through a receptor called GLUT4. While the number of GLUT4 receptors in people with diabetes does not increase in response to dietary glucose as much as it does in healthy people, it seems that this is not the major cause of hyperglycemia.

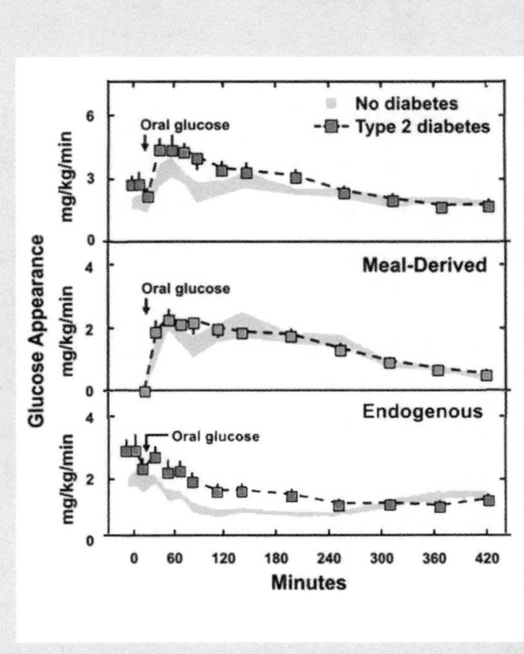


Figure 10-1. Source of blood glucose in people with and without type 2 diabetes. Top figure shows that after ingesting glucose, blood glucose remains higher in people with diabetes. The middle figure shows that people with diabetes and normals have similar responses to meals. The bottom panel shows that the people with diabetes are continuing to produce their own (endogenous) glucose from the liver. Re-drawn from Rizza [64].

People with diabetes still have enough of these receptors under most conditions. The major problem, as shown in **Figure 10-1**, appears to be the persistence of glucose production from the liver.

Under normal conditions, release of glucose from liver glycogen and gluconeogenesis are both regulated by insulin and glucagon. As glucose goes up, insulin goes up and glucagon goes down. In response, the liver stops producing additional glucose. A loss of this stimulus-response control over glucose production is one of the defects in people with diabetes. On the face of it, this suggests that it is a good strategy not to add dietary glucose which will simply sit on top of the unregulated level of built-in production.

## CAN YOU TREAT IT?

> "If low-GI is good, how about no-GI?."
>
> — Eric Westman

Dietary carbohydrate restriction has historically been a therapy for diabetes before and since the discovery of insulin [65]. And it is not really a new idea that blood glucose control has positive effects on all of the downstream effects of the disease, including lipid markers for and incidence of cardiovascular disease. For many diabetes sufferers, dietary carbohydrate restriction is all that is needed to improve symptoms and the benefits persist as long as carbohydrate intake is low. It becomes a semantic question whether they can be called cured if they have to stay on the diet but there is still the issue as to whether the low-carbohydrate diet, or the high-carbohydrate diet recommended by health agencies is the more extreme.

The coincidence of obesity and type 2 diabetes is well established. However the results of studies by Nuttall and Gannon, researchers at the University of Minnesota (**Figure 10-2**) provide strong evidence against the idea that there is a causal link between the two. Nuttall and Gannon have produced a series of well-designed, well-controlled experiments demonstrating the value of carbohydrate restriction in treating diabetes under conditions were no weight is lost. It is not easy to lose weight. While people on a low-carbohydrate diet frequently say that it is easy to lose weight that is really in comparison to other weight loss diets. This is an obvious advantage. From a theoretical standpoint, their studies support a mechanism by which both obesity and diabetes are reflections of a central cause, likely disruptions in the glucose insulin axis, rather than a direct causal effect of obesity on diabetes. Obesity and diabetes are more likely to stand in a parallel rather than serial relation to each other. More obvious evidence is that there are many people with both type 1 and type 2 diabetes who are not fat and, of course, most fat people do not have diabetes.

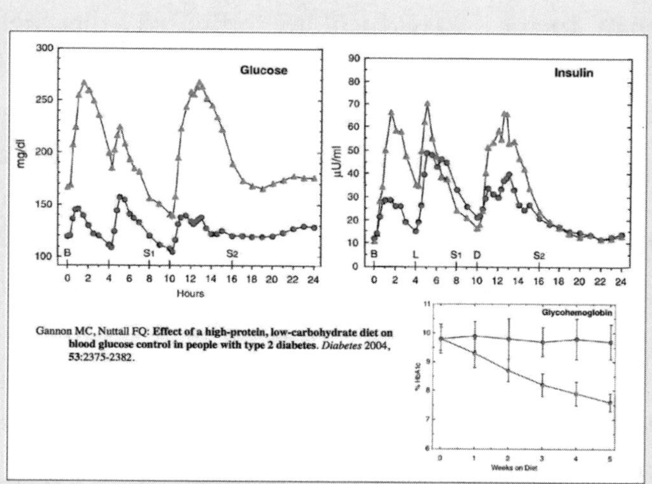


FIGURE 10-2. Comparison of blood glucose, endogenous insulin and glycosylated hemoglobin in six males with mild untreated type 2 diabetes fed a low-carbohydrate/ high-protein diet (non-ketogenic; 20% carbohydrate, 30% protein). Results are shown before (▲) and after (●) five-weeks.

The obstinate refusal of endocrinologists and diabetes educators to face this is a major hurdle to overcome in dealing with the current epidemic. Almost every statement from health agencies and individual experts emphasizes weight loss as the prime goal of diabetes treatment. Endocrinologists to whom these points are presented will generally follow the recommendation and target weight loss. It is simply that the scientific evidence on the subject is just not on their radar. Why not? One reason is that when you see how much endocrinologists do know, it is not surprising that they don't know about nutrition. As for those who act as if they know nutrition but refuse to consider low-carbohydrate diets — not that they have a refutation but rather simply ignore it — causes are unknown. For some, it is not that they love their patients less but that they love hating Dr. Atkins more.

The quotation about low-GI diets at the head of this section is from Eric Westman. In 2008, David Jenkins compared a diet high in cereal with a low glycemic index diet [66]. The glycemic index is a measure of the actual effect of dietary glucose on blood glucose. Pioneered by Jenkins and coworkers, a low-GI diet is based on the same rationale as a low-carbohydrate diet, that glycemic and insulin fluctuations pose a metabolic risk. GI emphasizes "the type of carbohydrate," that is, it offers a politically correct form of low-carbohydrate diet and as stated in the 2008 study: "We selected a high–cereal fiber diet treatment for its *suggested health benefits* for the comparison so that the *potential value of carbohydrate foods* could be emphasized equally for both high–cereal fiber and low–glycemic index interventions." (My *emphasis*).

The Conclusion of Jenkins's 24-week study was: "In patients with type 2 diabetes, 6-month treatment with a low–glycemic index diet resulted in moderately lower HbA1c levels compared with a high–cereal fiber diet." **Figure 10-3** shows the results for HbA1c and weight loss. They are modest enough.

By coincidence, on almost the same day, Eric Westman's group published a study that compared a low GI diet with a true low-carbohydrate diet [4]. The studies were comparable in duration and number of subjects and a direct comparison (**Figure 10-4**) shows the potential of low-carbohydrate diets.

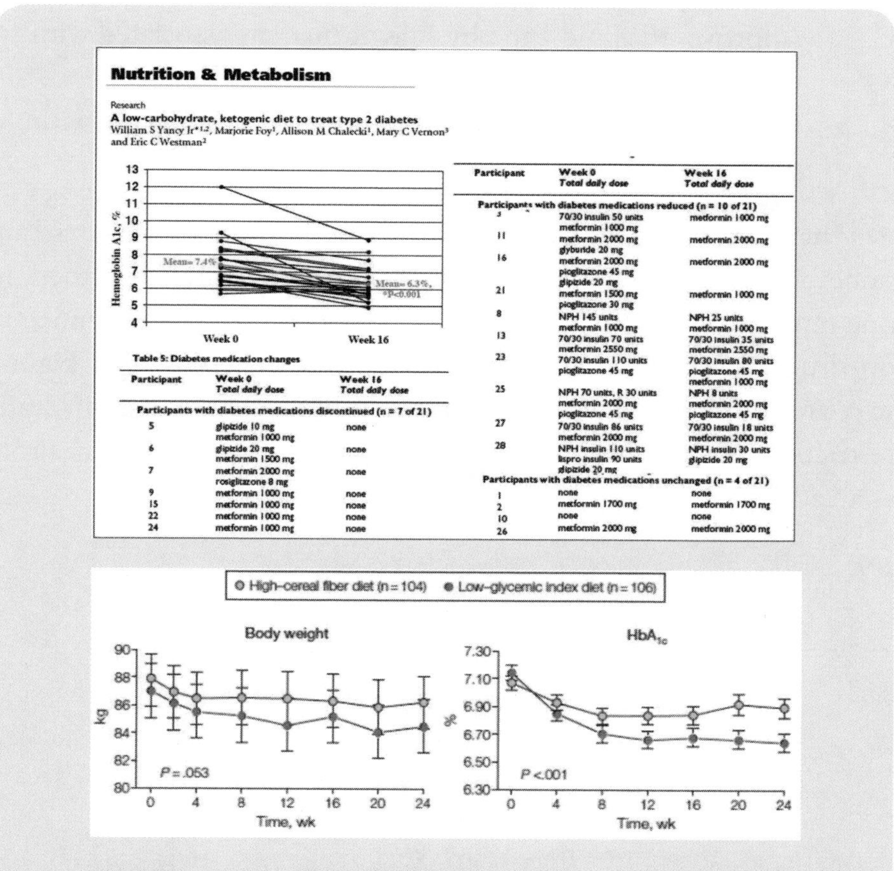

**Nutrition & Metabolism**

Research

**A low-carbohydrate, ketogenic diet to treat type 2 diabetes**

William S Yancy Jr*[1,2], Marjorie Foy[1], Allison M Chalecki[1], Mary C Vernon[3] and Eric C Westman[2]



**Table 5: Diabetes medication changes**

| Participant | Week 0 Total daily dose | Week 16 Total daily dose |
|---|---|---|
| **Participants with diabetes medications discontinued (n = 7 of 21)** | | |
| 5 | glipizide 10 mg<br>metformin 1000 mg | none |
| 6 | glipizide 20 mg<br>metformin 1500 mg | none |
| 7 | metformin 2000 mg<br>rosiglitazone 8 mg | none |
| 9 | metformin 1000 mg | none |
| 15 | metformin 1000 mg | none |
| 22 | metformin 1000 mg | none |
| 24 | metformin 1000 mg | none |
| **Participants with diabetes medications reduced (n = 10 of 21)** | | |
| 3 | 70/30 insulin 50 units<br>metformin 1000 mg | metformin 1000 mg |
| 11 | metformin 2000 mg<br>glyburide 20 mg | metformin 2000 mg |
| 16 | metformin 2000 mg<br>pioglitazone 45 mg<br>glipizide 20 mg | metformin 2000 mg |
| 21 | metformin 1500 mg<br>pioglitazone 30 mg | metformin 1000 mg |
| 8 | NPH 145 units<br>metformin 1000 mg | NPH 25 units<br>metformin 1000 mg |
| 13 | 70/30 insulin 70 units<br>metformin 2550 mg | 70/30 insulin 35 units<br>metformin 2550 mg |
| 23 | 70/30 insulin 110 units<br>pioglitazone 45 mg | 70/30 insulin 80 units<br>pioglitazone 45 mg<br>metformin 1000 mg |
| 25 | NPH 70 units, R 30 units<br>metformin 2000 mg<br>pioglitazone 45 mg | NPH 8 units<br>metformin 2000 mg<br>pioglitazone 45 mg |
| 27 | 70/30 insulin 86 units<br>metformin 2000 mg | 70/30 insulin 18 units<br>metformin 2000 mg |
| 28 | NPH insulin 110 units<br>lispro insulin 90 units<br>glipizide 20 mg | NPH insulin 30 units<br>glipizide 20 mg |
| **Participants with diabetes medications unchanged (n = 4 of 21)** | | |
| 1 | none | none |
| 2 | metformin 1700 mg | metformin 1700 mg |
| 10 | none | none |
| 26 | metformin 2000 mg | metformin 2000 mg |



FIGURE 10-3. Effect of high-cereal fiber or low-glycemic index diets on body weight and hHbA1c. Figure redrawn from reference [66].

**Figures 10-1, 10-2 and 10-4**, by themselves constitute the best evidence that a low-carbohydrate diet is the "default diet," the one to try first, for diabetes and metabolic syndrome. Dietary carbohydrate restriction:

- Improves glycemic and insulinemic control
- Doesn't require weight loss (although there is nothing better for losing weight)
- Improves the lipid and physiologic markers associated with the disease
- Reduces HbA1c, the best predictor of CVD in people with diabetes

There are hundreds of studies about all aspects of diabetes but none contradict the information in these three figures. But there is one more. A low-carbohydrate diet reliably reduces the dependence on drugs. Some people consider that the results shown in **Figure 10-5** are the single best reason for going with dietary carbohydrate restriction. In most diseases, we consider ability to reduce medication as an advance.

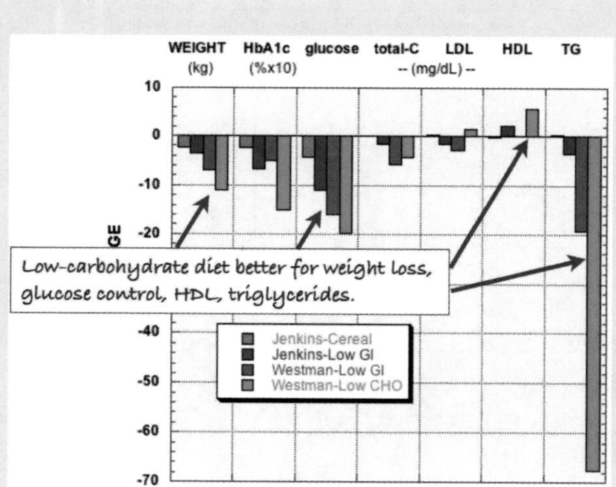


Figure 10-4. Comparison of low-glycemic index diet with high cereal diet, and of low-glycemic index diet with low-carbohydrate diet. Data from references [66] and [67].

Figure 10-5. Reduction of HbA1c and reduction in requirement for drugs. Data from Yancy, et al. [68]

Is that it? That's it. The hundreds of papers published provide information about the details of what is a complicated disease and the details of the response to the numerous drugs that are used as therapy. But the basic principles described here have never been refuted in any fundamental way. Diabetes is the necessary battleground in the new low-carb revolution and it is likely to provide a major victory. Scientifically, the burden of proof is on anybody who would say that it is a good idea for people with diabetes to have any significant amount of carbohydrate. Long-term random control (RCT) studies are a good thing although the people who insist on them for diabetes sit on panels that would never fund such a study if it included low-carbohydrate diets. But an RCT is not the best thing for everything. It is one kind of experiment. And all possibilities are not up for grabs in science. Diabetes is primarily about carbohydrate. For treatment, for however long it is tested, you have nothing better than reducing carbohydrate. Harm has not been demonstrated and, again, the burden of proof is on showing danger. Harm cannot be assumed in science. There is nothing in the outcome of low-carb trials of whatever length to suggest harm. Absolute dependence on arbitrary rules and "gold standards" causes harm.

## WHAT ABOUT CARDIOVASCULAR DISEASE?

The "concerns" about low-carbohydrate diets still revolve around the imagined risk of cardiovascular disease from fat in the diet despite the continued failure to show any risk. Carbohydrate restriction, however, improves the usual markers, notably HDL ("good cholesterol") and triglycerides. What about a long term trial to show that it prevents CVD? There is none but there are long-term trials of the effect of reducing fat. Many. They all fail to show any significant effect. Almost all fail to show any effect at all.

The problem is exacerbated in diabetes. There is a strong association between diabetes and the incidence of CVD. The largely discredit, or at least greatly exaggerated, diet-heart hypothesis and its proscriptions against dietary fat is what has caused us to ignore the carbohydrate elephant in the room. It turns out, however, that the best predictor of microvascular complications (blindness, amputations) and, to a lesser extent, macrovascular complications (heart attack, stroke) in patients with type 2 diabetes, is hemoglobin A1c, which is under the control of chronic dietary carbohydrate consumption. Data from the United Kingdom Prevention of Diabetes Study (UKPDS, [69]) shown in **Figure 10-6** provide support for this idea. In some sense, increased risk of CVD for people with diabetes is due simply to the diabetes itself.

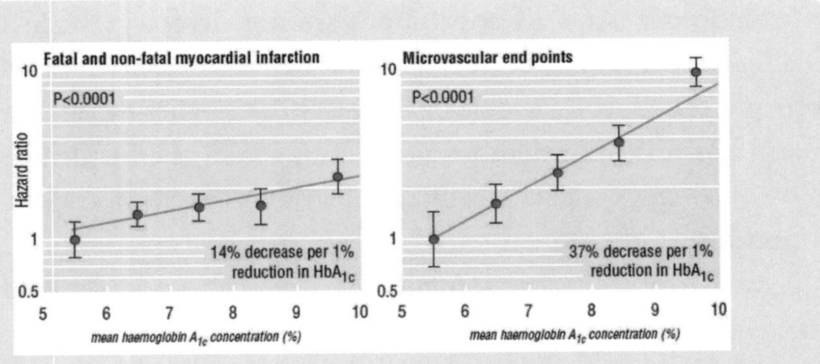


FIGURE 10-5. Dependence of risk of myocardial infarction and microvascular endpoints on HbA1c. Data adjusted for age at diagnosis of diabetes, sex, ethnic group, smoking etc. Data from reference [69].

## SUMMARY

Diabetes is a disease of carbohydrate intolerance. Type 1 is characterized by an inability to produce insulin in response to carbohydrate. In type 2, there is peripheral insulin resistance along with deterioration of the β cells of the pancreas. The most salient symptom (and a major contributor to the pathology) is high blood sugar which, not surprisingly, is most effectively treated by reducing dietary carbohydrates. The clinical measurements are 1) fasting blood glucose (sometimes written FBG; medicine is big on acronyms), 2) an oral glucose tolerance test (sometimes OGTT), the response in the blood to a dose of glucose, and 3) the percent of modified hemoglobin, hemoglobin A1c (HbA1c). It is not hard to guess the best treatment for a disease where the defect is a poor response to ingested carbohydrates but you do need to know if the theory will hold up in practice. A personal story may bring this into perspective. Next.

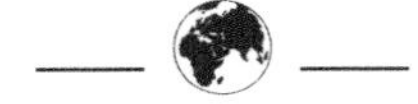

# Chapter 11

# Wendy's Story -The Uses Of Metabolic Adversity

---

Wendy Pogozelski is Professor and Chairman of Biochemistry at SUNY Geneseo in upstate New York. One of the people who has used low-carbohydrate diets to teach metabolism [1], she developed type 1 diabetes as an adult. In 2012, *ASBMB Today*, the house organ of the American Society of Biochemistry and Molecular Biology, started a series about challenges to biochemists. Wendy's story was their first publication in this series:

**The uses of metabolic adversity**

By Wendy Knapp Pogozelski

> **Sweet are the uses of adversity.**
> —William Shakespeare
> "As You Like It"

Blurred vision was the first sign that something was wrong. The front row of the freshman chemistry class I was teaching looked strangely fuzzy. Then, over the next few days, I was gripped by an unquenchable thirst and was constantly fatigued. Seemingly overnight I lost eight pounds. I recognized the symptoms of diabetes, but I was young(ish), slim(ish) and an avid kick-boxer. Mine was not the typical diabetic profile.

Despite my suspicion that I was experiencing raging hyperglycemia, the diagnosis — "You have diabetes" — was devastating. It marked the beginning of a lifestyle that is an enormous challenge. However, the journey has led me to an increased understanding of biochemistry, has enhanced my teaching and ultimately has cast me in a new role of helping others. It turned out that I had developed latent autoimmune diabetes in adults, or LADA, a subset of type 1 diabetes. LADA is due to an autoimmune reaction to pancreatic glutamate decarboxylase, or GAD65. While LADA has a slower onset than classic type 1, formerly known as juvenile diabetes, the two diseases follow a similar course and require injections of insulin.

Fortunately, I felt equipped to manage my condition. I teach metabolism to undergraduates using an approach that emphasizes insulin-dependent pathways as a unifying theme and one that offers an everyday context. I knew that carbohydrates, whether whole grain or highly processed, could raise my blood glucose to dangerous levels, so my response to the diagnosis was to reduce greatly carbohydrates in my diet. In addition, I was careful to monitor my blood sugar levels and insulin doses. The result was that my hemoglobin A1c (glycosylated hemoglobin, a measure of blood sugar control), was 5.4 percent, within the normal 4 percent to 5 percent range. My doctor said that I was his "best patient ever" and that I was achieving the blood sugars of a nondiabetic person.

Despite satisfaction with my glycemic control, my physician wanted me to see a dietitian. To my surprise, the dietitian was appalled by my diet. She said, "You have to eat a minimum of 130 grams of carbohydrates a day." I protested, but she recruited the rest of the medical team to endorse her position: "We all say you have to eat more carbs. The American Diabetes Association gives us these guidelines." One member of the team said, "I want you to eat chocolate. I want you to enjoy life."

As someone raised to be cooperative, and because I found it easy to embrace medical advice to eat chocolate, I agreed to eat more carbohydrates. The result was that my HbA1c rose above 7 percent. My blood sugar levels were frequently in the 200 to 300 mg/dl range (far above the normal level of about 85 mg/dl), even when I supplemented with extra insulin. My former dose of seven units of insulin per day increased to 30 units per day. The loss of control was immensely frustrating. My physician attributed my initial success to what is called the diabetes honeymoon. Often, when someone first begins taking insulin, there is a short-lived period during which β cells seem to recover a bit and secrete insulin. Regardless, it was clear that the dietitian's approach was not yielding the success I desired. I felt confused and uncertain as to what to do.

I decided to investigate for myself what my best diet should be. I studied the literature, I sought out researchers and physicians, and I attended countless metabolism-related talks. In addition, I connected with hundreds of people with diabetes. The most important contribution to my achieving clarity, however, was evaluating literature based on a molecular understanding of how metabolism works.

In my quest for answers, I found to my surprise that many dietitians and physicians were unable to explain the basis for the dietary recommendations they endorsed. Some did, however, express a desire for a better understanding or review of what they'd once learned. And in the general public, I encountered scores of diabetics and nondiabetics who also wanted tools to make sense of conflicting nutritional information.

I began to use what I had learned not only to expand and improve my teaching and research but also to step into the role of a nutrition explainer. First I was determined to see that none of my students would lack understanding of processes such as gluconeogenesis and the many pathways affected by insulin. I created new lecture topics and problem sets based on diabetes and nutrition applications. My students responded positively and appreciatively. There was a palpable increase in attention in class.

Students came to my office to chat about things that they had read. My class evaluations praised the use of nutritional context and often said, "This material could have been rather dull without all these great applications." I even heard (frequently) "I love metabolism!"

Beyond my student population, I engaged a world of bloggers, physicians and other people with diabetes, many of whom were eager to understand more deeply how things work metabolically. I now find myself being interviewed, quoted in papers, and invited to speak to groups of people, including physicians, who want to deepen their understanding of metabolic pathways. I am asked to share my nutrition-based teaching applications with other professors and with textbook publishers. In these efforts, I try to avoid dispensing nutritional advice; instead, I attempt to show how nutrient composition affects metabolic pathways so that my audience feels better able to evaluate nutritional recommendations.

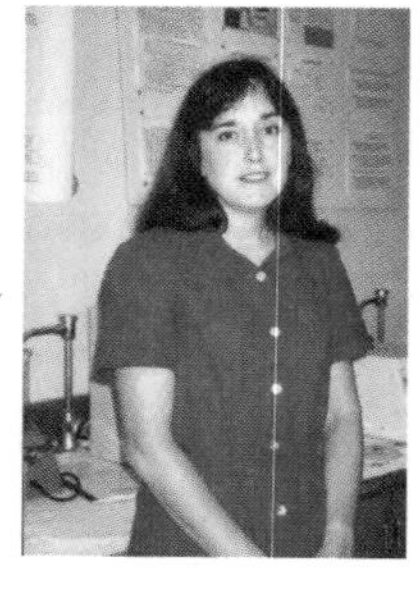

Wendy Knapp Pogozelski earned a B.S.from Chatham University and a Ph.D. in chemistry from Johns Hopkins University under the direction of Thomas Tullius. She spent two years as an Office of Naval Research postdoctoral fellow working at various sites in radiation biology. She is a professor of chemistry at the State University of New York (SUNY) College at Geneseo, where she has been since 1996. She teaches biochemistry, emphasizing medical and nutrition-based applications. Her current research focuses on radiation effects on mitochondrial function and mitochondrial DNA as well as on understanding how dietary strategies affect biochemical pathways.

Five years later, diabetes is still an immense mental and physical challenge, but I am grateful for the insight and tools that my education and training have provided me. Most importantly, if I am able to further the use of molecular science to help others find optimal dietary strategies, and if I can help the next generation, then my adversity will have had a positive outcome.

## Epilogue by Wendy Pogozelski

The story in *ASBMB Today* was written for a series on how scientists overcome hard times rather than as a treatise on how to manage diabetes. However, the essay was read by many folks who were interested from a standpoint of their own health concerns. I received many requests for an update, as people wondered if, after my foray into inclusion of carbohydrates, I returned to my low-carbohydrate style of eating. The answer is a resounding "yes". (With one small *caveat*, as you'll see below).

As I studied the scientific literature, I became more and more convinced that my absolute primary concern should be keeping my blood sugar levels as close to normal as possible. I saw that I achieve the flattest blood sugars when I keep my carbohydrate low and my insulin low. Dr. Richard Bernstein, a type 1 diabetic and engineer-turned physician who pioneered the use of glucose meters, calls this principle "the law of small numbers." Carbohydrate restriction results in minimization of errors. Hyperglycemia and hypoglycemia come from mis-estimation of carbohydrate amount, rate of carbohydrate absorption and insulin absorption and activity. These factors are nearly impossible to predict accurately. Many people who use large amounts of insulin to cover large amounts of carbohydrate in their diet frequently find themselves in dangerous situations (passing out, etc.) when the peak activity of the insulin occurs earlier than the peak absorption of the dietary carbohydrate. I have never passed out and my health care team has been astounded by my lack of hypoglycemic episodes. *Hyper*glycemia also needs to be avoided though. It is these high blood sugars that correlate with the long-term deleterious effects of diabetes. Observing the diabetic amputees at the endocrinologist's office and watching people painfully shuffle into the dialysis center has been strong motivation to avoid these high blood sugars.

What is the evidence for the effectiveness of a low-carb dietary approach with me? I was used as a test subject for "sensor" technology. This device consists of a needle, sensor and a transmitter worn on the body and it communicates with an insulin pump. When my results were printed out after the experiment, my health care team was astonished at how level my glucose readings were. I was the last appointment of the day and all the workers gathered around to admire the printout of the "beautiful" blood sugars and ask me how in the world I did that. (This was at the office where the team had insisted that I needed to eat carbohydrate. Yes, it was very satisfying).

It is worth noting too how well having level blood sugar makes me feel. When my blood sugar goes over 200 mg/dl, I start to feel melodramatic and have an elevated emotional response to even minor difficulties. Low blood sugar induces glucagon and epinephrine hormone release, which result in sweating and a feeling of panic as well as low energy. Both high and low blood sugar make my brain sluggish. Also, as a headache-prone person for much of my life, I found that my formerly frequent headaches nearly disappeared when I began to practice carbohydrate restriction.

When I keep my meal at less than 10 g of carbohydrate, my blood sugars rise by no more than 40 mg/dl; sometimes they rise as little as 10 mg/dl, but regardless, they return to normal within two hours – like a non-diabetic. I find that too much protein will elevate my blood sugar so I keep that amount moderate but I don't consciously restrict it, or my fat.

Despite my knowledge that carbohydrate restriction is best for me, I sometimes have deviated from this plan of attack. Particularly, since I became a mom, there has been a lot more carbohydrate in the kitchen tempting me. Couple that with the chronic exhaustion of motherhood and you've got a situation that makes reaching for carbohydrate much more likely. I rediscovered that M&Ms (used effectively for potty-training a toddler) are delicious, and my plans to eat no more than three have consistently been shown to be no match for whatever else is at work. (My theory is that there is an evil force activated when one eats M&Ms and he is only appeased when the bag is empty). Every time I have indulged, however, I have always concluded "It wasn't worth it" when I saw my high blood sugars or had to compensate for my over-estimation of my insulin.

I also decided that I really, really like dark chocolate and given that it is full of antioxidants, I do allow myself some. I save my carbs for it. The 85% variety I eat has 4g/square and is much more satisfying than milk chocolate, so it's possible to enjoy without over-indulging. There are days too when I decide that it's a "Carb Day". For example, one very hot day in the summer warrants my once-a-year small ice cream or custard cone. Or if some kind person makes me a birthday cake I'll eat a bit. I call these excursions "experimental error." I am not perfect, but I try to keep my carbohydrate intake under 50g/ day and ideally around 30g/day. For me, the lower my carbohydrate, the far better my control.

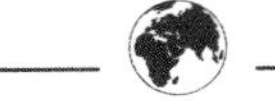

# Chapter 12

# Metabolic Syndrome - The Big Pitch

The last two chapters brought out the idea that diabetes represents the most clear-cut example of how the glucose-insulin axis affects health. This disease is at the center of nutritional thinking even if you are not a patient yourself. Even if you are primarily interested in weight loss or have concern about cardiovascular disease (CVD) or you are just interested in general good health, insulin metabolism is always in the foreground. A big focal point is the metabolic syndrome (MetS). Gerald Reaven's original observation[12, 70] was that overweight, high blood glucose, high blood pressure and the lipid markers assumed to indicate cardiovascular risk commonly appeared together in the same patient (**Figure 12-1**).

The concept has now been extended to include several other physiologic markers, inflammation and LDL particle size, that also seem to be tied together. Insulin is credited with control of the syndrome and Reaven currently insists on calling it insulin-resistance syndrome [71, 72].

*Metabolic Syndrome NCEP ATP III Definition*

**Subjects having 3 of the following criteria**

| | ***Men*** | ***Women*** |
|---|---|---|
| Abdominal obesity | waist circumference >102 cm | waist circumference >88 cm |
| Hypertriglyceridemia | >150 mg/dL | |
| Low HDL-C | <40 mg/dL | <50 mg/dL |
| High blood pressure | >130/85 mm Hg | |
| High fasting glucose | >110 mg/dL | |

NCEP=National Cholesterol Education Program; ATP=adult treatment panel; HDL-C=high-density lipoprotein cholesterol.

FIGURE 12-1. Definitions of metabolic syndrome. Different organizations have their own variations and other factors such as LDL-particle size have been included by some researchers.

## I MAY HAVE SAID SOMETHING SMART

The importance of metabolic syndrome came through to me a few years ago. It was a seminar on metabolic syndrome and the underlying cell biology. I don't remember the details of the presentation but I thought it was quite good. The speaker was also a doctor. In fact, he was Mike Huckabee's doctor. After the seminar, I asked him about low-carbohydrate diets and he unexpectedly went ballistic. "Go to the Atkins website. You can eat all the bacon you want. That's what it says." I was somewhat taken aback. Did I say Atkins? I didn't really know what to say. I noticed that he still had on the screen his last slide showing the metabolic syndrome (something like **Figure 12-1**).

Pointing to the screen, I said "you know, all of those markers are exactly the things that are improved by low-carb diets." He said, "Well, they're also improved by low calorie diets.," which is not true. Low-Fat diets, or at least high carbohydrate diets, will not improve triglycerides and, more likely, will make them worse.

The incident stuck in my head. A little later that day I thought "I may have said something smart." The features of MetS were known to be improved by carbohydrate restriction but it was not generally stated explicitly. Turning it around in your mind, you might say that the response to a low-carbohydrate diet could actually be the essential feature of metabolic syndrome, a kind of operational definition. This is important because some people said that MetS was not for real. They held that saying that your patient has the combination of markers of metabolic syndrome provides no more information than saying that they have several individual markers. What they mean is that the way to treat markers A, B and C (for example, obesity, diabetes and high cholesterol) is with a drug for A, a drug for B and a drug for C. In other words, they didn't have a drug for MetS. They only have drugs for each of the individual markers. The fact that A, B and C can all be treated with a single intervention, namely a low-carbohydrate diet, suggests that they all arise from a common cause: a disruption in the glucose-insulin axis, roughly described as insulin resistance. Other people had said this in other publications. I had even written a paper myself entitled "Metabolic Syndrome and Low-Carbohydrate Ketogenic Diets" in the Medical School Biochemistry Curriculum, but I hadn't really seen the impact. There is a step in the evolution of ideas where you realize that the comment you made in passing has important implications and has to be re-stated as a law.

If all the markers of metabolic syndrome could be improved by a low-carbohydrate diet, possibly even in the absence of calorie restriction, than what did that mean for the millions of people facing the risk predicted by these markers? What did it mean for the drugs that treat each individual condition but ignore the root cause? And what did it mean for those national authorities on health that were and are still recommending a low-fat, high carbohydrate diet? If the experimental data is there, would the nutritional establishment embrace it even though it contains the words "low-carbohydrate." It was 2005 and we really thought that they would. Talk about the naïveté of youth.

Jeff Volek and I went through the literature and tabulated the responses to low-carbohydrate and low-fat diets with respect to the markers of MetS. The results were as expected (**Figure 12-2**). We published the results in *Nutrition & Metabolism* [38]. I was the editor at the time and thought that the importance of the paper would improve the standing of our journal. We recognized that we were dealing with modern science where people don't even have time to read an abstract so we put the whole story in the title: "Carbohydrate restriction improves the features of Metabolic Syndrome. Metabolic Syndrome may be defined by the response to carbohydrate restriction." The data show that except for a couple of measurements (one on insulin, one of fasting glucose), the markers of MetS are improved much more by a low-carbohydrate diet, sometimes dramatically.

| Reference | # | Subjects | Duration | Diet | CHO (g/d) | CHANGE weight (%) | HDL (%) | TAG (%) | TAG/HDL (%) | Glucose (%) | Insulin (%) | DBP (mm Hg) |
|---|---|---|---|---|---|---|---|---|---|---|---|---|
| Brehm *et al*. 2003 | 1 | Obese Women | 6 mo | Low-CHO | 41-97 | -9.3 | 13.4 | -23.4 | -32.4 | -9.1 | -14.8 | -5 |
| | | | | LF | 163-169 | -4.2 | 8.4 | 1.6 | -6.3 | -4.0 | -23.0 | -1 |
| Soncike *et al*. 2003 | 2 | Overweight Adolescents | 12 wk | Low-CHO | 37 | -10.7 | 8.7 | -40.5 | -45.2 | | | |
| | | | | LF | 154 | -4.1 | 4.2 | -5.4 | -9.2 | | | |
| Samaha *et al*. 2003 | 3 | Obese Men/Women | 6 mo | Low-CHO | 150 | -4.5 | 0.0 | -20.2 | -20.2 | -8.6 | -27.3 | |
| | | | | LF | 201 | -1.4 | -2.4 | -4 | -1.6 | -1.6 | 5.6 | |
| Foster *et al*. 2003 | 4 | Obese Men/Women | 1 yr | Low-CHO | ad lib | -7.3 | 18.2 | -28.1 | -29.5 | | | |
| | | | | LF | ad lib | -4.5 | 1.4 | 0.7 | -2.6 | | | |
| Volek *et al*. 2004 | 5 | Overweight Women | 4 wk | Low-CHO | 29 | -3.9 | 1.3 | -23 | -28.3 | -3.8 | -8.8 | |
| | | | | LF | 186 | -1.4 | -8.6 | -11.2 | -4.2 | 1.3 | 23.2 | |
| Sharman *et al*. 2004 | 6 | Overweight Men | 6 wk | Low-CHO | 36 | -5.6 | -3.3 | -44.1 | -42.3 | -5.8 | -41.5 | |
| | | | | LF | 224 | -3.6 | -6.6 | -15 | -8.3 | -5.2 | -28.1 | |
| Brehm *et al*. 2004 | 7 | Obese Women | 4 mo | Low-CHO | 69 | -10.8 | 16.3 | -37.3 | -46.1 | | | -9 |
| | | | | LF | 174 | -6.8 | 4.5 | -10.3 | -14.2 | | | -3 |
| Meckling *et al*. 2004 | 8 | Obese Men/Women | 10 wk | Low-CHO | 59 | -7.7 | 12.2 | -29.4 | -37.1 | -8.0 | -28.7 | -6.1 |
| | | | | LF | 225 | -7.4 | -15.4 | -25.4 | -11.8 | -10.2 | -3.3 | -5 |
| Stern *et al*. 2004 | 9 | Obese Men/Women | 1 yr | Low-CHO | 120 | -3.9 | -2.8 | -28.6 | -26.8 | | | |
| | | | | LF | 230 | -2.3 | -12.3 | 2.7 | 29.6 | | | |
| Yancy *et al*. 2004 | 10 | Obese Men/Women | 24 wk | Low-CHO | 30 | -12.3 | 9.8 | -47.2 | -51.8 | | | -6 |
| | | | | LF | 198 | -6.7 | -2.9 | -14.4 | -12.1 | | | -5.2 |
| Aude *et al*. 2004 | 11 | Obese | 12 wk | Low-CHO | ad lib | -6.2 | -7.6 | -23.2 | -21.1 | | | |

FIGURE 12-2. Comparison of effects on markers of metabolic syndrome of low-carbohydrate and low-fat diets. Data from reference [38].

Probably the best indicator of CVD risk of commonly-measured parameters is the ratio of triglycerides:HDL where the reduction is typically 3-10 times greater in carbohydrate reduction.

## VOLEK'S TEST OF THE THEORY

Chapter 9 described the experiments in Jeff Volek's laboratory showing that saturated fat in the blood was *reduced* by a low-carbohydrate diet with high saturated fat compared to low-fat diet with low saturated-fat. The results on control of plasma saturated fat are critical since the presence of dietary saturated fat is still an objection to low-carbohydrate diets. It was also the magnitude of the effect that was surprising. The total SFA fraction in the low-carb arm was reduced by more than half, and this reduction was more than three times the average change in the low-fat arm. This study had a larger overall significance, however.

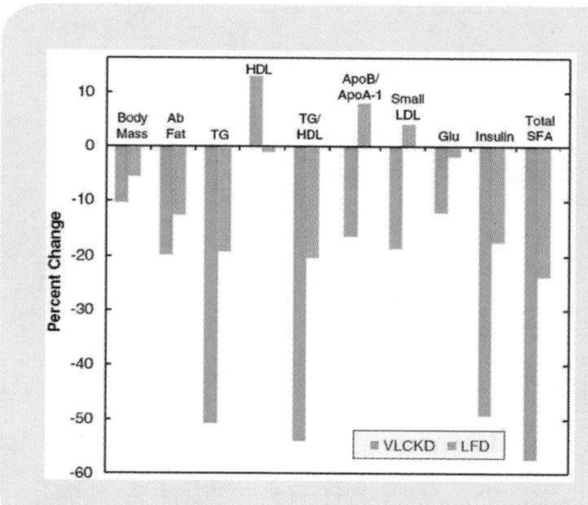


**FIGURE 12-3.** Summary of responses of 40 people with metabolic syndrome to very-low-carbohydrate ketogenic diet (VLCKD) or low-fat diet (LFD). Data from Volek, *et al.* [30, 31, 61].

The real power of Volek's experiments, however, is that the participants all fit the definition of metabolic syndrome and a wide variety of lipid, and physiologic parameters were measured. **Figure 12-3** shows you that everything got better: HDL, insulin, leptin and, most dramatically, triglycerides.

## THE PITCH

This chapter reinforces the big pitch: If metabolic syndrome (MetS) is a real thing, if seemingly different physiologic effects — overweight, high blood pressure, atherogenic dyslipidemia (high triglycerides, low HDL, high blood glucose, high insulin) — are all a reflection of a common underlying stimulus (proposed to be disruption in insulin metabolism), then if we can treat any one of those features, we can treat them all.

Nothing is better than low-carb for weight loss but lots of diets work. It's harder for women and it's harder as you get older but there are lots of ways to get thinner. We don't really have the answer on CVD. We know a lot of things that may be relevant but we don't really know the fundamental cause. We *do* know about diabetes. Cutting back on carbohydrate is the most effective treatment. For many it is a virtual cure. In the long term, it is better than drugs. So, if MetS is real, then effectively treating hyperglycemia will improve all of the features of MetS, that is, we have a prescription for general health.

## THE HEAD-AND-SHOULDERS EFFECT

In addition to metabolic effects, a low-carbohydrate diet will cure irritable bowel syndrome and related disorders in many people. (And cancer is waiting in the wings). In some sense, the problem with convincing people of the benefits of a reduced carbohydrate strategy is that it appears to be good for everything, good for what ails you. You can sound like a hard-sell pitchman. I call this the Head-and-Shoulders® effect. I don't know whether it is true but a rep from Proctor and Gamble once told me that when they first brought out the shampoo of that name, they advertised that it would cure your dandruff in three days. What their tests actually showed was that it would cure it in one day but they didn't think anybody would believe that.

## SUMMARY

Metabolic syndrome is a profound biological concept. We may

underestimate its importance because we've become used to the idea, but the fact that a group of clinical markers — overweight, high blood glucose, high insulin, high blood pressure and a group of lipid markers, high triglycerides, low HDL — should all have a high frequency of appearing together is unusual. They are not superficially similar. That they can all be brought under control by a single intervention, dietary carbohydrate restriction, suggests that they really are part of a syndrome with a common cause related in some way to the global effects of insulin. Volek's experiment is consistent with many studies in the literature but, because of the number of different parameters that were measured and because of the dramatic effects, it stands as a kind of classic experiment, under-appreciated but scientifically compelling.

The global effects of low-carbohydrate diets extend beyond metabolism and include a treatment for gastrointestinal problems [73]. There is also the well-known, if poorly investigated, effect on appetite. If there is confusion in metabolism, adding psychology into the mix can only make things worse since, in some sense, we don't even know what hunger is. The next chapter provides my take on things.

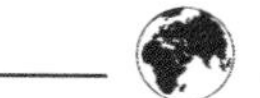

# Chapter 13

# Hunger: What It Is, What To Do About It

The reporter from *Men's Health* asked me: "You finish dinner, even a satisfying low-carb dinner" — he is a low-carb person himself — "you are sure you ate enough but you are still hungry. What do you do?" I gave him good advice. "Think of a perfectly broiled steak or steamed lobster with butter, some high protein, relatively high-fat meal that you usually like. If that doesn't sound good, you are not hungry. You may want to keep eating. You may want something sweet. You may want to feel something rolling around in your mouth, but you are not hungry. Find something else to do — push-ups are good. If the steak *does* sound good, you may want to eat. Practically speaking, you might want to keep hard boiled eggs, kielbasa, something filling, around (and, of course, you don't want cookies in the house)." I think this was good practical advice. It comes from the satiating effects of protein food sources, or perhaps the non-satiating, or reinforcing effect of carbohydrate. But the more general question is: what is hunger?

We grow up thinking that hunger is somehow our body's way of telling us that we need food but for most of us that is not the case. Few of us are so fit, or have so little body fat, or are so active, that our bodies start calling for energy if we miss lunch. Conversely, those of us who really like food generally hold to the philosophy that "any fool can eat when they're hungry." Passing up a really good chocolate mousse just because you are not hungry is like ... well, I don't know what it's like. Of course, if you are on a low-carb diet, you may pass it up for other reasons, or at least not want to eat too much.

Getting to the point here, if I presented you with a multiple choice question that asked what hunger is, the answer would be "all of the above." We feel hunger when we haven't eaten for a while. We may feel hunger if the food looks good or if we are in a social situation in which eating is going on, the spread of *petits fours* that were in the lobby at the break in an obesity conference, the congressional prayer breakfast or the Pavlovian lunch bell.

Or we may eat because we think it is time to eat. This point was made by the Restoration poet and rake, John Wilmot, Earl of Rochester. Rochester is famous for his bawdy poetry which is raunchy even by today's standards (you must be over eighteen to follow this link: http://bit.ly/1t9yvV1) but his *Satyr against Reason and Mankind*, which is more commonly included in texts on eighteenth century literature, makes fun of dumb rules and phony reason:

> My reason is my friend, yours is a cheat;
> Hunger calls out, my reason bids me eat;
> Perversely, yours your appetite does mock:
> This asks for food, that answers, "What's o'clock?"
> This plain distinction, sir, your doubt secures:
> 'Tis not true reason I despise, but yours."

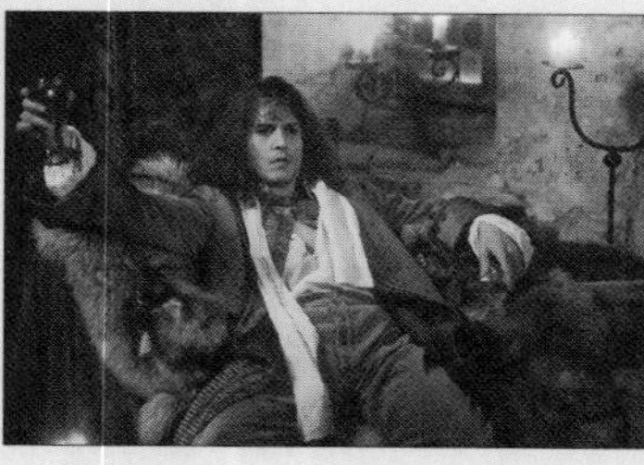

**Figure 13-1.** Johnny Depp as the Earl of Rochester (*The Libertine*, 2004).

Americans have not conquered this problem and may have made it worse. A diet experiment invariably includes a snack as if it has the same standing as breakfast, lunch and dinner, the first of which is itself of questionable generality. Visitors remark on how Americans are eating all the time, not just at meals. If you do do that, it doesn't take long until you are hungry all the time.

Different people have different responses to external cues. In experiments in which subjects are interrogated but incidentally have snacks available, it is not surprising that thin people regulate their intake by the clock on the wall. Overweight people, in distinction, are less sensitive to this input and dip into the snacks even if "it's almost dinner time." Similarly, at the Union Theological Seminary in New York, the school for training Rabbis, it is the overweight students who adhere better to fasting on high holy days. Consumption is less connected to internal (physiologic) cues and external (religious) reasons can have control.

The psychologist B. F. Skinner [74] described the problem in a typically dense way.

> "I am hungry" may be equivalent to "I have hunger pangs," and if the verbal community had some means of observing the contractions of the stomach associated with pangs, it could pin the response to these stimuli alone. It may also be equivalent to "I am eating actively." A person who observes that he is eating voraciously may say, "I really am hungry," or, in retrospect, "I was hungrier than I thought," dismissing other evidence as unreliable. "I am hungry" may also be equivalent to "It has been a long time since I have had anything to eat," although the expression is most likely to be used in describing future behavior: "If I miss my dinner, I shall be hungry."

What he is getting at here is that whatever the actual causes of eating behavior, the behavior itself may *precede* the description of the "motivation to eat." In other words, we tend to identify a feeling that is associated with eating behavior as the *cause* of the behavior.

> "I am hungry" may also be equivalent to "I feel like eating" in the sense of "I have felt this way before when I have started to eat." It may be equivalent to... "I am thinking of things I like to eat" or "I am 'eating to myself.'" To say, "I am hungry," may be to report several or all of these conditions. . . ."

The point is that "hungry" only means you are in a situation where you are used to eating. It doesn't mean that feeling hungry will make you eat, or, more important, that you have to eat.

## LESSONS FROM VAGOTOMY

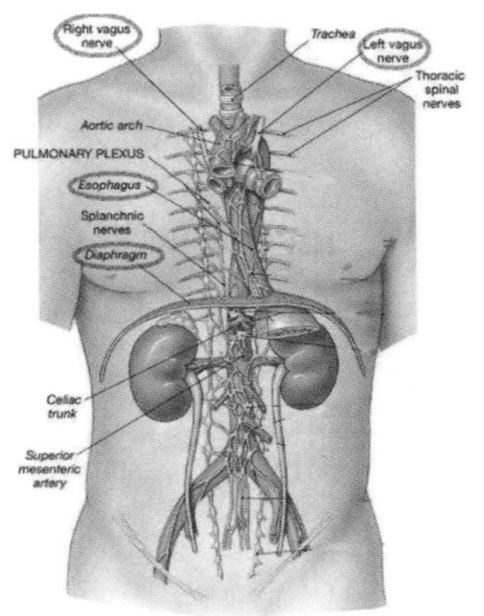


The vagus nerve contains many nerve fibers that provide communication between the brain and other parts of the body (a nerve is a collection of nerve cells or ne ur ons w hose l ong extensions or axons are referred to as fibers). Cells that send signals from the brain to distant organs are called efferent (pr. Ee-fer'-ent). Efferent fibers in the vagus nerve regulate the digestive tract — enlargement of the stomach, secretions from the pancreas, change to ac c om m oda te a lar ger volume of food (known to doctors as accommodation). However, most of the fibers in the vagus nerve are sensory afferents (afferents carry information from the body to the brain) providing sensations of satiety and hunger as well as feeling of discomfort when we are full.

Vagotomy, cutting the vagus nerve, was practiced as a means of controlling ulcers and is still a target, at least experimentally, for treating obesity. A surgeon, Dr. John Kral in the Department of Surgery at Downstate who had performed such operations described to me how patients complained that they had lost their appetite. He had to explain to them that you do not have to eat all the time, that nothing will happen if you miss a few meals.

Hunger is a signal that you are used to eating in a particular time or situation. You are not required to answer the signal.

## "You Eat Because You Are Fat"

In trying to go beyond energy balance, there is a tendency to think of hunger in terms of hormones, emphasizing regulation by the hypothalamus analogous to temperature regulation. The hormones are referred to as orexigenic, increasing appetite (from the Greek; the Greek equivalent of *bon appetit* is *kali orexi*), or anorexigenic, depressing appetite. While this is part of the picture, in the analysis of eating, it leads to some confusion because the endocrine approach emphasizes hormonal *output* from the fat cell and, in some sense, bypasses the question of how the fat cell got fat in the first place, that is, it bypasses metabolism. More important, in the end, for animals and humans outside of a laboratory setup, behavior trumps hormones. The analogy is also not entirely accurate in that animals (and humans) regulate their temperature hormonally only to a small extent. The major control of temperature is behavioral; we put on clothes and we hide in caves.

An important aspect of this problem is the attempt to understand the error in "a calorie is a calorie." One critique of the energy balance model runs something like this: dietary carbohydrate → insulin → ( other hormones →) increased appetite → greater consumption. In the extreme case, some explanations might boil down to "you don't get fat because you eat; you eat because you got fat." On the face of it, it doesn't make any sense (which is why I am not attributing it to anybody in particular). It sounds like one of the seemingly profound academic aphorism that Woody Allen was so good at parodying: "All of literature is just a footnote to Faust." I understand that it implies that the hormonal secretion from adipose tissue encourages eating. But again, it does not tell you why you got fat in the first place. It mixes up metabolism with behavior and has implicitly accepted the idea that calories are what counts, that is, macronutrients affect how much you eat (total energy), rather than how it is processed. Although macronutrients clearly differ in satiety, regardless of your hormonal state, if there is no food, you will not increase consumption. Also, the effects of insulin are not so clear-cut. Whereas metabolically, insulin is anabolic, at the level of behavior it is probably anorexigenic in most cases.

Why do we get fat? We get fat because we eat too much of the stuff that encourages excessive weight gain. We don't know what that is but we know that it is not fat *per se*. Given the unambiguous effectiveness of carbohydrate restriction in *reducing* excess weight, it would be surprising if carbohydrate weren't a big part of the picture.

The so-called metabolic advantage, less weight gain per calorie, where it exists, is a metabolic effect. The most likely mechanism is that, due to the effect of insulin on rates of reaction, anabolic (storage) steps may increase accumulation before competing feedback (breakdown) can catch up. Explained in the next chapter, it rests on non-equilibrium thermodynamics [75], which recognizes the importance of rates as well as energy.

## WHAT CAN YOU DO ABOUT IT?

The suggestion at the beginning of this section was to make sure you know what kind of hunger you are talking about. In this, behavioral psychology stresses the difference between "tastes good" and the technical term, reinforcing, which only means that the food increases the probability that you will keep eating. Anecdotally, we all have the experience of somebody (else?) saying "I don't know why I ate that. It wasn't very good."

However little you have to eat to answer feelings of hunger, it is certainly bad advice to eat if you are not hungry. Professional nutritionists, even the Atkins website, are always telling you to have a good breakfast. Why you would want to have a good anything if you are trying to lose weight is not easy to answer. They say that you will eat too much at the next meal as if, in the morning, you can make the rational decision to eat breakfast despite no desire for food while, at noon, you are suddenly under the inexorable influence of urges beyond your control. More reasonable might be: "If you find that you eat too much at lunch when you don't eat breakfast, then..." but that is not the style of traditional nutrition.

## MORE ON BEHAVIOR

The principle in behavioral psychology is that the time to reinforcement is more important than the quality of the reinforcer. Taste and mouth feel are so immediately reinforcing that probably only aversive stimulation works well. One positive take on hunger and what it means is that feeling hungry may mean that your diet is working and that you are really losing weight and therefore might stop eating before satiation. However encouraging that might be as a guide to action (or inaction), it usually can't compete well with even the smell of food. You need something strongly negative.

One of the more effective regimens is a diet strategy from Dr. Allen Fay, a psychiatrist in New York. It works like this:

1) You pick an amount of weight you want to lose in the next week; you can pick zero but, of course, you can't go up.

2) You write a check for $2, 000 to the Republican National Committee (in my case) and give it to Dr. Fay.

3) If, at the end of the week, you haven't hit the target, he mails the check.

In some cases, Dr. Fay said, you don't even need money. One patient wrote a letter to a right-to-life organization, telling them what a great job they were doing. The thought that she would get on their mailing list as a supporter was sufficiently aversive to keep her on target. You pick your own threat, of course. Dr. Fay suggested the American Nazi Party but I thought that they would only buy those shabby uniforms whereas, from my perspective, the Republicans would do real damage. My relation to Dr. Fay is partly professional (although he admits that there are people who are beyond psychotherapy) and partly friend. For the technique to work, you must be distant enough from the person holding the check so that they will actually mail it, but close enough that you will not consider physical violence if they do.

Imagery can help ... up to a point. A major problem situation for dieters is that they have eaten what they want and feel satisfied but there is still food on their plate and they pick at it until they feel sick. My approach, when I felt full, was to imagine spiders coming out of the food. This worked for a while but over time I noticed that I was losing my distaste of spiders. Eating has a very strong Pavlovian component. It is not nice to fool Mother Nature.

## EXERCISE

The only thing that people in nutrition agree on is the value of exercise. While it is not as important as diet for weight loss, it does interact with diet and has obvious benefit. One question is when to have meals in relation to exercise. Although outside my area of expertise and likely to be an individual thing, there is some good guidance in the following old joke.

The couple come to the doctor and don't want to have any more children but they don't want any artificial methods of birth control. The doctor recommends exercise.

Husband: Before or after?
Doctor: Instead of.

## SUMMARY

Hunger is poorly defined or, at least its relation to behavior and physiology is not simple. We have a sensation which may be tied to any number of things, food availability, meal-time, or even a real need for nourishment. The description that encompasses all the different things is that it means you are in a situation in which you are used to eating. So, in the search for causes of eating, what you come up with may only be a restatement of the behavioral observations. Knowing that it is a feeling that doesn't have to be answered may be helpful. Reduction in appetite is a major feature of carbohydrate restriction but the other end of weight loss is metabolic efficiency and the widely cited, if poorly understood, laws of thermodynamics. I try to shed some light on that. Next chapter.

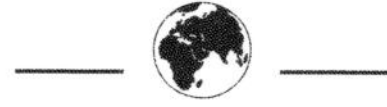

# CHAPTER 14

# "CALORIE IS A CALORIE," THERMODYNAMICS, AND ALL THAT

## "A CALORIE IS A CALORIE"

Can you lose more weight on one diet than another if they have the same number of calories? The question is usually about a low-carbohydrate diet where the so-called metabolic advantage promises you that cutting out carbs will lead to reduced efficiency in storing fat. Folks go crazy when you suggest it's true. Whenever a scientific paper presents data showing that such a thing really happens, showing that one (usually low-carb) diet, is more effective than another, somebody always jumps in to say that it is impossible, that it would violate the laws of thermodynamics. Like the cartoon characters who run out over the cliff and fall only when they realize that they are not on solid ground, somehow the data are expected to go away once thermodynamics is invoked.

Of course, the data can't violate the laws of thermodynamics. There is the possibility that the data really are accurate and that the critic doesn't get it. Thermodynamics, the physics of heat, work and energy, is a tough subject and it takes real *chutzpah* to jump in where many physicists fear to tread.

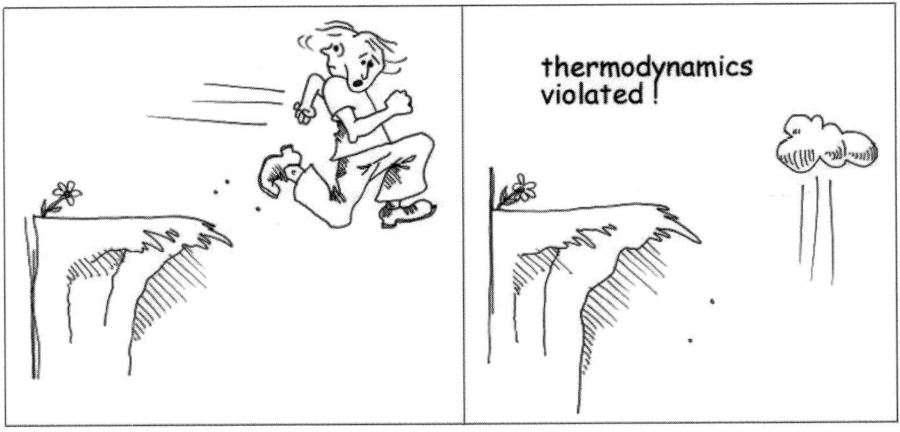


Thermodynamics, however, is interesting. It has been described as the first revolutionary science. You probably don't really need it to study nutrition but if you catch on to the basics, you will understand something that seems counter-intuitive to many people. It will explain how you get more bang for your nutritional buck, that is, how you lose more weight per calorie.

When you consider that the fundamental unit in nutrition is the calorie, a unit of energy, it seems likely that it would be worth knowing something about the physics of energy exchange.

TEXT BOX 14-1.

*Arnold Sommerfeld was one of the great physicists in the development of quantum mechanics (theory of atomic structure). He was also generally considered to be an expert on most areas of physics. His take on thermodynamics:*

*The first time I studied it, I thought that I understood it except for a few minor details.*

*The second time I studied it, I thought that I didn't understand it except for a few minor details.*

*The third time I studied it, I knew I didn't understand it but it didn't matter because I already knew how to use it.*

## BOTTOM LINE ON METABOLIC ADVANTAGE

Here are the four big questions and the answers. The rest of the Chapter will explain and justify these conclusions.

1. Metabolic advantage or, a better term, energy efficiency, is not contradicted by any physical law. Thermodynamics, in fact, more or less predicts variable energy efficiency. The way it has been discussed in nutrition is incorrect and does not conform to the way chemical thermodynamics is normally used.

2. Arguments against metabolic advantage often rely on practical considerations: how small the effect is. At the same time, the same critics espouse the value of cumulative small effects, operative in diets where you explicitly control calories, where 50 calories a day is supposed to add up over a year. It doesn't. Metabolism doesn't work like that. Homeostatic (stabilizing) mechanisms compensate for simple changes in calories unless they are the right kind of calories and, in fact, the effects of different macronutrients can be dramatic. In any case, if there really is any change at all, that should be a call to find out how to maximize it, not toss it.

3. Even if you aren't sure it's ever been demonstrated, it makes sense to try to make it work for you since, from the scientific standpoint, it is possible and the payoff is great.

4. Several mechanisms, particularly substrate cycling and gluconeogenesis, are involved. Experimentally, inefficiencies in digestion and metabolic processing, the so-called thermic effect of feeding, contribute as well.

## WHERE WE ARE GOING

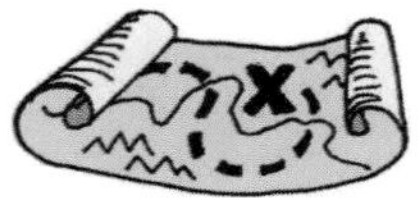


Many people find metabolic advantage counter-intuitive because of the idea of energy conservation. I will explain the fallacy. I will present some of the data and then explain how it could happen in terms of biochemical mechanisms.

## THE DATA

There are basically two kinds of diet experiments. Some clearly show energy balance and some clearly don't. On the one hand, if you take a normal person and keep them in a hospital room and feed them constant calories (top panel, **Figure 14-1**), you will find that "wide variations in the ratio of carbohydrate to fat do not alter total 24-h energy need [76]," their weight will stay roughly constant. The figure is an example of what is meant by "a calorie is a calorie." Common enough. Frequently, experimentally, a calorie *is* a calorie. It's the same in experiments comparing diets of different macronutrient composition. Two people who are roughly similar in age and health will respond similarly to two isocaloric (same calories) diets regardless of the diet composition (amount of fat, carbohydrate and protein). This means that yes, calories count. But, there are many exceptions.

The energy balance shown in the figure is achieved by biology, not the laws of thermodynamics. In those cases where everything balances out, it isn't physical laws but rather the unique characteristics of living systems that keep things constant (homeostasis). Big rule: in biology, almost everything is connected in feedback and homeostatic mechanisms compensate for chemical changes. In view of this, we should be asking "how is energy balance possible when it is not predicted from thermodynamics", not "how could there be different weight gain or loss for the same calories." So let's look at the exceptions, the second type of diet experiment seen in the literature.

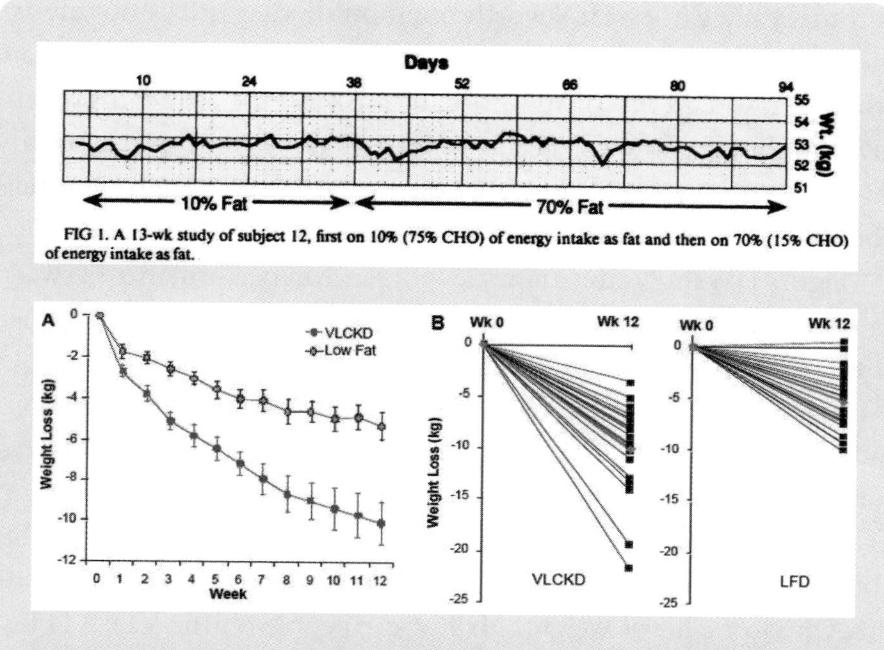


Figure 14-1. Comparison of diets. Data from references [30, 61].

The exceptions can be dramatic. **Figure 9-2.** Duplicated in the bottom panels of **Figure 14-1** show results of a study from the laboratory of Jeff Volek, then at the University of Connecticut. In this study, described previously in Chapter 9, there were 40 overweight men and women with metabolic syndrome (high triglycerides, low HDL or at least two of several other factors). They were assigned to one of two *ad libitum* diets, described previously, either a very low-carbohydrate ketogenic diet (VLCKD) designed to provide a distribution of macronutrients along the following lines: %CHO:fat:protein = 12:59:28, or a low-fat diet (LFD) with a distribution %CHO:fat:protein = 56:24:20. The experiment lasted 12 weeks. Although neither group was specifically told to reduce calories, both groups did show a spontaneous decrease in energy intake — it seems that if you sign up for a diet experiment you automatically eat less. It's worth mentioning that this is not always the way the experiment is set up — frequently the low-carbohydrate arm is allowed *ad lib* consumption of food as long as it conforms to low-carb but the low-fat diet to which it is to be compared explicitly regulates calories (e.g., [77]). That the low-carb diet usually wins tells you something right off.

**Figure 14-1** shows the dramatic difference in performance between the VLCKD and the low-fat diet. Part A indicates the average effect; weight loss on the VLCKD group was dramatically better. In reading the medical literature, however, it is important to ask about individual performance, especially when you are comparing different time points. People are different. Nobody loses an average amount of weight. People in both groups lost weight but what is remarkable about the figure is the number of people on the low-carbohydrate diet who lost a lot of weight. Half of the people on the VLCKD lost more than the single best person on the low-fat diet.

## CAN YOU TRUST DIETARY RECORDS?

Critics of this kind of experiment say that it relies on patient dietary records, which are known to be inaccurate. While this is true, such data are not *wildly* inaccurate. Values can be off by 20% not 50% and are unlikely to be sole cause of the differences. Also, ketone bodies were measured so at least the VLCKD group did what they were told. More important, if the differences were due to inaccurate reporting of dietary intake, that is, if the diets were truly different in caloric intake, the people on the VLCKD must have over-reported what they ate and the people on LFD must have under-reported what they ate, or both. From a practical standpoint, it might be encouraging to be on a diet where you think that you are eating more than you really are.

Low-carbohydrate diets almost always win in a face-off with low-fat diets. Establishment nutritionists take it as a win if there is a tie but you can do that for just so long. So if it is not just about the calories, where does thermodynamics really fit in? With the disclaimer in **Textbox 14.1**, I will give you a rough idea about how it's done in real biochemistry.

## THERMODYNAMICS

It is the physics of heat, work and energy. The subject is fundamentally down to earth. Its roots are in the attempt to find out just how efficient a steam engine you could build — thermodynamics comes from the industrial revolution where the efficiency of steam engines was a big deal. In weight loss, we are really asking how efficiently food is utilized. The other side of thermodynamics is that the methods are highly mathematical and arcane, even for scientists. Thermodynamics has been described as "the science of partial differential equations" which is not to everybody's taste. The results, however, give you very simple equations for predicting things. Heavy-duty theory and practical application. It's what people who do like thermodynamics like about it. That's the main theme of this book — science with direct applicability. You get an equation that tells you whether you have a good steam engine or, in fact, whether your food is fattening.

## THE LAWS OF THERMODYNAMICS

When people say the laws of thermodynamics, they usually mean the first law, the law of conservation of energy. However, "conservation of energy" can be a sound bite, at the level of "Einstein said that everything is relative." You have to know exactly what is being conserved. Precise definitions become very important. One of the many difficulties in understanding thermodynamics is that there are simple principles which seem obvious enough but their import is under-appreciated without a real example.

The first law says precisely that there is a parameter called the internal energy and the change (Δ) in the internal energy of a system is equal to the heat, q, added to the system minus the work, w, that the system does on the environment. (The internal energy is usually written as U so as not to confuse it with the electrical potential).

$$\Delta U = q - w \qquad (1)$$

This is how thermodynamics is taught. To go to the next step you need to understand the idea of a state variable. A state variable is a variable where any change is path-independent. For example, the familiar temperature T and pressure P are state variables. It doesn't matter whether you change the pressure quickly or slowly. The effect on the system is controlled by the difference between the pressure after the change minus the temperature before the change, that is, ΔP. The usual analogy is the as-the-crow-flies geographical distance, say, between New York and San Francisco. This is a state variable; it doesn't matter whether you fly directly or go through Memphis and Salt Lake City like the flights that I wind up on.

Now, U in equation (1) is a state variable. Any process that you carry out will have a change in U that depends only on the initial and final states. However, q and w are NOT state variables. How you design your machine will determine how much work you can get out of it and how much of the energy change will be wasted. Looking at the biological case, two metabolic changes with the same U have no theoretical reason why they should have the same relative amounts of heat and work, that is, the same efficiency (storing fat as compared to generating heat). Of course, they might but there is no theoretical barrier to difference. In this, the first law contains the suggestion of the second law. The second law is what thermodynamics is really about. The second law pretty much guarantees that you are not going to get all work. The likelihood that two diets have exactly the same inefficiency is extremely low.

There are four laws of thermodynamics and the first law only operates in concert with the others. (They *are* physical laws). The zeroth law and the third law are pretty much theoretical, defining thermal equilibrium and the condition of absolute zero of temperature. It is the second law that embodies the special character of thermodynamics. Described by Ilya Prigogine, the Nobel-prize winning chemist and philosopher of thermodynamics, as the first revolutionary science, it is the second law that explains how one diet can be more or less efficient that the other. The essential feature of the second law is the existence of a thing called entropy.

## ENTROPY

The entropy is traditionally defined with respect to a classic imaginary experiment. Although theoretical, it is clearly related to practical things. The experiment involves a creature referred to as the Maxwell's Demon who is capable of doing things perfectly smoothly and slowly without exerting any energy or creating any heat from friction (**Figure 14-2**). The apparatus is a box with a partition, a membrane that separates the box into two compartments, one that is filled with a dilute gas and one that is empty.

The demon very carefully and slowly removes the membrane so that no work is done and no heat is generated. Now, according to the first law, which specifies the need to conserve energy (the ability to do work) and heat, nothing has really happened. In a real experiment, you could make an electronic device to open a door into the compartment so efficiently that would hardly raise your electric bill, so effectively that energy is conserved and nothing should happen. Of course, you know that something will happen. The gas will fill up the whole box. Why? Because that's the way the world is according to the second law. The second law says that the entropy will always increase. The entropy is a measure of how disorganized a system is, that is, what its possibilities are. A box full of gas is a looser distribution than a gas confined to only one side of the box. Another description: you would not need a very good GPS to find out if the molecule is in New York City *vs* whether it is in Yankee Stadium.

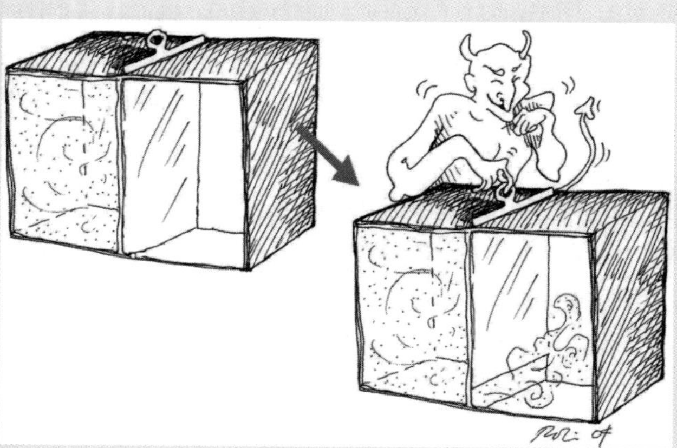

FIGURE 14-2. A "Maxwell's Demon" removes the partition between two compartments very slowly (does no work and generates no heat). The gas in the first compartment fills up both sides because the entropy will increase.

The gas fills up the whole box because it is the most probable way for the molecules to be distributed. The second law is about probability. Before the nineteenth century, physics held a view of a universe that was mechanical, a universe standing alone in time and controllable. The second law suddenly brought out the irreversible and statistical nature of things. It is not that nobody knew that time passes but the idea of physical processes running down like a clock was a revolutionary idea. The history of physics shows how hard it was for people, even very smart people, to understand and cope with the idea of probability. But, as it evolved, the second law became very practical and explained how energy can be used to do work and how chemical reactions occur. It is the key to understanding energy transformation in life.

## ENTROPY AND INFORMATION

Entropy is about information. It is frequently said that increased entropy means increased disorder but a more precise way to put it is that it means a less demanding way of arranging a system. It means higher probability. A straight flush has much lower entropy than two of a kind because there are fewer ways to get a straight flush. And entropy, that is, information, can overpower energy. A receiver in American football can catch a pass even though he is double-teamed (energy is compromised) because he (ideally) has the information as to where the ball will be thrown. The term entropy is also used in communications where it indicates the extent to which a message has been corrupted during transmission.

One formal way of stating the second law is that it is impossible to carry out an operation where the sole effect is to transfer heat from a cold body to a warm body. This is obvious enough but it may not be easy to explain why. After all, the ocean is cold but does have a huge amount of heat because it is so large. Why couldn't a ship exract a little bit of that heat to run its engines. That's the question Maxwell was really asking.

The original creature proposed by Maxwell was more sophisticated than the example above. It was only later that somebody else called it a demon. This demon sat on a membrane separating two compartments. One compartment had a hot gas and, the other, a cold gas. The partition had a little door, a very well-machined, well-oiled door whose openings and closings did not require any real amount of work and did not generate any heat. The demon would look into the cold gas and if he saw a fast moving particle, he would open the door and let the particle into the hot compartment. He could, similarly, let slow moving particles move from the hot gas to the cold gas. The net effect was to transfer heat from a cold body to a warm body, a clear no-no according to the second law. It was a thought experiment but you could make a really efficient door so why couldn't you make something at least close to this set-up? The ocean is cold but it is so far from absolute zero and it is so big that there is so much heat, why couldn't you make something like a Maxwell's demon to get some of it to power your ocean liner? What's wrong here? Was the second law not universal?

This paradox completely stumped physicists of the nineteenth century. It's because it's about probability and randomness and they were not used to thinking like that. The answer to Maxwell's paradox is that it is not really a paradox so much as another way of stating the second law. That's how the world is. Information costs. You can't make such a set-up. If you could use some fancy electronic device to set up a sensor to distinguish between fast and slow molecules, it would have to do work. The reason it gets confusing is that in the physical (real) world we are only used to dealing with gross collections of things and averages. If we want to get down to single molecules, we have to run a machine to do it. Another way of saying it is that the reason that we can't make anything perfectly efficient because you can't control individual molecules. Where we're going on this is that if you think of the work that you do that is powered by your food, you can't get it to work completely efficiently. Some part of the energy must be wasted. Of course, unlike an engineer, if you are trying to lose weight, the job of synthesizing and storing fat may be one that you want to run as inefficiently as possible.

## THE SECOND LAW AND METABOLIC ADVANTAGE

There are a lot of different ways of stating the second law but one version emphasizes the fact that all real engines, in fact, all processes in the real world, are inherently inefficient — not just practically, not because you can't machine them so carefully that there's no friction, but theoretically, absolutely — no escape from inefficiency. The second law says that a perfect engine, living or otherwise, is not possible (unless you could get one to run at the mysterious temperature called absolute zero; the third law does give you that).

Inefficiency depends on where you stand and what you are trying to accomplish. In a human being, sometimes keeping warm, that is, using food for heat, may not be considered inefficient but from the point of view of a machine that is trying to manufacture protein and other cell material, it is energy that is wasted. The heat generated in the processing of food is called either thermic effect of feeding (TEF) or diet-induced thermogenesis (DIT). (The old name was specific dynamic action). These measure energy wasted as heat. They are an expression of the inefficiency of the human machine. There are other ways to waste energy. The so-called NEAT, non-exercise activity thermogenesis which is the scientific name for fidgeting. The measured TEF of different macronutrients is different; protein is much greater than carbohydrate which is greater than fat. In other words, metabolic advantage is a well documented fact and the extent to which small changes add up is only a question of how you do the experiment. If you have to make glucose through the process of gluconeogenesis, rather than getting it from the diet, you are going to waste energy.

## Real Thermo. Beyond "Energy In = Energy Out"

Another simple idea that can lead to confusion — sometimes great confusion — and the major fallacy in thinking that thermodynamics ties you to "calories in, calories out" is the concept of system and environment. In chemical thermodynamics, we focus on the reaction, not the reaction plus the environment. We measure the extent to which reactions need or give off energy. It is not about conservation. It is about dissipation of energy. The 4 kcal/g that we assign to carbohydrate is the energy exported from the reaction of oxidation. That's what you do in chemical thermodynamics. Else, all food would have zero calories; the heat lost in oxidation is gained by the calorimeter. Calories in, equals calories out, but that literally leaves you with nothing.

What comes next shows you how real thermodynamics work. It is not mathematical. All you need is high school algebra but it is an explanation of what you might do in a chemistry course. You can see the beauty of thermodynamics and how it can tell you, right off, that it's not just calories in, calories out. You may like it. Or you can jump to the summary at the end.

The second law says, in essence, that all (real) systems are inefficient. In practice, the law can be used to tell you whether a chemical reaction actually produces energy or whether you will have to put in energy to make it go. This is the key thing in chemistry (or living systems): does the reaction go as written.

When we write A⟶B, we want to know whether the reaction will proceed from left to right spontaneously. "Spontaneously" means without the addition of energy. It does not mean fast, which is a separate question. The 4 kcal of energy that you measure in the calorimeter is both a measure of the tendency of the reaction to occur (oxidations generally produce energy) and also the maximum energy available to do work. They are very closely related because, although living systems do mechanical (muscle) work, the main use of the energy is in chemical work, synthesizing metabolites and cell material.

The second law leads to the definition of a number of different forms of the energy (which are used under different conditions). The particular form of the energy that is used under conditions of constant temperature and pressure (where biochemists usually work) is called the Gibbs Free Energy, almost always abbreviated with the letter G, and the change associated with chemical or other processes is written with the Greek delta, ΔG. The Gibbs Free Energy for a chemical is precisely defined as the maximum work you can get from running the reaction at constant temperature and pressure and it is identified with the tendency of the reaction to go in the forward direction. The 4 kcal produced by the oxidation of glucose tells you that that is the most you could get out of it in terms of work or driving other chemical reactions. In practice, some may be wasted as heat or other unproductive processes.

## REAL THERMODYNAMICS

You can gain some insight by going back to the beginning. A fundamental idea is a notion of system and environment. In fact, chemical thermodynamics tends to focus only on the system (the chemical reaction). Otherwise all food would have zero calories because when you measure combustion in the calorimeter (where calories are determined), the heat lost by combustion of the food would be equal to the heat gained by the calorimeter and so from direct application of conservation of energy, there are no calories to assign to the food. Chemical thermodynamics emphasizes the reaction of the system, not the whole universe. We want to know about the energy exchange when we burn food. The complete oxidation of glucose in the calorimeter *produces* 4 kcal. It is not about conservation. It is about dissipation of energy.

The word thermodynamics is thrown around a lot in nutrition, mostly by people who have no idea what it is about. Again, you don't need thermodynamics to do nutrition but if you do it, you have to do it right so, in case you want to see what people really do in chemical thermodynamics, I will present a good example.

The basic idea is that we identify the energy of a chemical reaction with spontaneity, that is, whether the reaction goes forward by itself or whether you have to do something to make it go. (Again, spontaneous does not mean fast but only that no energy has to be added to make things go). The rule is that if the Free Energy change is negative ($\Delta G < 0$) for the reaction, the reaction is downhill **(Figure 14-3)** will go by itself and will give off energy (which you may be able to capture by coupling it to another chemical reaction or to some mechanical, electrical or heat machine). The Gibbs Free Energy has two components, the heat of reaction, called **enthalpy** ($\Delta H$) and the entropy ($\Delta S$).

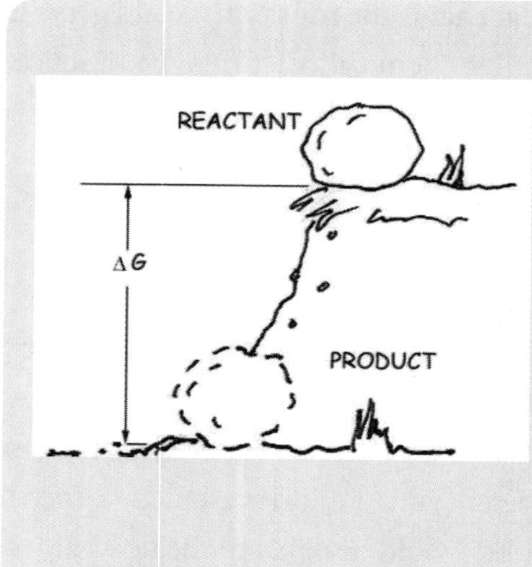


FIGURE 14-3. Chemical energy can be thought of as analogous to potential energy in physics. In the diagram, the boulder has potential energy by virtue of its height on the cliff. The conversion of reactant to product is down-hill ($\Delta G$ is (-)). Work can be done by pushing the boulder off the cliff. For the reverse reaction, you would have to do an amount of work equal to $+\Delta G$ to move the boulder up the cliff.

Here's a simple example of what you might do in real thermo. Suppose that you wanted to know about the formation of carbon monoxide (CO) and how much energy is given off if carbon is oxidized to CO. Generally thought of in the context of a poison, CO has other uses and, among other things, a small amount is produced in the human body (during the breakdown of heme from hemoglobin). So is the oxidation of carbon to CO uphill or downhill and by how much? To keep it simple, we'll take the heat of reaction, ($\Delta H$). We can do the experiment so that the entropy is not an important player (low temperature). The heat of reaction is easily measured.

In the case of oxidizing carbon, then, if heat is given off ($\Delta H$ = (-)) the reaction will be spontaneous and go by itself. The problem with trying to figure out how much energy you can get by burning carbon to carbon monoxide is that you can't really measure it. If you try to carry out the reaction, you always get some $CO_2$. So, what can you do?

Here's how we do it: We want to measure the heat of reaction for oxidation of carbon to CO. We can't measure that directly. However, we can measure the enthalpy of burning of carbon to $CO_2$. (A minus sign means heat is given off).

$C + O_2 \longrightarrow CO_2 \quad \Delta H = -94$ kcal

We also know the energy of burning CO to $CO_2$.

$CO + \frac{1}{2} O_2 \longrightarrow CO_2 \quad \Delta H = -68$ kcal

Another great simplifying feature of thermodynamics is that the energy for going the other way is the same numerically with the opposite sign, so:

$CO_2 \longrightarrow CO + \frac{1}{2} O_2 \quad \Delta H = +68$ kcal

State functions can be added just as in simple algebra. The associated energies add up too (**Figure 14-4**).

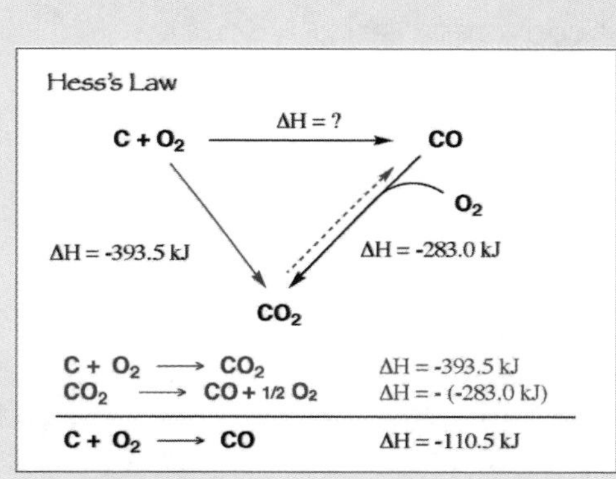


FIGURE 14-4. Calculating heat of reaction for formation of CO. Path of the blue arrows (measured) must equal the direct conversion to CO, so we just add them up. (Note: energies in figure in kJ = 4.28 kcal).

The beauty of thermodynamics — the attraction to those people, like Einstein, who like it — is that you can manipulate the results with elementary algebra. The great simplicity in this kind of calculation reflects its highly predictive power. What did we do? We had two different paths from carbon to carbon monoxide, one (two-step) path that we could calculate and one that we are trying to find out. They must be equal, as in **Figure 14-4**. The principle that allows you to add up heats of reaction is called Hess's law.

## HESS'S LAW SHOWS THAT "A CALORIE IS" NOT "A CALORIE"

What follows is a Hess's law analysis of "a calorie is a calorie." In the context of nutrition, the law implies that energy yield for metabolism will be path-independent, that is, the same for all diets and proportional to the calorimeter values. The calorimeter values say that energy yield for carbohydrate and for protein are equivalent fuels, ΔG (oxidation) = -4 kcal/mol as shown in Figure 14-5. Remember that a (-) sign means energy is given off and the process is spontaneous. The calories in food, again, is the energy for burning the food to $CO_2$ and water. Here's the plan. We make two paths for oxidizing protein: path 1 (direct) or path 2 + path 3 (first convert to carbohydrate).

Protein + $O_2 \longrightarrow CO2 + H2O \quad \Delta G1 = 4$ kcal/g
Carbohydrate + $O2 \longrightarrow CO2 + H2O\ \Delta G2 = 4$ kcal/g
Protein — *GNG* $\longrightarrow$ Carbohydrate + $O2 \longrightarrow CO2 + H2O\ \Delta G3 + \Delta G2 = ?$

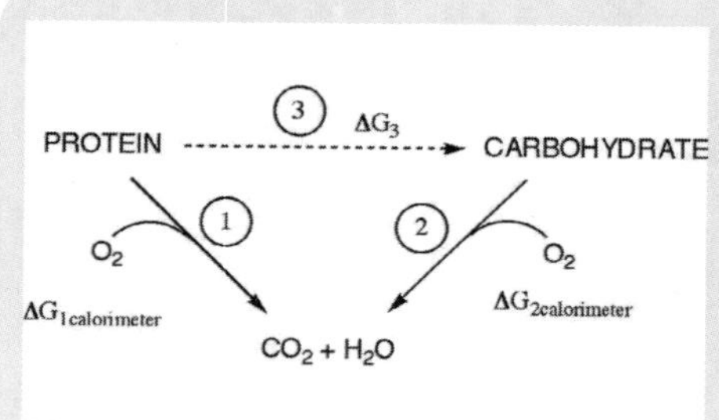


FIGURE 14-5. According to Hess's Law (adding up energies), the energy for path 1, $\Delta G_1$ should be equal to the energy for path 3 followed by path 2, $\Delta G_1 - \Delta G_2$. Using calorimeter values and the principle that a calorie is a calorie leads to a contradiction.

In path 1, we burn protein directly to $CO_2$. Now, because free energy is a state variable, the free energy $\Delta G_1$ must be equal to the sum of $\Delta G_2$, the energy for path 2 plus $\Delta G_3$, the energy for path 3. This means that $\Delta G_3$ for path 3 must be about zero. However, this is the process of gluconeogenesis. Students work very hard learning that gluconeogenesis is an endergonic process; it costs energy (about 6 ATP). Assuming that only the calories measured in the calorimeter are important leads to a contradiction.

## THE NON-EQUILIBRIUM PICTURE

One more level of sophistication. To some extent, it is not really about thermodynamics at all, or at least not equilibrium thermodynamics. Equilibrium thermodynamics is what is usually studied and we are taught that rates of reaction are considered separately from energy. The results of equilibrium thermodynamics tell us that amino acids are more stable than proteins. The rate of breakdown, however, is very slow. If you could keep the bacteria off your steak it would last for months or years. At the end of time it would be all amino acids (or even simpler things). In biochemistry, however, rates become important because living systems are not at equilibrium until they die. Things are moving forward. All the reactions in biology are catalyzed by enzymes which control the *speed* of a reaction, not the energetics. A better way to put it might be to say that the key players in all this are hormones and hormones generally affect enzymes which, in turn, affect rates, not energy.

Living systems are not at equilibrium. Living systems, in fact, maintain themselves very far from equilibrium. They are characterized by an in-and-out flux of material and energy. In a dietary intervention, material fluctuates around a level far from equilibrium. In other words, changes with time become important and changes may be controlled by the presence of catalysts, that is, enzymes, or other factors that affect the rate of reaction.

**Figure 14-5** shows the theoretical fluctuations of fat within a fat cell. The key idea is that the reactions, breakdown and re-synthesis, are very far from equilibrium where you would have little fat, mostly fatty acid.

Looking at fat gain and loss (**Figure 14-5**), adipocytes cycle between states of greater or lesser net breakdown of fat (lipolysis and re-formation) depending on the hormonal state which, in turn, is dependent on the macronutrient composition of the diet. A hypothetical scheme for changes in adipocyte TAG and a proposal for how TAG gain or loss could be different for isocaloric diets with different levels of insulin is shown in the figure. The basic idea is that fat fluctuates but if you slow storage enough that it hasn't had a chance to break down before you come in with another meal, fat will accumulate whatever the caloric input.

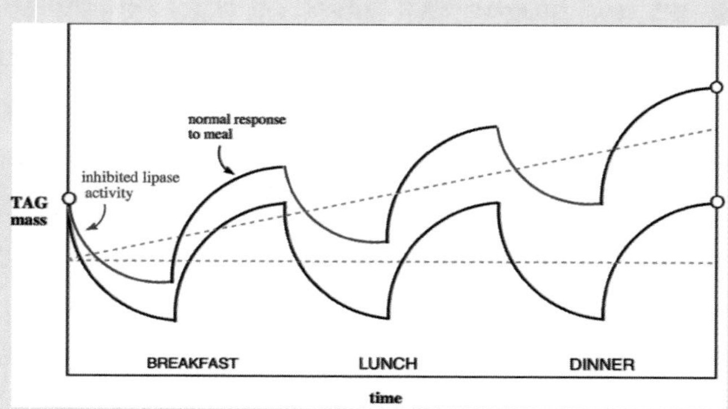


FIGURE 14-6 Hypothetical model for the effect of insulin on efficiency of storage. Black line indicates response under conditions of weight maintenance, fluctuates but averages to no change. The upper blue line shows the effect of added insulin on hormone-sensitive lipase activity. The important point is that the energy differences are very small compared to the equilibrium value, which would be very far below the figure. The system is not controlled by energy but by rates.

Under normal control conditions of weight maintenance, the breakdown and utilization of TAG follows a pattern of lipolysis (fasting) and intake plus re-synthesis (meals). To make it simple, we assume a sudden, instantaneous spike in food at meals. Then the curves represent the net flow of material within the adipocyte. This averages out to a stable weigh maintenance (lower red dotted line in **Figure 14-6**). If we keep each meal at constant calories but increase the percentage of carbohydrate or otherwise generate a higher insulin level, the hormone-sensitive lipases, the enzymes that break down fat will be inhibited (blue line in the Figure). Re-synthesis of TAG is less affected by the elevated insulin (may actually slow down). The net effects are changes in the direction of accumulation of TAG. It is theoretical but the model shows you how kinetics (how fast it's happening) may be more important than thermodynamics.

## Summary

Metabolic advantage, or energy efficiency, is not contradicted by the laws of thermodynamics. The second law is more important than the first and it emphasizes inefficiency. There are several biochemical mechanisms, thermic effect of feeding, gluconeogenesis and substrate cycling that account for the observed variable efficiency which, in humans, generally supports the advantages of low-carbohydrate diets. Because it is physically possible to have variable weight gain and because the experimental observations in people favor carbohydrate restriction, it is worth a shot. The insistence that only calories count is one of the bad ideas that has held back research and limited the ability of individual dieters to get good advice and it has to be addressed before we can move on. It is not the only bad idea, however. These should also be addressed. Next chapter.

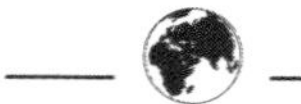

# Chapter 15

# Summary: Bad Ideas

A summary so far is that nutritional thinking has followed two really bad ideas: "You are what you eat," and "a calorie is a calorie." If you want to pick just two things that account for the nutritional mess in this country and around the world, these would be it. The ideas are, on the face of it, contradictory — if eating fat makes you fat or puts fat in your arteries, then fat is bad. If all calories are the same, then fat is neither good nor bad.

## Bad Idea: "You Are What You Eat."

At least unconsciously, people really do hold to the idea that food gets packaged into your body as in refrigerator woman and we really do go with the assumption that fat makes you fat and that saturated fat clogs your arteries because it is greasy. These ideas are the first thing to get rid of if we are to make progress in dealing with nutrition. "You are what you eat" is not a real biological idea. *You are what your body*, that is, your metabolism, *does with what you eat* is the better principle. Your body is not a storage container. It is a machine. Not one that grinds everything

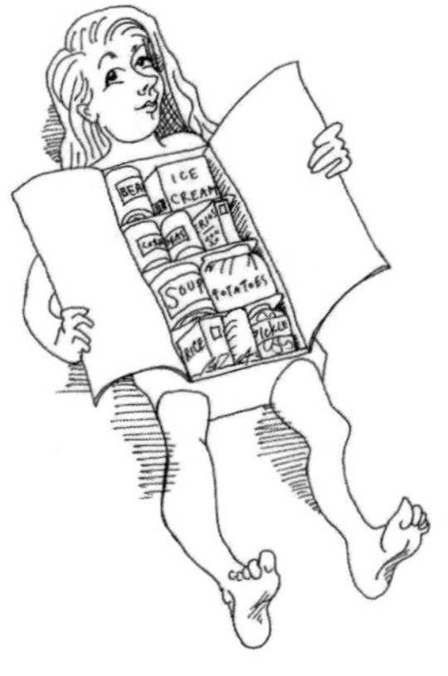

down to calories, but a chemical machine. The input to the machine is the digestive tract but even the digestive system is more than simple plumbing.

Within the cells of the intestine, between the absorption of food and the entry into the circulation, transformations are taking place. The nutrients that intestinal cells process, for their own metabolism and those that ultimately wind up in the blood, may be very different from what you ate. For example, the components of protein, the individual **amino acids**, are re-shuffled and processed even in the cells of the intestine. The particular arrangement of amino acids for particular proteins that is encoded in your DNA determines the biologic activity of those proteins. There are about twenty amino acids all together. During digestion, protein is broken down to the component amino acids which are absorbed. Ten of the amino acids, the essential amino acids, are required in the diet. The others are inter-convertible. A re-shuffling of some of the amino acids by the process known as **transamination** provides the right mix of amino acids for any particular protein in any particular tissue. So this process of interconversion of amino acids is going on all the time and as early in metabolism as the cells of the intestine. Beyond building blocks for proteins, amino acids take part in metabolism on their own. The amino acid alanine, for example, is a key player in metabolism providing carbons for gluconeogenesis. Described in Chapter 6, the process connects protein, carbohydrate and energy metabolism. The amount of alanine leaving the intestine is typically three times the amount that came in. Providing amino acids for carbohydrate is, again, part of why you don't have to *consume* any; the glucose that the brain requires can come from amino acids such as alanine or other metabolites. **Gluconeogenesis** is one of the transformations going on all the time in your body (mostly in the liver where Claude Bernard found it originally). Sometimes described as a "last resort" for production of glucose, gluconeogenesis, like the interconversion of amino acids, goes on all the time. Your body does not need any dietary glucose. You are not what you eat.

## ALSO NOT GOOD: "A CALORIE IS A CALORIE."

The previous chapter described how little can be expected from the idea that "a calorie is a calorie," that is, that the energy (calories) supplied in food is all the same, that it doesn't matter whether the calories come from *To urnedos Rossini*, Twinkies® or from whole grain cereal. The implication is that if two people do the same amount of exercise, that they will gain or lose the same amount of weight, calorie for calorie. Despite arguments of the type we went through, many people feel that the idea makes sense and that it is perfectly intuitive. A tip-off on what's wrong with the idea that "a calorie is a calorie" is that, if the scientific evidence really supported it, people wouldn't still be trying to prove it, and there probably wouldn't be any professors of biochemistry, not even one, who claimed that the idea is false.

## OTHER BAD IDEAS AND THE NUTRITION MESS

It's hard not to see a total nutritional mess in the population. Most people have the vague idea that eating a low-fat diet must be good in some way even though one scientific study after another shows that this is not true and the dire predictions on dietary fat have never panned out. Some of the experts are backing down on this; the American Heart Association quietly removed any recommendation on total dietary fat in 2000. What? You didn't know that? Their webmeister doesn't know that either. Their websites, for example, "The American Heart Association's Diet and Lifestyle Recommendations" at http://bit.ly/1nJnjwh continue to recommend low-fat. The AHA is officially down only on saturated fat and, of course, *trans*-fats. The dietary guidelines from the government also say that they don't put any limits on total fat but their recommendations are for low-fat milk, lean meat, etc. So, low-fat or not low-fat? And if it's not low-fat, why is everybody recommending it?

## A SIMPLE PROBLEM

When people tell you that a problem is very complex, there's a good chance that what they mean is that they don't want to face the part of it that is really simple. And a lot of it really is simple. If you look around, you see that people are fatter than they used to be. Reliably fatter. Not everyone. Not everyplace. Much less in New York City or Vermont. But in what New Yorkers call America (starts someplace in New Jersey), people really are fatter, sometimes obese. Overweight is a real burden. Not that it's a health risk the way they say it is. What the data show is that life expectancy is not really dependent on how much you weigh except at the very extremes. It is true that the things that make you fat can also make you susceptible to disease or metabolic disturbances but weight *per se* is not a health risk. It is, however, a tremendous psychological burden. For many people, it colors their whole life. It's a constant strain. Every meal is a battle and there is a constant, unwelcome overtone of bad vibes in eating. The sense of control is the key variable. It's not really your social life, at least for men. It's not just the subtle prejudice against fat people. All those count, but it's more that people who might otherwise have great ability to plan their daily actions and to determine the course of their lives, can't seem to get control over their own body.

The causes are simple. We followed a false star in nutrition. The fat people you see in the mall were encouraged to believe that fat was an enemy. Worse, they were encouraged to believe that the things that were hurting them, things like bread and potatoes were neutral, were part of life, were maybe even "healthy." You may see them eating a sandwich just at the moment you think about how everybody is fat.

Most of all, it is not just people with a weight problem but people with diabetes, people with a disease of carbohydrate intolerance.

People with diabetes were encouraged and are still encouraged to believe that carbohydrates were a necessary part of life. Most nutritionists and an unknown number of physicians still believe in the low-fat dogma despite the absolute contradictory results from all kinds of experiments, large and small, and despite the one over-powering fact that sits on top of all this: what happened in the thirty or forty years of the epidemic of obesity and diabetes was a dramatic increase in the consumption of carbohydrate. Fat consumption, if anything went down. In the face of all the contradictory evidence, the Dietary Guidelines for Americans, the advice for the population sanctioned by the US Department of Agriculture (USDA) states flatly that "healthy diets are high in carbohydrates." Diets high in carbohydrate may be healthy if you are already healthy or, more important, if you think that you have control over your weight and associated health problems. But, for most people, it's wrong and many people know it's wrong. Many physicians and scientists know it's wrong: they may not say it out loud because there is a lot of group-think out there and few of us are up to fighting with the group.

## HOW COULD THEY ALL BE WRONG?

The Harvard School of Public Health is very prestigious. How could they all be wrong? How could it be as bad as the critics say? Isn't there peer review? And what do they have to gain? Won't it all come out in the end? It is a tough question to answer but the next section will show you that it is bad, very bad, however hard it is to say why. It may be a field that is hopelessly corrupt intellectually. I have always drawn the analogy to alchemy. As a student, I could never understand how alchemy could persist for as long as it did. We were taught that alchemy was the quest for transmutation, the creation of gold from baser metals or other stuff which, of course, is not possible. How could the alchemists have kept going in the face of failure? Part of the answer is that there was more to alchemy than transmutation. The alchemists contributed to pharmacology and metallurgy, for example. The story on gold, however, is probably that there were simply people who wanted to think that they owned gold. There were also people who were willing to certify that the "gold" that people had was genuine even if it was simple copper-plate. Finally, there were the makers of gold whose reputation might go up if they appeared to create gold even if they themselves knew that they were only doing some copper-plating. As long as no one broke into the circle, everything was smooth.

In a controversial field, there are few researchers with real neutrality but if you sit on a granting agency study section or you are the editor of a journal, you are supposed to have self-awareness and know when you are unfairly squelching the opposite point of view. Most of the establishment in medical nutrition seems incapable of this behavior. Like the alchemists, the editors of the prestigious medical journals, *The Journal of the American Medical Association* and *The New England Journal of Medicine*, are quite willing to certify that researchers with like opinions have produced confirmation. The panel at the granting agency is willing to say that peer-reviewed publication means that the work (which is consistent with their point of view) deserves continued funding and it has proved very difficult to break into the circle. The media, in turn, pay attention only to these journals. The next section examines in detail some of the alchemists' "gold" in nutrition. The point is that these studies are poor and the conclusions are unjustified. On the positive side, it is informative to understand why it was done wrong and, therefore, what it would have taken to do it right. From the point of view of sociology and health, this bad practice should be swept away. This is unlikely to happen and it is important for individuals to understand how bad it is.

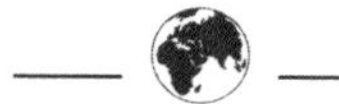

# Part 2

---

# Policy And The Mess In Nutrition

---

# Chapter 16

# The Medical Literature: A Guide To Flawed Studies

**Doctor:** Therein the patient
Must minister to himself.
**Macbeth:** Throw physic [medicine] to the dogs; I'll none of it.

— William Shakespeare, Macbeth

Nutrition in crisis. Almost every day "a new study" shows that you are at risk for diabetes or cardiovascular disease or all-cause mortality brought on by a newly appreciated toxin which turns out to be something that you just had for lunch. It is not clear that any of these studies were subject to any kind of serious critical peer review and, for the curious, they are frequently dismembered by the bloggers. The continuous cycle of weak studies and their deconstruction goes beyond time wasting. People are hurt because bad recommendations are left out there even when research shows that they are inappropriate. And science takes a big hit. Peer review by technical and medical journals is supposed to be the gate-keeper on scientific evidence but papers showing very weak associations or even ones that are grossly misleading are accepted. And the media, which might be expected to help us, makes it worse. It's not really their fault. A science reporter could not reasonably have the time to read the original in detail and must accept the conclusions in the abstract and so the message is transmitted through mass media. And when you do explain to the reporter how misleading these reports are and how people will be hurt, they are truly concerned and sympathetic but they don't always have complete editorial control. In any case, they would like to help, but tomorrow they have to cover a story that may be even worse. It is really hard for the consumer. This post from Facebook probably tells the story:

> So epically confused about diet. Everything I read is contradictory on epic proportions. About the only consistencies are low-sugar raw veggies and water. How in the world is a girl to sort it out, other than try everything and see what works for me?
>
> And I hesitate to even ask, as diet has become as controversial as religion and politics -but wouldn't you think that all of this would be easily testable and provable, in a way that religion and political opinions are not? People are different, but shouldn't it be possible to come up with a system that takes inputs of body stats and genetic history, and outputs a general reasonable diet to follow? Any insight on getting clarity here?

It is likely that the population at large is not any more comfortable. I wrote to her off-list and re-iterated the first three rules: 1. If you are okay, you are okay, 2. If you want to lose weight don't eat; if you have to eat, don't eat carbs, if you have to eat carbs, eat low glycemic index carbs, and 3. If you have diabetes or metabolic syndrome, you have to try a low carb diet first.

It is likely that many people wind up believing nothing or believing that everything is exaggerated although I think that there is a popular notion that "maybe fat is bad and maybe I should not put so much salt on my food." And then there is the progression of raspberry-ketones, resveratrol and *trans*-fats and methylglyoxal, each of which will either kill you or save you from being killed by the others.

Most discouraging are the health agencies. The American Diabetes Association (ADA) wants people with diabetes to have a lot of carbohydrates. They keep saying that they don't have a diet and, that they're not opposed to low-carb diets (for weight loss) and, as described above, they continually stress "individualization" but there are no indications as to which individuals benefit from which intervention. What criteria for what diet? Despite the disclaimers, it is for sure that the ADA is *perceived* as opposing low-carbohydrate. And it seems clear they are responsible for that perception. The evidence that weight loss is not required for improvement in diabetes, from the work of Nuttal and Gannon [78], for example, is not mentioned. They know about that evidence. I know because I have told members of the committee personally. The ADA guidelines do not cite important scientific work showing that weight loss is not required for improvement in diabetes. People who are not scientists ask me: "Can you do that? Are you allowed not to cite other people's work?"

The ADA websites are clear on the necessity for including carbohydrate in your diet. All of the contradictory evidence does not seem to make any real impact. **Figure 16-1**, from *The Food Navigator*, the food industry house organ, says it all: "Meanwhile, a growing body of research has suggested that replacing fat with carbohydrates could increase the risk of heart disease but consumers are still focused on low-fat food and beverage products..."

There is a daily progression of sweeping statements that go way beyond the published data. There what is perceived as an inability or —one doesn't know the motivation — an unwillingness to zero in on real factors and, again, the unwritten rule to avoid mentioning the value of carbohydrate restriction.

The literature, especially major medical publications are still subscription based, that is, not directly accessible to many who are interested. The results are then fed downstream to the media, who take at face value anything it is fed and will pass it on to the general public.

Rigid dogma has reached Galilean proportions. Fructose and sugar are bad (unless you try to lump them in with all carbohydrates). If you want your paper on fructose to be published, begin with: "Because of the deleterious effects of dietary fructose, we hypothesized that..." Never start with "Whether dietary fructose has a deleterious effect..." I know. Our paper on fructose ([79] was published with "whether..." as the opening sentence but only after a rebuttal of reviewers' criticisms that turned out to be 15 pages long. And if you even mention low-carbohydrate, you are guaranteed real grief. When JAMA published George Bray's "calorie-is-a-calorie" paper [80] and I pointed out that the study more accurately supported the importance of carbohydrate as a controlling variable, the editor refused to publish my letter. In this, the blogs have performed a valuable service in providing an alternative POV but if unreliability is a problem in the scientific literature, that problem is multiplied in internet sources. In the end, the consumers may feel that they are pretty much on their own.

It does take some confidence, especially for the lay person, to feel that their intuitive understanding that the difference between white rice and brown rice is so small that it really doesn't matter what Harvard's computer says. Most researchers are very much disinclined to get into a shooting match, or worse, whistle-blowing. The long blue line is a strong force in repressing investigation, not because the police think corruption is okay, but because scandal reflects badly on everybody. Whistle-blowing in this field is especially weird because sometimes the transgressions are right out in the open. Figures are published showing marginal associations and the text says that they are significant and therefore you should change your diet accordingly.

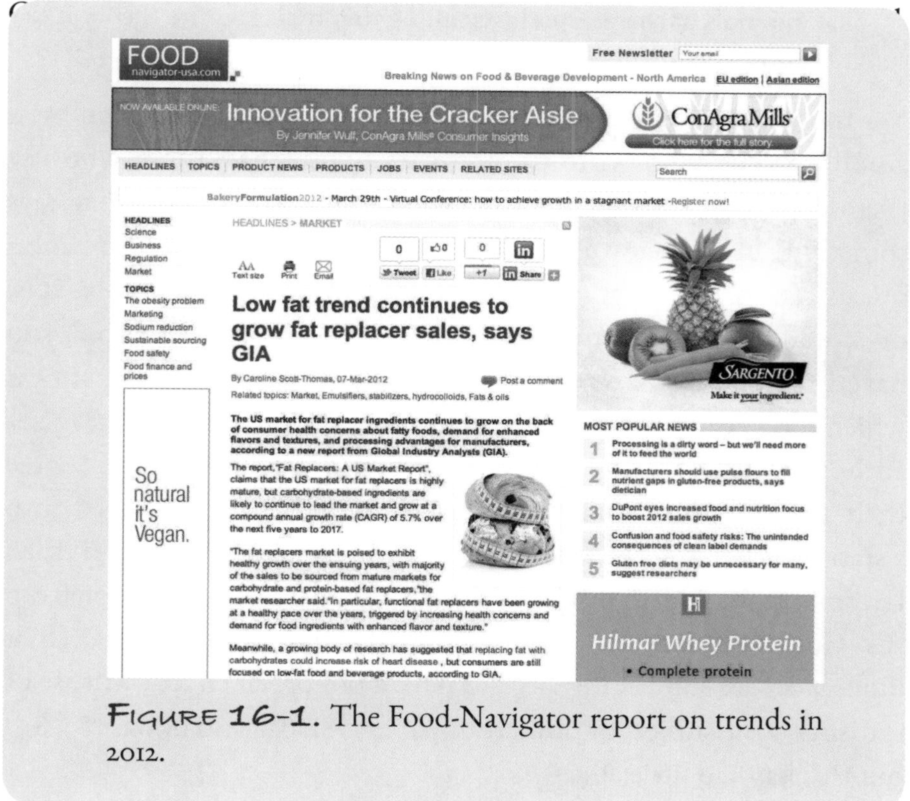

FOOD navigator-usa.com

Free Newsletter

Breaking News on Food & Beverage Development - North America EU edition | Asian edition

NOW AVAILABLE ONLINE: Innovation for the Cracker Aisle
By Jennifer Wulf, ConAgra Mills® Consumer Insights
ConAgra Mills
Click here for the full story

HEADLINES | TOPICS | PRODUCT NEWS | PRODUCTS | JOBS | EVENTS | RELATED SITES

BakeryFormulation2012 - March 29th - Virtual Conference: how to achieve growth in a stagnant market -Register now!

HEADLINES
Science
Business
Regulation
Market

TOPICS
The obesity problem
Marketing
Sodium reduction
Sustainable sourcing
Food safety
Food finance and prices

So natural it's Vegan.

HEADLINES > MARKET

**Low fat trend continues to grow fat replacer sales, says GIA**

By Caroline Scott-Thomas, 07-Mar-2012

Post a comment

Related topics: Market, Emulsifiers, stabilizers, hydrocolloids, Fats & oils

**The US market for fat replacer ingredients continues to grow on the back of consumer health concerns about fatty foods, demand for enhanced flavors and textures, and processing advantages for manufacturers, according to a new report from Global Industry Analysts (GIA).**

The report, "Fat Replacers: A US Market Report", claims that the US market for fat replacers is highly mature, but carbohydrate-based ingredients are likely to continue to lead the market and grow at a compound annual growth rate (CAGR) of 5.7% over the next five years to 2017.

"The fat replacers market is poised to exhibit healthy growth over the ensuing years, with majority of the sales to be sourced from mature markets for carbohydrate and protein-based fat replacers," the market researcher said. "In particular, functional fat replacers have been growing at a healthy pace over the years, triggered by increasing health concerns and demand for food ingredients with enhanced flavor and texture."

Meanwhile, a growing body of research has suggested that replacing fat with carbohydrates could increase risk of heart disease, but consumers are still focused on low-fat food and beverage products, according to GIA.

SARGENTO
Make it your ingredient.

MOST POPULAR NEWS

1 Processing is a dirty word – but we'll need more of it to feed the world
2 Manufacturers should use pulse flours to fill nutrient gaps in gluten-free products, says dietician
3 DuPont eyes increased food and nutrition focus to boost 2012 sales growth
4 Confusion and food safety risks: The unintended consequences of clean label demands
5 Gluten free diets may be unnecessary for many, suggest researchers

Hilmar Whey Protein
• Complete protein

FIGURE 16-1. The Food-Navigator report on trends in 2012.

## STATISTICS: DEATH OF THE MEDICAL LITERATURE.

Many scientists believe that if you do a good experiment, you don't need statistics. David Colquohon, a well known neuroscientist and critic of poor scientific method, agrees. Colquohon is the author of an excellent, if technical, statistics book (free download from his website *DC's Improbable Science*) and the introduction to his book points out:

> "... the snag, of course, is that doing good experiments is difficult. Most people need all the help they can get to prevent them

making fools of themselves by claiming that their favorite theory is substantiated by observations that do nothing of the sort."

This kind of circumspection is, unfortunately, more common among people who write the statistics books than those who use them. A good statistics book will have an introduction that says something like "what we do in statistics, is we try to put a number on our intuition." In other words, it is not really, by itself, a science. It is, or should be, a *tool* for the experimenter's use and, like any tool, you have to know how to use it. And there is not always agreement on which tool. All statistics is interpretation. The problem is that many authors of papers in the medical literature allow statistics to become their master rather than their servant; numbers are plugged into a statistical program and the results are interpreted in a cut-and-dried fashion. Statistical significance (that two sets of data are not from the same population) is confused with clinical significance (that differences are sufficiently large to have a biological effect). Misuse of statistics is the subject of numerous papers [81, 82] and books [83, 84] but this has had little effect.

## THE GOLDEN RULE OF STATISTICS (GRS)

Here's the Golden Rule for reading a scientific paper, from the book *PDQ Statistics* by Norman & Streiner [85]:

> "The important point ... is that the onus is on the author to convey to the reader an accurate impression of what the data look like, using graphs or standard measures, before beginning the statistical shenanigans. Any paper that doesn't do this should be viewed from the outset with considerable suspicion."

In other words, explain things clearly to the reader. There are complicated ideas in science but the often quoted statement (only once before in this book) from Einstein that you should make it simple but not too simple is a reasonable demand for you the reader to make of the scientific literature.

## STATISTICAL SHENANIGANS VS COMMON SENSE

So, how do you deal with the reports in the press that tell you that white rice will give you diabetes but brown rice won't? The principle is that biochemistry is not separate from anything else we do. It can have subtleties and it can rely on mathematics but it uses the same rules of logic as daily life. So, the first question you have to ask is whether it makes sense; how is it possible that white rice is so different from brown rice. A moment's thought suggests that the major difference is in stuff that isn't even digested, the fiber. On the other hand, they are always pushing fiber, whole grain and all that, so you might want to hear their case, but there is the possibility that the entire fiber thing itself is questionable or at least exaggerated. And the Asian societies that are always invoked to tell us how much we need grain never eat brown rice. Never. So, common sense makes you suspicious.

## HABEAS CORPUS DATORUM

Science is an extension of common sense but there are revolutionary ideas. In fact, the revolutionary ones are usually the most important. How do you deal with that? You want to be suspicious if it violates common sense but you can't throw out the idea just for that reason. The solution is simple if not always easy to implement. If it is a reasonable conclusion, you can cut the author some slack. If the idea is far out, you need to see the data. All the data. Not the hazard ratio, not just the conclusions from the computer. My new grand principle of doing science: *habeas corpus datorum*, let's see the body of the data. If the conclusion is non-intuitive and goes against previous work or common sense, then the data must be strong and all of it must be clearly presented.

So, how should you read a scientific paper? I usually want to see the pictures first. In a scientific paper, they are called figures but it's not just saving a thousand words. (I get a thousand emails every week or so). It's about presentation of the data. It's about the GRS: "convey to the reader an accurate impression of what the data look like, using graphs or standard measures, before beginning the statistical shenanigans." In fact, it's really not "or." Figures are so much better than tables that a whole book "Medical Illuminations" has been written about the idea [84]. Many of us write scientific papers the same way. We make the figures first and then try to explain what they say. The principle: a scientific paper is supposed to explain. I tell graduate students that if you do an experiment and you don't explain it well, it is as if you had never done it. In teaching students how to present their work, I ask them: "Describe what you are supposed to do in a scientific seminar or other presentation." Sometimes they try but I usually make it worse by adding: "No. In one word. What are you supposed to do? One word." Having reached an appropriate level of annoyance they will be relieved to hear the answer: "Teach." You want to explain things to your audience. The same is true of a scientific paper. Again, the GRS: "The onus is on the author."

## CAVEAT LECTOR

A scientific paper is also selling. Scientific papers are rarely just data. They have an idea that they are trying to sell. Teach and sell are the two things you do in science. The reader has to be an educated consumer however. As a consumer, you should be suspicious of overselling. One good indicator is the use of value judgements as if they were scientific terms. "Healthy" (or "healthful") is not a scientific term.

If a study describes a diet as "healthy," it is almost guaranteed to be a flawed study. If we knew which diets were "healthy," we wouldn't have an obesity epidemic. A good example is the paper by Appel [86] on the DASH diet which has as its main conclusion:

"In the setting of a healthful diet, partial substitution of carbohydrate with either protein or monounsaturated fat can further lower blood pressure, improve lipid levels, and reduce estimated cardiovascular risk."

It's hard to know how healthful the original diet could have been if removing carbohydrate improved everything. In addition, not only was this about a "carbohydrate-rich diet used in the DASH trials" but it is " ... currently advocated in several scientific reports." Another red flag is when they tell you how widely accepted their idea is.

Understatement is good. One of the more famous is from the classic Watson & Crick paper of 1953 [87] in which they proposed the DNA double helix structure. They said, "It has not escaped our notice that the specific pairing we have postulated immediately suggests a possible copying mechanism for the genetic material." A study that contains the word "healthy" is an infomercial. A paper that says it is "evidence-based" is patting itself on the back.

## Looking for the Figures

Presentation in graphic form usually means the author wants to explain things to you, rather than snow you. The Watson-Crick paper cited above had the diagram of the double-helix, which essentially became the symbol of modern biology. It was drawn by Odile, Francis Crick's wife, who is described as being famous for her nudes, only one of which I could find on the internet. Odile's original DNA structure, however, is still widely used in textbooks.

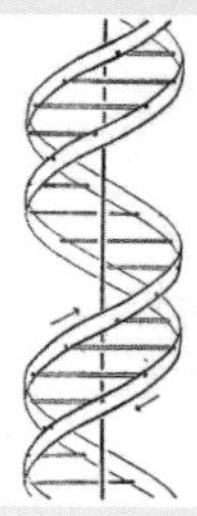

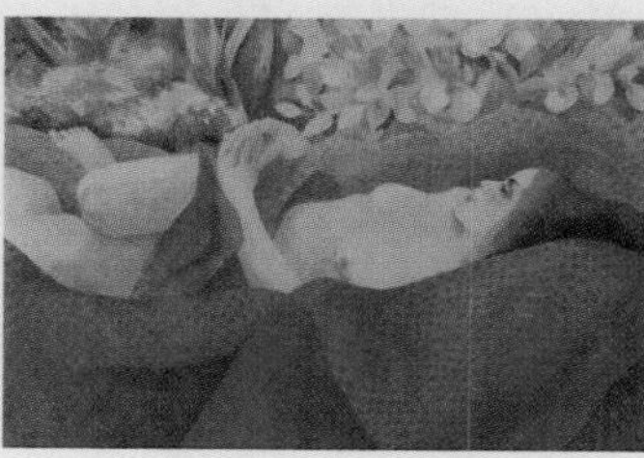

Figure 16-2. The Original DNA Structure from Watson and Crick and Nude by Odile Crick.

## WHAT'S WRONG WITH THE LITERATURE? WHAT'S RIGHT?

What's right is that there are many published papers in the nutritional literature that are informative, creative and generally conform to the standards of good science. Naturally, like any scientific literature, most of the papers are pretty much routine, of specialized interest or, as described in one of the choices on the checklist for referees when you review manuscripts: "Of interest to other workers in the field." It is not the mediocre papers but rather a surprising number of really objectionable papers. The medical literature is full of papers bordering on fraud, or at least, misrepresentation. There are many papers that are full of fundamental errors and total lack of judgement in interpretation. Worse, many give you the feeling that somebody is going to get hurt because of bad medical advice that follows from the misinterpretations.

Most work in most fields, more or less by definition, is mediocre. But unlike the preponderance of detail that makes run-of-the-mill papers so boring, papers in medical nutrition make drastic claims about saving hundreds of thousands of lives by scaling up to everybody, a result that had hardly any effect to begin with. If a conclusion is shaky, applying it to the whole population is in violation of the definition of zero: X x 0 = 0, X real.

It is difficult to face the fact that so much of the medical literature is published by people who are not trained in science, which means they don't know the game, they haven't seen much of it and don't know it when they see it. Now, there is no real training in science. You can learn techniques but it's not about cyclotrons, it's about ideas. There is no reason why a physician can't do real scientific thinking but, at the same time, there is no reason why they can. An MD degree is not a guarantee of any expertise outside your area of specialty.

The irony is that the practice of medicine can be highly scientific.

Differential diagnosis and the experience in recommending the right drug is the kind of things that are part of scientific disciplines. The same physician who will intuitively solve a medical mystery, though, will assume that, for scientific research, things are different, that there are somehow arbitrary rules and that brute force application of statistics will tell you whether what you did is true.

Chapters to follow detail the failures, ranging from the slightly inaccurate — "association does not imply causality" (sometimes it does and sometimes it doesn't), to the idiotic — you must do intention-to-treat; if you assign people to take a drug and they don't take it, you have to include their data with those who did. ("If you only report compliers you introduce bias.").

And then there are "levels of evidence," arbitrary rules that get incorporated into tables, the top of which is always some kind of "gold standard." The odd thing about levels of scientific evidence is that nobody in any physical science would recognize them. They are, in fact, the creation of people who are trying to do science but don't know it when they see it, fundamentally amateurs who have arbitrary rules along the lines of the apocryphal story about Mozart:

> A man comes to Mozart and wants to become a composer. Mozart says that they have to study theory for a couple of years, that they should study orchestration and become proficient at the piano, and goes on like this. Finally, the man says "but you wrote your first symphony when you were 8 years old." Mozart says "Yes, but I didn't ask anybody."

So what are the mistakes? I will list these and each of the following chapters will discuss them. Some are general kinds of mistaken notions although most are misapplications of normally acceptable practice, particularly statistics.

**Chapter 17:** Observations generate hypotheses. Observational studies test hypotheses. Association implies causality. (Sometimes).

**Chapter 18:** Red meat and the new puritans. Studies in relative risk.

**Chapter 19:** Crimson slime. Making Americans afraid of red meat.

**Chapter 20:** Uses and misuses of group statistics. Bill Gates walks into a bar...

**Chapter 21:** The seventh egg. More statistical shenanigans vs common sense.

**Chapter 22:** Intention-to-treat.

**Chapter 23:** The fiend that lies like truth. Summary on how to read the medical literature

## SUMMARY

The book *PDQ Statistics* gives us the Golden Rule: In a scientific paper, "the onus is on the author to convey" (and the reader has the right to expect) "an accurate impression of what the data look like using graphs or standard measures." To understand research in nutrition or, really, any science, one has to be prepared to question the "experts." If a paper does not adhere to this Golden Rule and is too quick to begin "the statistical shenanigans," it "should be viewed from the outset with considerable suspicion."

The bottom line is that you have to expect real communication from the author of a scientific paper. The problem, for many people, is believing, that the best and the brightest are at fault. But it is not hard to find examples of experts making mistakes. The low standards in nutrition mean that you are substantially on your own. There is help. The next few chapters give you some principles and things to look for.

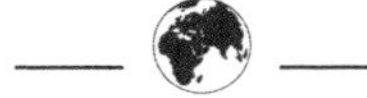

# Chapter 17

# Observational Studies, Association, Causality

" ... 789 deaths were reported in Doll and Hill's original cohort. Thirty-six of these were attributed to lung cancer. When these lung cancer deaths were counted in smokers versus non-smokers, the correlation virtually sprang out: all thirty-six of the deaths had occurred in smokers. The difference between the two groups was so significant that Doll and Hill did not even need to apply complex statistical metrics to discern it. The trial designed to bring the most rigorous statistical analysis to the cause of lung cancer barely required elementary mathematics to prove his point."

Siddhartha Mukherjee —*The Emperor of All Maladies*

Scientists don't like philosophy of science. It is not just that pompous phrases like "hypothetico-deductive systems" are such a turn-off but that we rarely recognize descriptions in philosophy articles as what we actually do. In the end, there is no definition of science any more than there are definitions for music or literature. Scientists have different styles and it is hard to generalize about actual scientific behavior. Research is a human activity and precisely because it puts a premium on creativity, it defies categorization. As the physicist Steven Weinberg put it, echoing Justice Stewart on pornography:

> "There is no logical formula that establishes a sharp dividing line between a beautiful explanatory theory and a mere list of data, but we know the difference when we see it — we demand a simplicity and rigidity in our principles before we are willing to take them seriously [88]."

We know that what we see in the current state of nutrition is not it. This forces us to consider what science really is — what is it that makes nutritional medical literature so bad? If we can identify some principles, maybe we can penetrate the mess and see how it could be fixed. One frequently stated principle is that "observational studies only generate hypotheses." There is the related idea that "association does not imply causality," usually cited by those authors who want you to believe that the association that they found does imply causality.

These ideas are not exactly right or, at least, they insufficiently recognize that scientific experiments are not so easily wedged into categories like "observational studies." The principles are also widely invoked by bloggers and critics to discredit the continuing stream of observational studies that make an association between the favored targets, eggs, red meat, sugar-sweetened soda, which can be "tied to" prevalence of some metabolic disease or cancer. In most cases, the original studies are getting what they deserve but the bills of indictment are not accurate and it would be better not to cite absolute statements of scientific principles. It is not simply that these studies are observational studies but rather that they are *bad* observational studies and, in many cases, the associations that they find are so weak that the study really constitutes an argument for a *lack* of causality. On the assumption that good experimental practice and interpretation could be even roughly defined, I laid out in my blogpost a few principles that I thought were a better representation, if you can make any generalization, of what actually goes on in science:

Observations generate hypotheses.

Observational studies *test* hypotheses.

Associations do not *necessarily* imply causality.

In some sense, all science is associations.

Only mathematics is axiomatic (starts from absolute assumptions).

If you notice that kids who eat a lot of candy seem to be fat, or even if you notice that you yourself get fat eating candy, that is an *observation*. From this observation, you might come up with the hypothesis that sugar causes obesity. An observation generates hypotheses. A *test* of your hypothesis would be to carry out an *observational study*. For example, you might try to see if there is an association between sugar consumption and incidence of obesity. There are different ways of doing this — the simplest epidemiologic approach is simply to compare the history of the eating behavior of individuals (insofar as you can get it) with how fat they are. When you do this comparison you are *testing your hypothesis*.

You must remember that there are an infinite number of other things, meat consumption, TV hours, distance from the French bakery, grandfather's waist circumference that you could have measured as an independent variable. You have a hypothesis that it was candy. What about all the others? Mike Eades described falling asleep as a child by trying to think of everything in the world. You just can't test them all. As Einstein put it "your theory determines the measurement you make." If you found associations with everything, would anything be causal?

## ASSOCIATIONS CAN PREDICT CAUSALITY

In fact, association can be strong evidence for causation and frequently an association can provide support for, if not absolute proof, of the idea to be tested. Hypotheses generate observational studies, not the other way around. A correct statement is that association does not *necessarily* imply causation. In some sense, all science is observation and association. Even thermodynamics, the most mathematical and absolute of sciences, rests on observation. As soon as somebody builds a perpetual motion machine that works, it's all over.

Biological mechanisms, or perhaps all scientific theories, are never proved. By analogy with a court of law, you cannot be found innocent, only not guilty. That is why excluding a theory is stronger than showing consistency. The grand epidemiological study of macronutrient intake vs diabetes and obesity, that is, all of the data on what Americans ate in the last forty years, shows that increasing carbohydrate is associated with increased calories even under conditions where fruits and vegetables also go up and fat, if anything goes down. The data on dietary consumption and disease in the whole population describes an observational study but it is strong because it gives support to a *lack* of causal effect of increased carbohydrate and decreased fat on positive outcome. Again, in science, finding a contradiction has greater impact than merely finding a consistent result It is now clear, that prospective experiments (where you pick the population first and see how people do on your variable of interest) have shown in the past, and will undoubtedly continue to show, the same negative outcome. But will anybody give up on saturated fat? In a court of law, if you are found not guilty of child abuse, people may still not let you move into their neighborhood. My point here is that saturated fat should never have been indicted in the first place.

An association will tell you about causality if 1) the association is strong and 2) if there is a plausible underlying mechanism and 3) if there is not a more plausible explanation. The often cited correlation between cardiovascular disease and number of TV sets does not imply causality because, although principle 1 is observed, there is no logical direct underlying mechanism. Countries with a lot of TV sets have modern life styles that may predispose to cardiovascular disease. TV does not cause CVD. Interestingly, in CVD, where there has been so many papers published, where there is so much medical interest, it is not obvious that we yet have a good underlying mechanism.

## RE-INVENTING THE WHEEL. ME AND BRADFORD HILL

This chapter is a re-working of a blogpost that I published in 2013. The post included the previous paragraphs where I tried to lay out a few principles for dealing with the kind of observational studies that you see in the scientific literature. I was speaking off the top of my head, trying to describe the logic that scientists use in interpreting data. It was an obvious description of what is done in practice. I didn't think it was particularly original and, again, I don't think that there are any hard and fast principles in science. When I described what I had written to my colleague Gene Fine, his response was "aren't you re-inventing the wheel?" He meant that Bradford Hill, pretty much the inventor of modern epidemiology, had already established these and a couple of others as principles. Gene cited *The Emperor of All Maladies* [89], an outstanding book on the history of cancer. I had, in fact, read *Emperor* on his recommendation. I remembered Bradford Hill and the description of the evolution of the ideas of epidemiology, population studies and random controlled trials. The story is also told in James LeFanu's *The Rise and Fall of Modern Medicine* [90], another captivating history of medicine.

I thought of these as general philosophical ideas, rather than as grand scientific principles. Perhaps it is that we're just used to it, but saying that an association has to be very strong to imply causality is common sense and not in the same ballpark with the Pythagorean Theorem. It's something that you might say over coffee or in response to somebody's blog. Being explicit about it turns out to be very important but, like much in philosophy of science, it struck me as not of great intellectual import. It all reminded me of learning, in grade school, that the Earl of Sandwich had invented the sandwich and thinking "this is an invention?" Woody Allen thought the same thing and wrote the history of the sandwich. He recorded the Earl's early failures — "In 1741, he places bread on bread with turkey on top. This fails. In 1745, he exhibits bread with turkey on either side. Everyone rejects this except David Hume."

In fact, Hill's principles are important even if they do seem obvious. Simple ideas are not always accepted. The concept of the random controlled trial (RCT), randomly assign people to the drug or behavior that you're testing or to a group that is the control, obvious to us now, was hard won. Proving that any particular environmental factor — diet, smoking, pollution or toxic chemicals — was the cause of a disease and that, by reducing that factor, the disease could be prevented, turned out to be a very hard sell, especially to physicians whose view of disease may have been strongly colored by the idea of an infective agent.

*The Rise and Fall of Modern Medicine* describes Bradford Hill's two important contributions [90]. He demonstrated that tuberculosis could be cured by a combination of two drugs, streptomycin and PAS (*para*-aminosalicylic acid). Even more important, he showed that tobacco causes lung cancer. Hill was Professor of Medical Statistics at the London School of Hygiene and Tropical Medicine but was not formally trained in statistics and, like many of us, thought of proper statistics as simply applied common sense. Ironically, an early near-fatal case of tuberculosis prevented formal medical education. His first monumental accomplishment was, in fact, to demonstrate how tuberculosis could be cured with

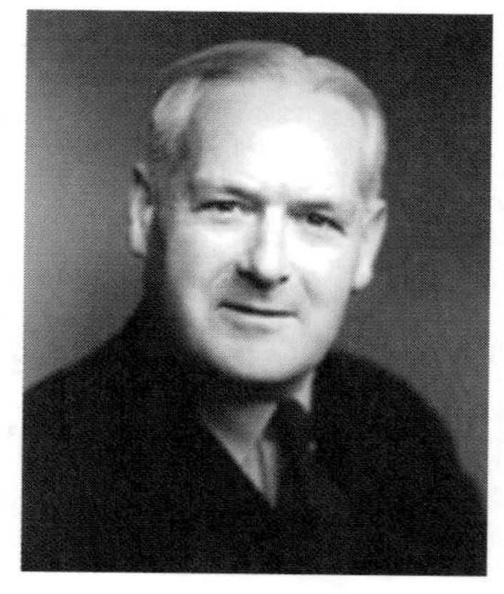

the streptomycin-PAS combination. In 1941, Hill and his co-worker Richard Doll undertook a systematic investigation of the risk factors for lung cancer. His eventual success was accompanied by a description of the principles that allow you to say when association can be taken as causation.

> Wiki says: "In 1965, built upon the work of Hume and Popper, Hill suggested several aspects of causality in medicine and biology ... ", but his approach was not formal — he never referred to his principles as criteria — he recognized them as common sense behavior and his 1965 presentation to the Royal Society of Medicine is a remarkably sober, intelligent document. Although described as an example of an article that, as here, has been read more often in quotations and paraphrases, it is worth reading the original even today. http://epiville.ccnmtl.columbia.edu/assets/ pdfs/Hill_1965.pdf

Note: "Austin Bradford Hill's surname was Hill and he always used the name Hill, AB in publications. However, he is often referred to as Bradford Hill. To add to the confusion, his friends called him Tony." (This comment is from Wikipedia, not Woody Allen).

---

*Meeting January 14 1965*

**President's Address**

**The Environment and Disease: Association or Causation?**

by Sir Austin Bradford Hill CBE DSC FRCP(hon) FRS (*Professor Emeritus of Medical Statistics, University of London*)

Amongst the objects of this newly-founded Section of Occupational Medicine are firstly 'to provide a means, not readily afforded elsewhere, whereby physicians and surgeons with a special knowledge of the relationship between sickness and injury

observed *association* to a verdict of *causation*? Upon what basis should we proceed to do so?

I have no wish, nor the skill, to embark upon a philosophical discussion of the meaning of 'causation'. The 'cause' of illness may be immediate and direct, it may be remote and indirect underlying the observed association. But with the aims of occupational, and almost synonymously preventive, medicine in mind the decisive question is whether the frequency of the undesirable event B will be influenced by a change in the environmental feature A. *How* such a

## ASSOCIATION AND CAUSALITY. THE NINE CRITERIA

Bradford Hill described the factors that might make you think that an association implied causality. The criteria are still perfectly reasonable. In the current medical literature, they are probably much more widely practiced in the breach than the observance. There is the possibility that the application of Hill's principle to the medical literature would substantially reduce the size of that literature:

(1) **Strength.** "First upon my list I would put the strength of the association." This, of course, is exactly what is missing in the continued epidemiological scare stories whose measures of relative risk are so small. Hill describes:

> " ... prospective inquiries into smoking have shown that the death rate from cancer of the lung in cigarette smokers is nine to ten times the rate in non-smokers and the rate in heavy cigarette smokers is twenty to thirty times as great."
>
> "On the other hand the death rate from coronary thrombosis in smokers is no more than twice, possibly less, than the death rate in nonsmokers. Though there is good evidence to support causation it is surely much easier in this case to think of some features of life that may go hand-in-hand with smoking — features that might conceivably be the real underlying cause or, at the least, an important contributor, whether it be lack of exercise, nature of diet or other factors."

## RELATIVE RISK

Hill expressed doubts about a **relative risk** of two or less. Criticized elsewhere in this book, relative risk (RR) is what it sounds like; the ratio of the risks from two outcomes. Risk is the probability of an outcome. For example; if you were to compare a group of factory workers in a chemical plant, say, to the general population and you found that, for every 1000 workers, 26 developed cancer, then the probability of cancer is 26/1000, 0.026 or 2.6%. If you found in the general population that there were only 13 cases of cancer for every thousand people, then the risk for the population is 13/1000, 0.013 or 1.3%. The RR is (26/1000)/(13/1000) = 2:1. This might be considered evidence for environmental hazard although, as Hill says, it would be better if the RR were 10, but 2 is considered grounds for taking the results seriously (or taking the factory owner to court). RR, however, is relative. It hides information. The RR would still be 2 if there were 26 out of a *million* workers getting sick and 13 out of a million in the population. The absolute risk is the difference between the probabilities. Absolute risk in the example is small (2.6% -1.3% = 1.3%). Less than 2 % more of the workers got cancer than in the general population. If you did take the factory owner to court, the judge might ask for additional evidence.

This is what are we up against. The abstract from a study on eating breakfast [91] found that: "Men who skipped breakfast had a 27% higher risk of CHD compared with men who did not (relative risk, 1.27...)" By Hill's standards, or by common sense, a relative risk of 1.27 would not make you want to eat breakfast if you are not hungry (presumably the major reason people don't eat breakfast). Describing the results as "27% higher risk" might influence your behavior more but, given everything that we know, it is hard to see how eating more food is going to have a great benefit for heart disease. Reporting relative risk so as to make the effect larger is the single most prevalent mistake in the medical literature and the media that report on that literature.

So, a high relative risk is no guarantee of causality but if it's low, that's definitely suspicious. Back to Hill's criteria.

(2) **Consistency**. Hill listed the repetition of the results in other studies, under different circumstances, as a criterion for considering the extent to which an association implied causality. We expect results to be reproducible and a weak association may gain some strength if the observation is reproduced. Consistency of strong results, however, is what we want to see. Criterion 2 is not independent of criterion 1.

The last point, that strength and consistency are not independent criteria, was not mentioned by Hill but is of great importance. Consistently weak associations do not generally add up to a strong association. If there is a single practice in modern medicine that is completely out of whack with respect to careful consideration of causality, it is the meta-analysis where studies with marginal strengths are averaged to create a conclusion that is stronger than the majority of its components. In fact, many meta-analyses may include studies that have not shown any association at all and average them with a couple that have, reporting the average as significant. Averaging studies without significant outcomes and expecting to get an effect is as foolish as it sounds, but it is widely practiced.

(3) **Specificity**. Hill was circumspect on this point, recognizing that we should have an open mind on what causes what. On specificity of cancer and cigarettes, Hill noted that that the two sites in which he had showed a cause and effect relationship, were the lungs and the nose.

(4) **Temporality.** Obviously, we expect the cause to precede the effect or, as some wit put it, "which got laid first, the chicken or the egg?" Hill recognized that it was not so clear for diseases that developed slowly. "Does a particular diet lead to disease or do the early stages of the disease lead to those peculiar dietetic habits?" Of current interest are the epidemiologic studies that show a correlation between diet soda and obesity. These studies are quick to see a causal link but there is always a question of which way causation proceeds. One might reasonably ask "what kind of people drink diet sodas?"

(5) **Biological gradient.** The association should show a dose-response curve. In the case of cigarettes, the death rate from cancer of the lung increases linearly with the number of cigarettes smoked. A subset of the first principle, that the association should be strong, is that the dose-response curve should have a meaningful slope, that is, the difference between the numbers at the beginning and the end of the scale should be big.

(6) **Plausibility.** On the one hand, this seems critical — the association of egg consumption with diabetes is obviously foolish — but the hypothesis to be tested may have come from an intuition that is far from evident. Hill said, "what is biologically plausible depends upon the biological knowledge of the day." Here, Hill's emphasis on effect size is important. If the association is far-fetched, unexpected or derived from a less-than-obvious idea, the association should be strong.

(7) **Coherence.** Data, according to Hill, "should not seriously conflict with the generally known facts of the natural history and biology of the disease." The natural history of diabetes is the effect of carbohydrate not fat.

(8) **Experiment.** It was another age. It is hard to believe that it was in my lifetime. "Occasionally it is possible to appeal to experimental, or semi-experimental, evidence. For example, because of an observed association some preventive action is taken. Does it, in fact, prevent?" The inventor of the random controlled trial would be amazed how many try to take preventative action and how many, in fact, don't prevent. And, most of all, he would have been astounded that it doesn't seem to affect the opinion of the medical community. The progression of failures, from Framingham to the Women's Health Initiative, the lack of association between low-fat, low saturated fat and CVD, is strong evidence for the *absence* of causation.

(9) **Analogy:** "In some circumstances it would be fair to judge by analogy. With the effects of thalidomide and rubella before us, we would surely be ready to accept slighter but similar evidence with another drug or another viral disease in pregnancy."

The final word on what has come to be known as Hill's criteria for deciding about causation:

> "Here then are nine different viewpoints from all of which we should study association before we cry causation. What I do not believe — and this has been suggested — is that we can usefully lay down some hard-and-fast rules of evidence that must be obeyed before we accept cause and effect. *None of my nine viewpoints can bring indisputable evidence for or against the cause-and-effect hypothesis and none can be required as a sine qua non.* What they can do, with greater or less strength, is to help us to make up our minds on the fundamental question — is there any other way of explaining the set of facts before us, *is there any other answer equally, or more, likely than cause and effect?*" (My *emphasis*).

This may be the first critique of the still-to-be-invented Evidence-based Medicine.

## NUTRITIONAL EPIDEMIOLOGY

There are many critics of current nutritional epidemiology and most of us don't understand how the field could persist with so many weak results. Partly, it is precisely that the results are weak and since they are usually derived from large numbers of subjects, they are hard to contradict. More generally though, the answer is that statistics is not data and it is not a science as such. Statistics comes from a particular person's opinion on how the data should be interpreted. Conflict comes from different opinions. How can you adjudicate between these two principles: "The risk is small but when you scale it up to the whole population, you will save thousands of lives," and my own description of the theory (and opinion of its value) "when risk is small, there is low predictability of outcome. You can't scale up bad data."

The real impact of Hill's criteria is that they provide standards for interpreting epidemiologic studies. They are standards that still have a good deal of subjectivity but they are standards. In nutrition, they are simply ignored. They are ignored by authors and, most important, they are ignored by reviewers and editors who are expected to be the gatekeepers on solid science. In the end, the decision that an observational study implies causation is another way of saying that it is meaningful, that it is not an outcome of mathematical juggling, that it is, you know, science. *Emperor* described Hill's criteria as principles "which have remained in use by epidemiologists to date." But have they? Many have voiced criticisms of epidemiology as it's currently practiced in nutrition. One way to look at the current problems in nutrition is that we have a large number of research groups doing epidemiology in violation of most of Hill's criteria.

## IS IT SCIENCE?

Science is a human activity and what we don't like about philosophy of science is that it is about the structure of science rather than about behavior, that is, what scientists really do, and so there aren't even any real definitions. One description that I like, from Izja Lederhandler, a colleague at the NIH: "What you do in science is, you make a hypothesis and then you try to shoot yourself down." A good experiment puts the experimenter's theory to the test. An experiment whose outcome only shows consistency is not strong.

One of the most interesting sidelights on the work of Hill and Doll, as described in *Emperor*, was that during breaks from the taxing work of analyzing the questionnaires that provided the background on smoking, Doll himself would step out for a smoke. Doll believed that cigarettes were unlikely to be a cause — he favored tar from paved highways as the causative agent — but as the data came in, "in the middle of the survey, sufficiently alarmed, he gave up smoking." In science, you try to shoot yourself down and you go with the data. The mass of papers demonizing fat and the current flood of papers demonizing sugar, fail most of Hill's criteria. A major reason that they fail is that they set out to show consistency of the data with their theory, rather than to really challenge the theory, that is, they don't really try to shoot themselves down. As part of that they do not ask what else would equally explain the data.

## SUMMARY

The goal here is to help the consumer and perhaps other scientists read scientific publications. There really are no set principles of science. The existence of a "gold standard," that is, the one best type of experiment that answers all questions, is not recognized in most sciences. Observational studies are appropriate and imply causality if they show strong associations and if they have underlying mechanisms in basic chemistry or biology.

Bradford Hill laid down principles for dealing with observational studies which he recognized as attempts to turn common sense into practice. Hill's criteria:

1. Strength.
2. Consistency.
3. Specificity.
4. Temporality.
5. Biological gradients.
6. Plausibility.
7. Coherence
8. Experiment.
9. Analogy.

Hill showed a causal link between cigarettes and cancer because he found that deaths from lung cancer for cigarette smokers was nine to ten times that of non-smoker, a ratio that went up to twenty for heavy smokers compared to non-smokers. He was less sure about coronary thrombosis because the relative risk (RR) was in the range of 2 to one. This standard is not even proposed in modern nutritional experimentation. A nearly continuous flow of papers in the medical literature showing that something that you eat will cause some disease you don't want to have, with RR of 1.3, has marred the field substantially. Most epidemiologic studies, in fact, violate most of Hill's criteria.

The really important feature of scientific behavior is the mind-set. Good description: "What you do in science is you make a hypothesis and then you try to shoot yourself down." This is consistent with the general principle that excluding a hypothesis is always stronger than showing consistency. The problem in nutrition is that experimenters are trying to prove things, instead of trying to *dis*prove things. The next few chapters consider nutritional studies that claim to show adverse effects of red meat, fructose and eggs. I will go through these in detail because they represent different examples of what's wrong in the medical nutrition literature and what you need to know to read such studies constructively. A good place to start is the attack on red meat. That's next.

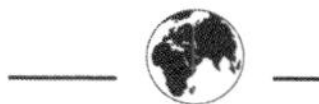

# Chapter 18

# Red Meat And The New Puritans

> "Dost thou think, because thou art virtuous, there shall be no more cakes and ale?"
>
> — William Shakespeare, *Twelfth Night.*

Experts on nutrition are like experts on sexuality. No matter how professional they are in general, in some way, they are always trying to justify their own lifestyle. They are sure that their own choices are the ones that everybody else should follow and they are always tempted to save us from our own sins, sexual or dietary. The new puritans want to save us from red meat. It is unknown whether Michael Pollan's *In Defense of Food* [5] was reporting the news or making the news but its coupling of not eating too much and not eating meat is common. *Vegetarian Times* says that 3.2 % of the US population are vegetarians and the media seem to think that they are the righteous few.

Meat is a favorite target for this new breed of puritans. There are good reasons for avoiding meat — better not to kill anything — but, for most people, the health angle is not one of them. We are also suspicious when they do protest too much. Protein is chemically complex, or more precisely, there are hundreds of different proteins that may have opposite effects in the body. There are twenty amino acids and they have many individual effects and some work together with the others. On the whole human level, it is not even clear that most of us eat a lot of meat. Protein tends to be a stable part of the diet. There was no change in protein consumption in the last forty years, the period of the obesity and diabetes epidemic. We may eat more than recommended by health agencies but they are not necessarily experts. In fact, many, particularly the elderly, frequently don't get enough. Given the complexities, it seems that the burden of proof should be on those who want to show risk. Both the scientific and popular press, however, give you the idea that meat can be considered guilty until proven innocent.

Red meat, in particular, is "linked to" just about any disease including diabetes where, if anything, it is likely to be beneficial. The major approach is epidemiological and the numerous papers have a common theme. Weak associations are found and it is claimed that if the low risk is multiplied by the whole population, we will save thousands of lives. Here, again, I am asking you to accept the idea that the best and the brightest are not doing acceptable science. Using the principles from the previous chapters, I will analyze a couple of specific papers. These reports have particular errors that you can look for when you try to decide if a scientific paper is valid or not.

One important idea: all statistics is subjective. Assumptions are made and numbers are calculated from those assumptions. The numbers are meaningful only if the assumptions fit the question to be answered. One simple idea to keep in mind: statistical significance is a mathematical term meaning that differences between an experimental group and their controls did not arise by chance. It does not mean that those differences are of sufficient magnitude or are of sufficient relevance that they have any practical or clinical significance. I'll begin with an older red meat study which illustrates the limitations of relative risk and odds ratio. This particular case has a punch line and I'll show you that the whole paper was probably some kind of flim-flam.

## RED MEAT SCARE OF 2009

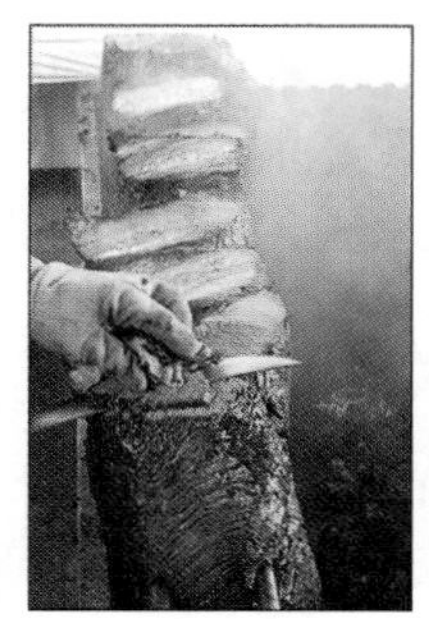

"Daily Red Meat Raises Chances Of Dying Early" was the headline in *The Washington Post* [92]. This scary story was accompanied by a photo of a gloved hand slicing beef with a scalpel-like knife, probably intended to evoke a CSI autopsy, although, to me, it still looked pretty good if slightly over-cooked. I don't know the reporter, Rob Stein, but I think we are not talking Woodward and Bernstein. For those too young to remember Watergate, the reporters from the Post were encouraged to "follow the money" by Deep Throat, their anonymous whistle-blower. The movie Fat Head suggests the variation that we "follow the data."

In the strange world of nutrition, scandalous behavior is right out in the open. Researchers don't like to be whistle-blowers because, unless the issue has some major impact, a breakdown in research principles makes us all look bad. The missteps in published papers in nutrition, however, require no insider information. The study that the Washington Post story was based on, "Meat Intake and Mortality," was published in the professional medical journal, *Archives of Internal Medicine* by R. Sinha and coauthors [93]. It got a certain amount of press at the time but, following the usual pattern, it soon disappeared from view to be simply cited as part of the "accumulating evidence" that meat would kill you. Nobody looked at it closely. Certainly not Rob Stein. To be fair, how could he? It is not his fault. It takes time to analyze such papers and he was likely to be assigned to a flower show the next day. It is not unreasonable that he take the authors at their word. It is worth looking at the details, however. All cause mortality, is what you really want to ask about, and so we should be sure that this is for real. The conclusion will be that there is nothing in this paper to make you think that any danger of red meat has been demonstrated and, in fact, its greatest virtue may be in showing you how to see through the flawed papers that populate the literature. Principles for reading that literature will be **highlighted**.

## COMMON SENSE AND EXPERIENCE FIRST

Your best bet in dealing with potential bias is to demand that, no matter how complicated the statistics, the results should not violate common sense (unless it can be explained). The salient fact about red meat is that during the thirty years that we describe as the obesity and diabetes epidemic, protein intake overall has been relatively constant but red meat consumption went down. As shown above, almost all of the increase in calories has been due to an increase in carbohydrates. Fat, if anything, went down. However, during this period, consumption of almost everything went up (**Figure 5-8B**). Wheat and corn, of course went up, but so did fruits and vegetables. The two things whose consumption went down were red meat and eggs. In addition, we need to remember that much research shows the benefits of replacing carbohydrate with protein, especially for the elderly [94-98]. So, here's something that you can use as a rule in analyzing papers in the literature.

> **Principle 1. Biology, common sense and experience comes before statistics. Do the results make sense?**

## SIMPLE STATISTICS. WHO'S LIKELY TO DIE?

The paper by Sinha and coworkers [93] is an observational study of the type discussed in the previous chapter, that is, they tried to match up outcomes for different groups in an existing population. In terms of informing the public, the report in *The Washington Post* is quite a bit more accessible than the original paper. It says;

> " ... researchers analyzed data from 545,653 predominantly white volunteers, ages 50 to 71, participating in the National Institutes of Health-AARP Diet and Health Study. In 1995, the subjects filled out detailed questionnaires about their diets, including meat consumption. Over the next 10 years, 47,976 men and 23,276 women died."

So the risk, or probability, of dying if you were in the study population is easy to calculate from *The Washington Post* report. Overall probability = (number of people who died) / (all the people in the study). That is equal to (47,976 + 23, 276) /545,653 = 0.13 or 13 %. This is a good reference point, something that we're sure of before anybody starts doing the statistics. The risk is not great. Only slightly more than one in ten people died in the course of the experiment. The article goes on to say that:

> "... those who ate the most red meat — about a quarter-pound a day— were more likely to die of any reason, and from heart disease and cancer in particular, than those who ate the least — the equivalent of a couple of slices of ham a day.
>
> Among women, those who ate the most red meat were 36 percent more likely to die for any reason, 20 percent more likely to die of cancer and 50 percent more likely to die of heart disease. Men who ate the most meat were 31 percent more likely to die for any reason, 22 percent more likely to die of cancer and 27 percent more likely to die of heart disease."

This sounds fairly scary, but is it? Let's do what scientists call a back-of-the-envelope calculation. You can skip this if you don't like math but it is just high-school algebra. (You can skip it if you didn't like high school algebra). We have the overall risk of mortality: 13 %. Now, for both men and women, the increase from eating meat is about 33 % so if N people died who ate low meat, then 1.33 x N is the number for meat eaters. We don't yet know the size of the meat eating group *vs.* the non-meat-eaters but let's do a rough calculation of the overall probability.

We add up how many died in each group and divide by the total number of people. That should be equal to 13 %. If there are N in the low meat group and 1.33 N in the high meat group, we have: 2.33 x N = 13% and N is equal to 0.0558 or about 5.6 % for the low-meat group and 13 -5.6 = 7.4 % for the fraction of high-meat eaters who died. So the absolute difference in risk = 7.4 -5.6 = 1.8 %. Before you even look at the original paper, we are now talking about a difference in risk in the ball park of a few percent. Your steak is already sounding a lot better.

What we are trying to do is to go beyond relative risk. The dire warning that "... those who ate the most red meat were 36 percent more likely to die for any reason," lost its kick when we did an absolute risk calculation. Why? Obviously, when it is a case of relative anything, you need to know: relative to what? While none of us is going to get out of this alive, in ten years a small fraction of a random collection of people will die. The bottom line:

**Principle 2. Are the results meaningful, that is, large numbers? Technically, this is called the effect size. Is the effect size large?**

## WHAT WAS MEASURED?

Other problems are that the paper says "A 124-item food frequency questionnaire ... was completed at baseline." Many people are suspicious of food questionnaires. They are often criticized because people may not accurately report what they ate, although this is a limitation of many nutritional studies. While this can be a source of error, the amount of error depends on how the data is interpreted. All scientific measurements have error. Here, the problem is the word "baseline". The study was started in 1995, continued for ten years, and mortality was followed during this period. This means that some people died as much as ten years after their reported food intake. This has to be considered along with the previous rule, whether we are looking at big changes. The take-home message here:

**Principle 3. If the effect is not large, then the data have to be very reliable. Conversely, if the data have big potential error, then the conclusion must be substantial.**

Are you eating the same thing you were eating ten years ago? More to the point, with all the *kvetching* about red meat in the media, is there any chance somebody in this study reduced red meat consumption? Any chance they did it half way through the study and would have appeared in a different group if data had been collected for them at that point? I guess I am wondering whether, if I get sick, it is due to the junk I ate in college.

But, let's take them at their word and assume the study is okay. What do we learn from the outcome? I will go through the reasoning in detail. Again, the math is simple but you can skip ahead.

## You in Las Vegas -Understanding OR, RR and HR

The damned statistics, as Mark Twain might have called them, go like this: the study population of 322, 263 men and 223, 390 women was broken up into five groups (quintiles) according to meat consumption, the highest group taking in about 7 times as much as the lowest group (big differences). The groups were compared according to a statistic called hazard ratio (HR). The authors report that the HR for eating red meat every day compared to eating red meat rarely is 1.44. First, I'll explain the different terms for expressing risk. HR is slight variation of relative risk (RR) so I'll explain that first.

The probability of an event happening is simply:

Probability = number of particular events / total number of events.

Probability in many medical tests is called risk. So,

Probability, or "risk" of getting a "6" with a fair die is 1/6.

If you have two groups, for example, meat eaters and vegetarians and you want to compare their risk, you report relative risk or (RR):

RR = risk (meat group) / risk (vegetarians).

It is important to realize that when you calculate RR, you have lost the information as to how much the risk was to begin with. If they tell you the RR of a disease, you don't know whether it is a rare disease or one that everybody has.

A problem in a medical experiment may be deciding when the experiment is over and a related measure is the hazard which is the same as the probability but measured over a fixed time intervals, that is, a rate.

Hazard is more complicated and technical, but it doesn't hurt to consider hazard as the same as probability. When you compare two groups, you report the HR. The interpretation is like the RR, relative probability of occurrence.

In some cases, rather than the probability, the odds might be reported. Odds are slightly different from probability.

Odds = (number of ways of winning)/(number of ways **not** winning).

Odds of getting a "6" with a fair die is 1/5. You would usually say that the odds are "1 to 5," or "5 to 1 against." As the probability gets smaller, the odds and the probability become closer together and in conversation are used similarly.

The probability of getting the ace of spades from fair deck = 1/52 = 0.0192.

Odds of getting the ace of spades = 1/51 = 0.0196

Odds ratio (OR) is what it says, the ratio of the odds of two different events. Again, you don't know whether the odds were good or bad only their relation to each other. An OR of 1 means that there is no difference in the likelihood of two events. It is sometimes said "50-50" or "equal odds."

Bottom line: in reading a scientific paper, you can take RR, HR and OR as roughly the same, telling you the comparison between how likely two events are to occur. The big caveat: you have to make sure you know what the individual probabilities are. The problem described in a narrative:

You are in Las Vegas. There are two black-jack tables and, for some reason (different number of decks or something), they have different probabilities of paying out. The probability of winning at Table One is 1 in 100 hands, or 0.01 or 1 %. At Table Two, the probability of winning is 1 in 80 or about 1.27%. The ratio of the probabilities is 1.27/1.0 = 1.27. (A ratio of 1 would mean that there is no difference between the tables). Right off, something is wrong: you lost a lot of information. One gambling table is definitely better than the other but the odds aren't particularly good at either table. But you had to know that in advance; you can't tell from the probability ratio because the information about the real payoff is lost. Suppose, however, that you did get a glimpse at the real info and you could find out what the absolute odds are at the different tables: 1 % at Table One, 1.27 % at Table Two. Does that help? Well, it depends on who you are. For the guy who is sitting at the black-jack table when you go up to sleep in your room at the hotel, and who is still there when you come down for the breakfast buffet, things are going to be much better off at the second table. He will play hundreds of hands and the better odds ratio of 1.27 is likely to pay off. Suppose, however, that you are somebody who will take the advice of my cousin, the statistician, who says to just go and play one hand for the fun of it, just to see if the universe loves you (that's what gamblers are really trying to find out). You're going to play the hand and then, win or lose, you are going to do something else. Does it matter which table you play at? Obviously it doesn't. The odds ratio doesn't tell you anything useful because your chances of winning are pretty slim either way. Put another way, if you buy two lottery tickets instead of one, your chances of winning are doubled, but does that make you want to play?

## TELL ME THE DIFFERENCE IN ABSOLUTE RISK

Going over to the original red meat paper (skip to the next paragraph if you just want the conclusion), there are a number of different "models" (reworking of the data) and there are mind-numbing tables giving you the different hazard ratios. Using the worst case HR between high and low red meat intakes for men, we get HR = 1.48 or, as they like to report in the media 48 % higher risk of dying from all causes. Sounds bad. But wait, what is the absolute difference in risk? Well, the paper says that the whole group of 322, 263 men was divided into five sub-groups (quintiles) of 322, 263/5 = 64, 453 people. The people who don't eat much red meat had 6,437 deaths or 10.0 %. The big meat eaters must have had 14.8 % deaths. That's an absolute difference of 5 % and it's the very worst conclusion correcting for some variables. The authors, however, corrected for other things that might have contributed to the outcome. Correcting for all variables, the difference for men goes down to 3 %.

Bottom line: There is an absolute difference in risk of about 3 %. How much would you change your life for that benefit? And remember, this is for big changes, like 6 or 7 times as much meat. So, what is a meaningful HR? For comparison, the HR for smoking *vs.* not smoking and lung disease was about 20. For smoking heavily, the HR was about 30. Going back to Bradford Hill's criteria: "First upon my list I would put the strength of the association," again, the effect size. Relative risk does not have meaning by itself. You must know the changes in absolute risk.

Another way of looking at the data is the number needed to treat (NNT), which is the reciprocal of the absolute risk or 20-30 people that you would have to treat to save one life. That's not great but it's something. Or is it?

## WHAT ABOUT PUBLIC HEALTH? GOOD NEWS OR NOT?

Okay. The odds are not very good. Many people would say that, sure, for a single person, red meat might not make a difference but if the population reduced meat by half, we would save thousands of lives. At this point, before you and your family take part in a big experiment to save health statistics in the country, you have to apply Principles 2 and 3. You have to ask how strong the relations are. To understand how good the data is you must look for things that would *not* be expected to have a correlation. "There was an increased risk associated with death from injuries and sudden death with higher consumption of red meat in men but not in women", which sounds like we are dealing with a good deal of randomness.

More important, what is the *risk* in *reducing* meat intake. The data don't really tell you that. Unlike cigarettes, where there is little reason to believe that anybody's lungs really benefit from cigarette smoke, we know that there are many benefits to protein especially if it replaces carbohydrate in the diet, especially for the elderly, especially for all kinds of people. So with odds ratios around one — remember that an odds ratio of one means that there is no difference between no red meat and lots of red meat — you are almost as likely to *benefit* from adding red meat as you are reducing it. Technically, it is called a two-tailed distribution, that is, things can change in both directions. The odds still favor things getting worse but it really is a risk in both directions. You are at the gaming tables. You don't get your chips back. If you bet on reducing red meat and it does not reduce your risk, it may increase your risk.

## THE FINE PRINT -THE SMOKING GUN

What's written above is approximately what I wrote as a blogpost. In turning it into this chapter, I went back to the original paper to check the calculations. I had used the numbers for men since it was a worst case (and it still has the problems that I described) but in re-calculating things, I looked at the numbers for women. The data are shown below:

**Multivariate Analysis Red, White, and Processed Meat Intake and Total and Cause-Specific Mortality in Women**

| Mortality in Women (n=223 390) | Quintile | | | | |
|---|---|---|---|---|---|
| | Q1 | Q2 | Q3 | Q4 | Q5 |
| | | Red Meat Intake[b] | | | |
| All mortality | | | | | |
| Deaths | 5314 | 5081 | 4734 | 4395 | 3752 |
| Basic model[c] | 1 [Ref] | 1.11 (1.07-1.16) | 1.24 (1.20-1.29) | 1.43 (1.38-1.49) | 1.63 (1.56-1.70) |
| Adjusted model[d,e] | 1 | 1.08 (1.03-1.12) | 1.17 (1.12-1.22) | 1.28 (1.23-1.34) | 1.36 (1.30-1.43) |
| Cancer mortality | | | | | |
| Deaths | 2134 | 1976 | 1784 | 1687 | 1348 |
| Basic model[c] | 1 [Ref] | 1.07 (1.01-1.14) | 1.15 (1.08-1.23) | 1.34 (1.26-1.43) | 1.42 (1.33-1.52) |
| Adjusted model[d,e] | 1 | 1.02 (0.96-1.09) | 1.06 (1.00-1.14) | 1.20 (1.12-1.28) | 1.20 (1.12-1.30) |
| CVD mortality | | | | | |
| Deaths | 1173 | 1155 | 1101 | 1027 | 900 |
| Basic model[c] | 1 [Ref] | 1.15 (1.06-1.25) | 1.32 (1.22-1.44) | 1.54 (1.41-1.68) | 1.82 (1.66-1.98) |
| Adjusted model[d,e] | 1 | 1.13 (1.04-1.23) | 1.26 (1.16-1.37) | 1.39 (1.27-1.52) | 1.50 (1.37-1.65) |

The population was again broken up into five groups or quintiles. The lower numbered quintiles are for the lowest consumption of red meat. Looking at all cause mortality, there were 5,314 deaths and when you go up to quintile 05, highest red meat consumption there are 3,752 deaths. What? The more red meat, the lower the death rate? Isn't that the opposite of the conclusion of the paper? And the next line has relative risk which now goes the other way: higher risk with higher meat consumption. What's going on? As near as one can guess, "correcting" for the confounders changed the direction. The confounders are listed in the legend to the figure. For the "basic model," the data were corrected for race and total energy intake and risk went up. Why? We can't tell if we can't see what the effect was.

A useful way to look at this data is from the standpoint of conditional probability. We ask: what is the probability of dying in this experiment if you are a big meat-eater? The answer is simply the number of people who both died during the experiment and were big meat-eaters (Q5) divided by the number in Q5 = 3752/(223,390/5) =

0.0839 or about 8%. If you are **not** a big meat-eater, your risk is (5314 + 5081+ 4734 + 4395)/(0.8 x 223, 390) = 0.109 or about 11%.

This paper tested the hypothesis that red meat is associated with all cause mortality. The data showed that it wasn't. That's what it showed. It wasn't unless you drag in other factors, education, marital status, family history of cancer body mass index, smoking history using smoking status (never, former, current), time since quitting for former smokers, physical activity, alcohol intake, vitamin supplement user, fruit consumption and vegetable consumption have to be added in to make it true. What makes anybody think that red meat among these other ten inputs is the key variable? Wouldn't it be better to find out which of these had the biggest effect? Maybe we're looking at the effect of smoking (known risk) corrected by all the others.

What I offer here is a professional scientist's view and I try to make my description dispassionate and not insulting but what is this but flim-flam?

## WHAT ABOUT RED MEAT?

Red meat isn't a chemical. What is it about the red meat? The meat? The red? To be fair to the authors, they also studied white meat which was mostly beneficial. But what about potatoes? Cupcakes? Breakfast cereal? Are these completely neutral? If we ran these through the same computer, what would we see? Unspoken, in everybody's mind is saturated fat, that Rasputin of nutritional risk factors who will come after you despite enough bullets in its body to have killed several scientific theories. Maybe it wasn't the red meat *per se* but the way it was procured. Maybe it's ritual slaughter that conferred eternal life (or lack of it) on the consumer — nothing is as harrowing as the Isaac Bashevis Singer stories equating meat eating with other sins of the flesh. Finally, there is the elephant in the room: carbohydrate. Basic biochemistry suggests that a roast beef sandwich may have a different effect than roast beef in a lettuce wrap.

## SUMMARY

Rules for dealing with the scientific literature:

1. Do the results make sense? Biology comes before statistics. Experience comes before statistics.
2. Is there a big effect. Are we talking about meaningful, that is, large numbers?
3. What was measured? If the effect is not large, then the data have to be very reliable. If the data have big potential error, then the conclusion must be substantial.

In nutrition, as in other fields, recommendations are often tinged by the personal preferences of those dishing them out. In combination with the dogmatic state of government and private recommendations, it takes some work to know if you are reading a meaningful study. The points in this chapter are that you have the right to ask for and the author has the obligation to provide clear explanations. The practical application of Hill's criteria is that results should make sense in terms of magnitude and what you know about biology. You should also be very suspicious if only relative risk is reported even if just in the Abstract. Remember, Alice has 30 % more money in the bank than Bob, but we don't know whether she is rich.

You can usually calculate absolute risk (the number of cases divided by the number of participants) so you can see if the report is about something that is very rare. The specific case in this chapter, the effect of red meat, fails to meet the criterion of meaningful effects and seems to be deployed to distract from the real culprit, the real elephant in the room: carbohydrate.

It's not over. Red meat is still a target. The next Chapter describes yet another case of how relative risk is used to paint an exaggerated picture of the effects of red meat consumption. It will also introduce the idea of confounders, factors that may influence the interpretation of the outcomes of an experiment. I will describe, too, the dangers in their misuse.

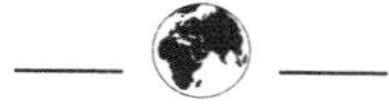

# Chapter 19

# Harvard -Making Americans Afraid Of Meat

---

> **TIME:** You're partnering with, among others, Harvard University on this. In an alternate Lady Gaga universe, would you have liked to have gone to Harvard?
>
> **Lady Gaga:** I don't know. I am going to Harvard today. So that'll do.
>
> — Belinda Luscombe, *Time Magazine*, March 12, 2012

There was a sense of *déja-vu* about the paper by Pan, *et al.* [99] entitled 'Red meat consumption and mortality: results from 2 prospective cohort studies.', that came out in April of 2012." That's what I wrote in May of 2012. The red meat problem was described in the previous chapter and I had written a blogpost about it but it wasn't long before the Pan paper from Harvard was published. Other bloggers worked it over pretty well so I ignored it. Then, I came across a remarkable article from the Harvard Health Blog. It was entitled "Study urges moderation in red meat intake." It was about the Pan study and it described how the "study linking red meat and mortality lit up the media ... Headline writers had a field day, with entries like

'Red meat death study,' 'Will red meat kill you?' and 'Singing the blues about red meat."' This was too much for me and what follows is another blogpost, pretty much as I wrote it then.

What was odd about the post from the Harvard blog was that the field day for headline writers was all described from a distance as if the study by Pan, *et al.* (and the content of the Harvard blogpost itself) hadn't come from Harvard but was rather a natural phenomenon, similar to the way every seminar on obesity begins with a graphic of the state-by-state progression of obesity as if it were some kind of meteorologic event.

The reference to "headline writers," I think, was intended to conjure images of sleazy tabloid publishers like the ones who are always pushing the limits of first amendment rights in the old *Law & Order* episodes. The Harvard Blogpost itself, however, is not any less exaggerated. (My friends in English Departments tell me that self-reference is some kind of hallmark of real art). It is not true that the Harvard study was urging moderation. In fact, the article admitted that the original paper "sounded ominous. Every extra daily serving of unprocessed red meat (steak, hamburger, pork, etc.) increased the risk of dying prematurely by 13%. Processed red meat (hot dogs, sausage, bacon, and the like) upped the risk by 20%." That is what the paper urged. Not moderation. Prohibition. "Increased the risk of dying prematurely by 13%." Who wants to buck odds like that? Who wants to die prematurely?

It wasn't just the media. Critics in the blogosphere were also working over-time deconstructing the study. Among the faults that were cited, a fault common to much of the medical literature and the popular press, was the reporting of relative risk.

The limitations of relative risk or odds ratio were discussed before. Relative risk is relative. It doesn't tell you what the risk is to begin with. Relative risk destroys information. The extreme example: As before, you can double your odds of winning the lottery if you buy two tickets instead of one, or Alice has 30 % more money than Bob but they may both be on welfare. So why do people keep reporting it? One reason, of course, is that it makes your work look more significant. But, if you don't report the absolute change in risk, you may be scaring people about risks that aren't real. The nutritional establishment is not good at facing their critics but, in this case, Harvard admitted that they don't wish to contest the issue.

## NOLO CONTENDERE

"To err is human, said the duck as it got off the chicken's back."

— Curt Jürgens in ***The Devil's General***

Having turned the media loose to scare the American public, Harvard now admitted that the bloggers are correct. The Harvard Health News Blog allocuted to having reported "relative risks, comparing death rates in the group eating the least meat with those eating the most. The absolute risks ... sometimes help tell the story a bit more clearly. These numbers are somewhat less scary." Why not try to tell the story as clearly as possible in the original article? Isn't that what you're supposed to do in science?

Anyway, there was a table in Harvard's Health News Blog:

| | **Deaths per 1,000 people per year** | |
|---|---|---|
| | 1 serving unprocessed meat a week | 2 servings unprocessed meat a day |
| Women | 7 | **8.5** |
| | 3 servings unprocessed meat a week | 2 servings unprocessed meat a day |
| Men | **12.3** | **13** |

This is the raw data. This is what you need to know. Unfortunately, the Harvard Blog doesn't actually calculate the absolute risk for you. You would think that they would want to make up for Dr. Pan's scaring you; an allocution is supposed to remove doubt about the details of the crimes. Let's calculate the absolute risk. It's not hard. Risk is a probability, that is, number of cases divided by total number of participants. Looking at the data for the men first, the risk of death with 3 servings per week is equal to the 12.3 cases per 1000 people = 12.3/1000 = 0.1.23 = 1.23%. Now going to 14 servings a week (the units in the two columns of the table are different) is 13/1000 = 1.3% so, for men, the absolute difference in risk is 1.3-1.23 = 0.07, less than 0.1%. Definitely less scary. In fact, not scary at all. Put another way, you would have to drastically change the eating habits of 1, 429 men (from 14 down to 3 servings of red meat) to save one life. In statistics it's called effect size and it is, just as you would think, just as Bradford Hill told us, the most important value in any experiment scientific or financial, or whatever. Less than 0.1% is pretty poor.

Still, it's something, at least according to the public health professionals. For millions of people, it could add up. Or could it? We have to step back and ask what is predictable about showing a change of less than one tenth of 1% risk. Couldn't it mean that if a couple of guys got hit by cars in one or another of the groups that that might throw the whole thing off. How many other things have a less than one tenth of 1% risk that weren't considered? Or, maybe a handful of guys in an upscale, vegetarian social circles lied about their late night trips to Dinosaur Barbecue. When can you scale up a small effect size?

If the effect size is small, and you want to scale it up, it must be secure, that is, it must not have much room for error. The Salk vaccine had an absolute benefit of only about 0.02%. Of the 400, 000 people in the test, the difference in the number of people who got the disease in the unvaccinated group compared to those who were treated was only 85 people. Obviously, it was a good idea to scale things. Such a small number could be scaled up because it was real, that is, very accurate. You knew who got the vaccine and who didn't. Nobody "may" have gotten the vaccine. Pan, *et al* don't really know, for sure, who ate what. The error in a food questionnaire data is tolerable if the outcome is a knock-out, like cigarettes and lung cancer. The red meat risk means nothing at all. Effect size is the name of the game.

There is an underlying theme here. There is the possibility that the mass of epidemiology studies from the Harvard School of Public Health and other groups are simply not real. The whole thing. Poor understanding of science, cognitive dissonance or something else may be the cause. Whatever it is, the progression of epidemiologic studies showing that meat causes diabetes, that sugar causes gout, all with low hazard ratios, that is, small effect size, may be meaningless. Discouraging and almost impossible to believe. A big piece of medical research is a house of cards.

## OBSERVATIONAL STUDIES, AGAIN

We made the point in the previous two chapters that when you compare two phenomena, when you do an observational study, you usually have an idea in mind (however much you keep it unstated). It is not bird watching. Pan, *et al* were *testing* the hypothesis that red meat increases mortality. If they had done the right analysis, they would have admitted that the test had failed, that the hypothesis was not true. To be precise, technically speaking, they could not reject the null hypothesis, that there is no discernible connection between eating red meat and premature death. The association was very weak and the underlying mechanism was, in fact, not borne out. As suggested before, in experimental research there really is only association. God does not whisper in our ear that the electron is charged. We make an association between an electron source and the response of a detector. Association does not *necessarily* imply causality, however; the association has to be strong and the underlying mechanism that made us make the association in the first place, must make sense.

What is the mechanism that would make you think that red meat increased mortality?, One of the most remarkable statements in the paper:

> "Regarding CVD mortality, we previously reported that red meat intake was associated with an increased risk of coronary heart disease and saturated fat and cholesterol from red meat may partially explain this association. The association between red meat and CVD mortality was moderately *attenuated* after further adjustment for saturated fat and cholesterol, suggesting a *mediating* role for these nutrients." (My *emphasis.*)

This bizarre statement — that saturated fat in the red meat played a role in increased risk because including saturated fat *reduced* risk — was morphed in the Harvard School of Public Health Newsletters plea bargain to "the authors of the Archives paper suggest that the increased risk from red meat may come from the saturated fat, cholesterol, and iron it delivers", although the blogger forgot to add "... although the data show the opposite. Reference (2) cited above had the conclusion that "consumption of processed meats, but not red meats, is associated with higher incidence of CHD and diabetes mellitus." In essence, the hypothesis is not falsifiable — any association at all will be accepted as proof. The conclusion may be accepted if you do not look at the data.

## THE DATA

In fact, the data are not available. The individual points for each people's red meat intake are grouped together in quintiles (broken up into five groups) so that it is not clear what the individual variation is and therefore what your real expectation of actually living longer with less meat is. Quintiles are, in my view, some kind of anachronism presumably from a period when computers were expensive and it was hard to print out all the data (or a representative sample). If the data were really shown, it would be possible to recognize that it had a shotgun quality, that the results were all over the place and that whatever the statistical correlation, it is unlikely to be meaningful in any real world sense. But you can't even see the quintiles, at least not the raw data. The outcome is corrected for all kinds of things, smoking, age, etc. This might actually be a conservative approach — the raw data might show more risk — but only the computer knows for sure.

## CONFOUNDERS

> "... mathematically, though, there is no distinction between confounding and explanatory variables."
>
> — Walter Willett, *Nutritional Epidemiology, 2nd edition.*

A "multivariate adjustment for major lifestyle and dietary risk factors" has many assumptions. Right off, you assume that what you want to look at, red meat in this case, is the one that everybody wants to look at, and that other factors are to be subtracted out. However, the process of adjustment is symmetrical: a study of the risk of red meat corrected for smoking might alternatively be described as a study of the risk from smoking corrected for the effect of red meat. Given that smoking is an established risk factor, it is unlikely that the odds ratio for meat is even in the same ballpark as what would be found for smoking. **Figure 19-1** shows how risk factors follow the quintiles of meat consumption. If the quintiles had been broken up according to the factors themselves, we would have expected even better association with mortality.

Another assumption in this kind of analysis is that there are many independent risk factors all of which contribute in a linear way. If, in fact, they interact, the assumption of linearity is not appropriate. You can correct for "current smoker," but, biologically speaking, you cannot correct for the effect of smoking on an increased response to otherwise harmless elements in meat, if there actually were any. And, as pointed out before, red meat on a sandwich may be different from red meat on a bed of cauliflower puree.

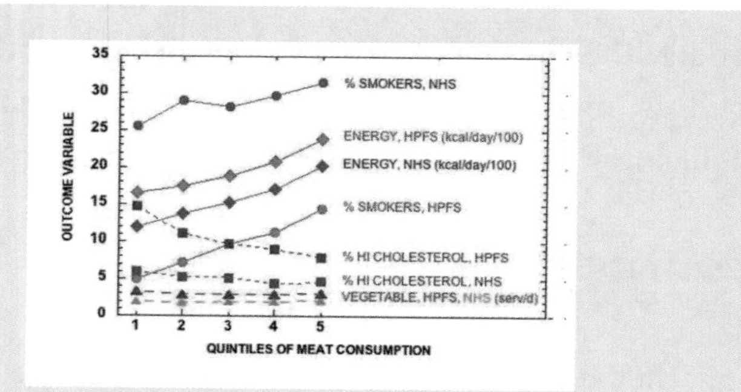


FIGURE 19-1. Effect of different parameters on outcome. Data from Pan, et al. [100].

This is the essence of it. The underlying philosophy of this type of analysis is "you are what you eat." The major challenge to this idea is that carbohydrates, in particular, control the response to other nutrients but, in the face of the plea of *nolo contendere*, it's all moot.

## WHO PAID FOR THIS AND WHAT SHOULD BE DONE

We paid for it. Pan, *et al.* was funded in part by 6 NIH grants and they're still paying for it. The latest production from this group now emphasizes the "change in meat consumption." [101] Remarkably, my objections to this paper were published as a letter to the editor [102]. My main point was that "Red meat consumption decreased as T2DM increased during the past 30 years." The journal does not allow figures in Letters to the Editor but I included it in my blogpost (**Figure 19-2**).

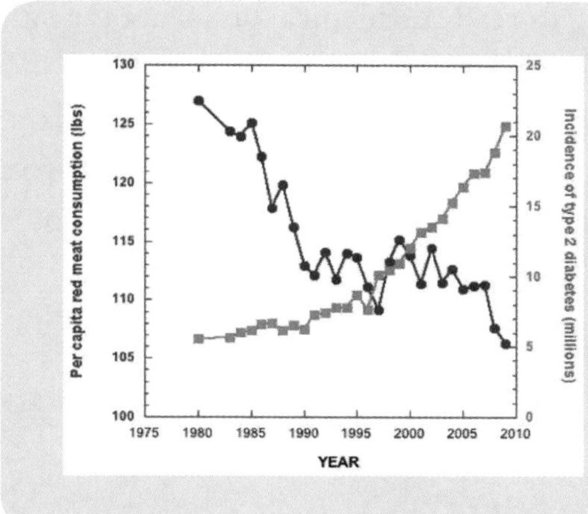


FIGURE 19-2
Red meat consumption and incidence of type 2 diabetes.

It is hard to believe with all the flaws pointed out here and by others and, in the end, admitted by the Harvard Health Blog, that this work was subject to any meaningful peer review. A plea of no contest does not imply negligence or intent to do harm but something's wrong. On the other hand, there is the clear attempt to influence the dietary habits of the population. This cannot sensibly be justified by an absolute risk reduction of less than one-tenth of one percent, especially given that others have made the case that some part of the population, particularly the elderly, may not get adequate protein. The need for an oversight committee of impartial scientists is the most reasonable deduction from Pan, *et al.* I will suggest it to the NIH.

## SUMMARY

What did we learn here? First, a paper that claims to show a decreased mortality from red meat, on analysis shows nothing. The risk is infinitesimal by the admission of the Harvard School of Public Health where the study was done — the absolute difference in risk is about one-tenth of one percent. A careful analysis shows that even this is meaningless. There is no risk from red meat.

The lesson for people trying to read the medical literature is again that statistics cannot be taken at face value and Hill's First Criterion kicks in. If the effect is weak, there must not be much error in the data. If the data have large error, the conclusion must be very strong. If you have a method with a lot of error and you get a weak association, it doesn't mean anything.

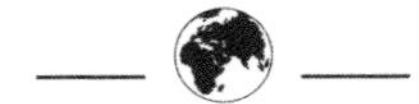

# Chapter 20

# Group Statistics -Bill Gates Walks Into A Bar...

Everybody has their favorite example of how averages don't really tell you what you want to know or how they are inappropriate for some situations. Most of these are funny because they apply averages to cases where single events are important. I'll list a few in the text boxes in this chapter. From the title: Iif Bill Gates walks into a bar, on average, everybody in the bar is a millionaire. Technically speaking, averages start with the assumption that there is a kind of "true" value and that deviations are due to random error. If we could only control things well — if there were no wind resistance and all balls were absolutely uniform — all of the balls would always fall in the same place; any spread in values is random rather than systematic. The familiar bell-shaped curve that illustrates

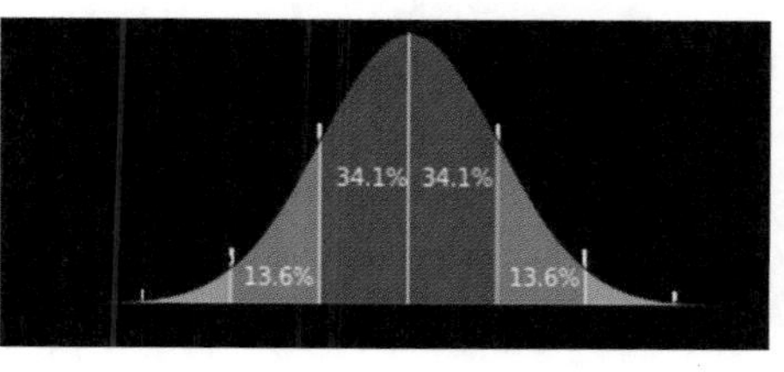


the mean (average) value and deviations from the mean is referred to as the normal distribution or Gaussian or, in some cases, the similar but not precisely the same, Poisson distribution. The distance marked σ (sigma) is called the standard deviation or SD and it is supposed to give you a feel for how the real points deviate from the mean. The area of the colored section in the figure shows the percentage of points that are one (dark blue) or two (lighter blue) SD away from the mean and what percentage of the points fall in that region.

So, from the standard deviation, you can tell how reliable the data are. A low standard deviation means that the mean value can be expected to be a reliable indication of what the actual data look like. A high standard deviation means that the data can be expected to be spread out.

> *The average resident of Dade County, Florida is born Hispanic and dies Jewish.*

There are many examples. The textbooks cite the blitz in London in WWII where the V-1 "flying bombs" were distributed in a characteristic random pattern. ("Aiming" was presumed due to fixed launch sites and fixed fuel; deviations came from wind resistance and other random factors). You can see a pretty good fit to the 3-D version of, in this case, the Poisson distribution.

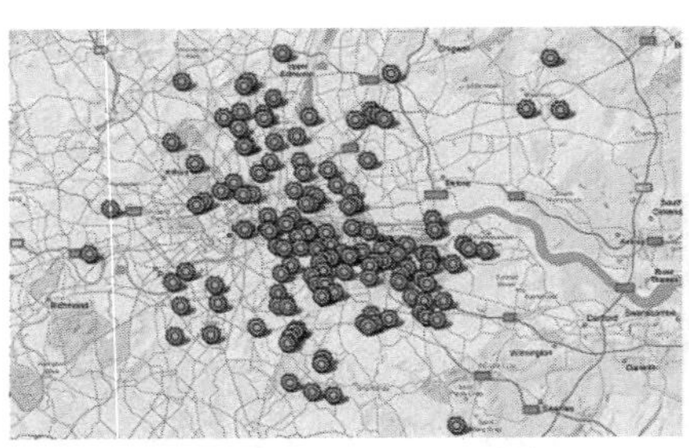

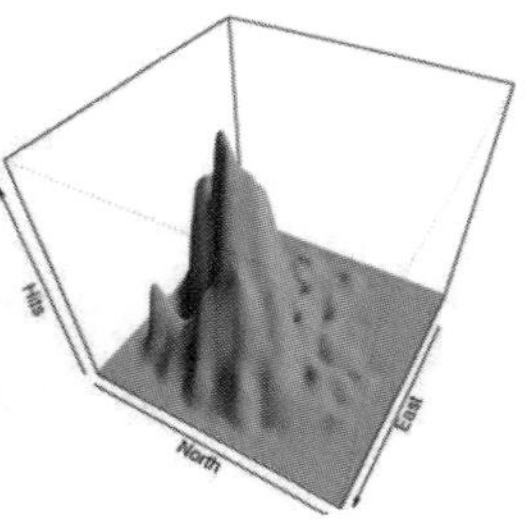


On the other hand, Allied bombing of the German town of Aachen destroyed much of the city while leaving intact the famous cathedral where Charlemagne was crowned. The joke was that the cathedral was unharmed because that's what we were aiming at. It is generally assumed that what is good enough for bombing is good enough for the social and biological science. But is it? Going from a large collection of individual points to two mathematical parameters (the mean and standard deviation), you obscure a good deal of information. A literally infinite number of different arrangement of points will give you the same mean and standard deviation.

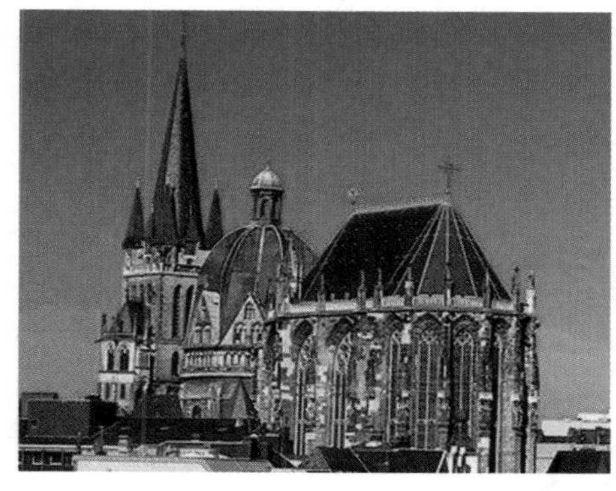

Even more important, are you really sure that your data is uniform, that is, as the statisticians describe, that they come from the same population. Getting to the point, how are group statistics used in nutrition and medicine? The underlying principle is usually stated as the idea that "one size fits all." But is this a good idea? When we see a spread in weight loss on different diets, for example, is that due to minor individual variations (one subject always goes to the gym right after breakfast)? Or is it due to fundamental differences between people? For example, might there be two classes of people, like insulin-sensitive and insulin-resistant?

> *Three statisticians go duck hunting. A duck flies overhead.*
> *The first statistician fires but the shot is a foot to the left.*
> *The second statistician fires, but the shot is a foot to the right.*
> *The third statistician says "got 'im."*

## NOBODY LOSES AN AVERAGE AMOUNT OF WEIGHT

Use of averages depends on a uniformity in the population. But in diet, we don't really believe that. Calling attention to all the people who eat more than you do and gain less weight than you do is considered an anecdotal observation. (The fact that you don't want to believe it adds some credibility). But there are experiments. David Allison's group [103] studied a number of identical twins, put them all on a weight reduction diet for a month and saw how much weight they lost. They calculated an energy deficit (differences in calories in and calories out) and compared that to the actual energy deficit, that is, weight loss minus food intake.

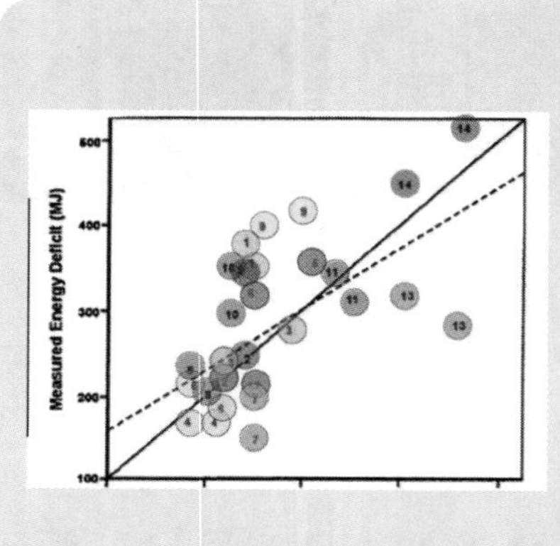


FIGURE 20-1. Relationship of estimated and measured energy deficit for 14 twin pairs (same numbers and color). Dotted line = regression of estimate on measured energy deficit; solid line represents identity (measured deficit = estimated). Subjects above solid line (of identity) are absolutely less efficient than those below. Data from Hainer, et al. [103].

Pairs of twins in **Figure 20-1.** were similar in their energy deficit, but there was big variation *between* twins. The study was carried out in a hospital but given the possible random variations of 28 people over the course of a month, this is pretty good evidence for what is popularly called "metabolic advantage" (people below the solid line) or maybe metabolic "disadvantage" (people above).

## SUMMARY

Group statistics hide information. Many different collections of individual data will give the same averages and the same statistical error. Well-controlled experiments with twins show big differences between pairs of twins but much smaller differences within twin pairs. In a diet experiment, if only group statistics are used, be suspicious.

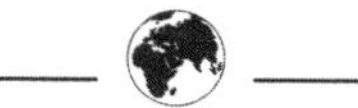

# Chapter 21

# The Seventh Egg

## WHAT DID YOU HAVE FOR BREAKFAST?

Stepping back and looking at the recent nutritional literature, I am struck by the miracle of life. How could humans have evolved in the face of threats from red meat, from eggs, even from the dangers of shaving? (If you write about nutrition you have to create a macro that types out "I'm not making this up:" the Caerphilly Study [104] shows you the dangers of shaving ... or is it the dangers of not shaving?). With 28% greater risk of diabetes here, 57% greater risk of heart disease there, how could our ancestors have ever come of child-bearing age? With daily revelations from the Harvard School of Public Health showing the Scylla of saturated fat and the Carybdis of sugar between which our forefathers sailed, it is amazing that we are here.

These studies that the media writes about, are they real? They are, after all, based on scientific papers. Although not all the media can decipher them, reporters generally talk to the researchers. The papers must have gone through peer review. The previous chapters suggest that the gatekeepers, as we think of peer reviewers, are less vigilant than they should be. In fact, many papers that are published in the major medical journals defy common sense. Is this possible? Can the medical literature have such a high degree of error? Could there be such a large number of medical researchers who are not doing credible science? How can the consumer decide? I am going to try to give an additional example that may help. When people ask questions like "could the literature be wrong?", the answer is usually "yes." I will try to explain what's wrong and how to read the nutritional literature in a practical way. I will make it simple. It is science, but it is accessible science. I am going to illustrate the problem with the example of a paper by Djoussé, "Egg consumption and risk of type 2 diabetes in men and women" [105]. But first, a joke.

> It was a dumb joke. In my childhood, there was the idea, undoubtedly politically incorrect, that Indians, that is, Native Americans, always said "how" as a greeting. The joke was about an Indian reputed to have a great memory. He is asked what he had for breakfast on New Year's day the previous year. He says "eggs." They are then interrupted by an earthquake or some natural disaster. The interviewer and the Indian do not meet again for ten years. When they meet, the interviewer says "how." The Indian answers "scrambled."

If the interviewer had been an epidemiologist, he might have asked if he had developed diabetes. In the study by Djoussé, *et al.* [105] participants were asked how many eggs they ate and then, ten years later, it was determined whether they had developed diabetes. If they had, it was assumed to be because of the number of eggs. Is this for real? Do eggs cause changes in your body that accumulate until you develop a disease, a disease that is, after all, primarily one of *carbohydrate* intolerance? **Type 2 diabetes**, recall, is due to impaired response of the body to the insulin produced by beta cells of the pancreas as well as a progressive deterioration the insulin-producing cells. Common sense says that it is a suspicious idea that eggs would play a major role. It is worth trying to understand the methodology and see if there is a something that justifies this obvious departure from common sense. Again the principles may be generally useful.

What did the experimenters actually do? First, people were specifically asked "to report how often, on average, they had eaten one egg during the past year," and "classified each subject into one the following categories of egg consumption: 0, < 1 per week, 1 per week, 2-4 per week, 5-6 per week, and 7+ eggs per week." They collected this data every two years for ten years. With this baseline data in hand they then followed subjects "from baseline until the first occurrence of one of the following a) diagnosis of type 2 diabetes, b) death, or c) censoring date, the date of receipt of the last follow-up questionnaire" which for men was up to 20 years. Thinking back over a year: Is there any likelihood that you might not be able to remember whether you had 1 vs. 2 eggs on average during the year? Is there any possibility that some of the men who were diagnosed with diabetes ten years after their report on eggs changed their eating pattern in the course of ten years? Are you eating the same food you ate ten years ago? Quick, how many eggs/week did you eat last year?

## THE GOLDEN RULE AGAIN

So right off, there is a problem in people reporting what they ate. This is a limitation of many, probably most nutritional studies and, while it can be a source of error, it is really a question of how you interpret the data. All scientific measurements have error. You simply have to be sure that the results that you are trying to find do not depend on any greater accuracy than the data that you have collected.

Eye-balling the paper by Djoussé, et al., we see that there are no figures. A suspicious sign. A graph of the number of eggs consumed vs the number of cases of diabetes is what would be expected. The results, instead, are stated in the Abstract of the paper as this mind-numbing conclusion. (Don't try to read this):

> Compared with no egg consumption, multivariable adjusted

> hazard ratios (95% CI) for type 2 diabetes were 1.09 (0.87-1.37), 1.09 (0.88-1.34), 1.18 (0.95-1.45), 1.46 (1.14-1.86), and 1.58 (1.25-2.01) for consumption of <1, 1, 2-4, 5-6, and 7+ eggs/ week, respectively, in men (p for trend <0.0001). Corresponding multivariable hazard ratios (95% CI) for women were 1.06 (0.92-1.22), 0.97 (0.83-1.12), 1.19 (1.03-1.38), 1.18 (0.88-1.58), and 1.77 (1.28-2.43), respectively (p for trend <0.0001).

What does all this mean? In fact, it means very little. These "statistical shenanigans" are, in fact an argument *against* a correlation. If you look at the paragraph, almost every number that you see is very close to 1. Without going through a detailed analysis, you can simply extract from the tables some simple information. There were 1, 921 men who developed diabetes. Of these, 197 were in the high egg consumption group, or about 1 in 10. For women, there were 2,112 cases of whom 46 were high egg consumers or a little more than 2 % of the diabetes cases were big egg-eaters. To me this suggests that diabetes is associated with something else than eggs and it is probably unjustified of the authors to conclude: "These data suggest that high levels of egg consumption (daily) are associated with an increased risk of type 2 diabetes in men and women."

What I described are the raw data and as we saw in Chapter 19, we have to consider confounders. In fact, if we analyzed the data in detail, we would find that the conclusion is actually poorly supported by the data but let's take the authors' conclusion at face value.

## THE SEVENTH EGG

If the authors' conclusion is correct, this means that there was no risk of diabetes from consuming 1 egg/week compared to eating none. Similarly, there was no risk in eating 2-4 eggs/week or 5-6 eggs/week. But if you upped your intake to 7 eggs or more per week, that's it. Now, you are at risk for diabetes.

Since I like pictures, I will try to illustrate this with a modified still from the movie, the *Seventh Seal* directed by Ingmar Bergman. Very popular in the fifties and sixties, these movies had a captivating if pretentious style; they sometimes seemed to be designed for Woody Allen's parodies. One of the famous scenes in the *Seventh Seal* is the protagonist's chess game with Death. A little PhotoShop and we have a good feel for what happens if you go beyond 5-6 eggs/week.

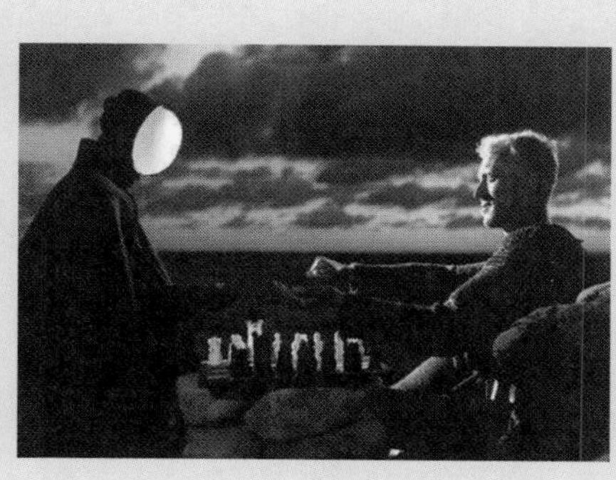

Figure 22-1.
The Seventh Egg.

## Summary:

A study of 20,703 men and 36,295 women makes a very weak case that eggs have anything at all to do with type 2 diabetes. Few of the people who developed diabetes were big egg eaters. Correction for confounders showed greater risk for this group but common sense says that this is absurd and that if you have to do so much work to show risk, it is not important. The problem is the mindless use of statistics. If the statistics go against common sense, then the authors should explain why. In detail. In the Abstract.

Sometimes, you can get a sense of how real the statistics are by looking for simple things. How many people were in the study and how many got sick, that is, are we talking about a rare disease or one that had low probability, that is, in the experiment: diabetes is a major health risk but if you take 1, 000 men for ten years, only 1 in

10 may develop diabetes so you need to be sure there is a big difference between the group that followed the behavior you are looking at and those who didn't.

The cases that we have looked at are from major institutions and well-known researchers. The studies had an impact when first published. We do have a problem in the medical literature. The best and the brightest are doing dumb things. Nothing shows how bad things are in academic medicine than intention-to-treat. That's next.

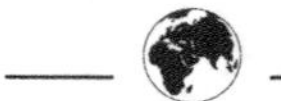

# Chapter 22

# Intention-To-Treat: What It Is And Why You Should Care

---

The medical literature has some strange things but nothing beats intention-to-treat (ITT), the strange and mostly not amusing statistical method that has appeared recently. According to ITT, the data from a subject assigned at random to an experimental group must be included in the reported outcome data for that group even if the subject does not follow the protocol, or even if they drop out of the experiment. In other words, it doesn't matter if you eat what the experimenter told you to eat, your lipid profile has to be included in the final report. At first hearing, the idea is counter-intuitive if not completely idiotic – why would you include people who are not in the experiment in your data? – suggesting that a substantial burden of proof rests with those who want to employ it. No such obligation is felt and, particularly in nutrition studies, such as comparisons of isocaloric weight loss diets, ITT is frequently used with no justification at all. Astoundingly, the practice is sometimes actually demanded by reviewers in the scientific journals. As one might expect, there is a good deal of controversy on this subject. Physiologists or chemists, hearing this description, usually walk away shaking their head or immediately come up with one or another obvious *reductio ad absurdum*, e.g. "You mean, if nobody takes the pill, you report whether or not they got better anyway?" That's exactly what it means.

On the naive assumption that some people really didn't understand what was wrong with ITT — I've been known to make a few elementary mistakes in my life — I wrote a paper on the subject. It received negative, actually hostile, reviews from two public health journals — I include an amusing example at the end of this chapter. I even got substantial grief from reviewers at *Nutrition & Metabolism*, where I was the editor at the time, but where it was finally published. I'll describe a couple of interesting cases from the medical literature and one relatively new instance — Foster's two year study of low-carbohydrate diets — to demonstrate the abuse of common sense that is the major characteristic of ITT.

The title of my paper was "Intention to Treat. What is the question?" The point was that there might be nothing inherently wrong with ITT if you are explicit about what you are trying to find out. If you use ITT, you are asking: What is the effect of *assigning* subjects to an experimental protocol? If you are very circumspect about that question, then there is little problem. But is anybody really interested in what the patient was *told* to do rather than what they actually did? The practice comes from clinical trials where you can't always tell whether patients have taken the recommended pills, just as in the real situation where you never know what people will do once they leave the doctor's office. In that case, you do an analysis based on your intention, that is, you have no other choice than to call the experimental group those who were assigned to the intervention. That's what we always did without giving it a special name. When you do know, however, there are two separate questions: Did they take the pill and is the pill any good? That's the data. You have to know both and if you want to collapse them into one number, you have to be sure you make clear what you are talking about. You lose information if you collapse efficacy and adherence into one number. It is common for the **Abstract** of a paper to correctly state that the results are about "assigned to a diet" but by the time the **Results** are presented, the independent variable has become not "assignment to the diet," but "the diet" which most people would assume meant what people ate rather than what they were told to eat. *Caveat lector.*

My paper on ITT was a kind of over-kill and I made several different arguments. The common sense argument gets to the heart of the problem. I'll describe that first and also give a couple of real examples.

## Common Sense Argument Against Intention-to-Treat

Consider an experimental comparison of two diets in which there is a simple, discrete outcome, e.g. a threshold amount of weight lost or remission of an identifiable symptom. Patients are randomly assigned to two different diets; diet A or diet B and a target of, say, 5 kg weight loss is considered success. As shown in **Table 22-1**, half of the subject in diet A are "compliers," able to stay on the diet. For whatever reason, half are not. The half of the patients in diet A who were compliers were all able to lose the target 5 kg, while the non-compliers did not. In diet B, on the other hand, everybody stays on the diet but, somehow, only half are able to lose the required amount of weight. An ITT analysis shows no difference in the two outcomes — half of group A stayed on the diet and all lost weight, while in study B, everybody complied but only half had success.

| | Diet A | Diet B |
|---|---|---|
| Compliance (of 100 patients) | 50 | 100 |
| Success (reached target) | 50 | 50 |
| ITT success | 50/100 = 50% | 50/100 = 50% |
| "per protocol" (followed diet) success | 50/50 = 100% | 50/100 = 50% |

Table 22-1. Hypothetical results for the thought experiment for analysis of diets A and B.

Now, you are the doctor. With such data in hand, should you advise a patient: "Well, the diets are pretty much the same. It's largely up to you which you choose." or, looking at the raw data (both compliance and success), should the recommendation be: "Diet A is much more effective than diet B but people have trouble staying on it. If you can stay on diet A, it will be much better for you so I would encourage you to see if you could find a way to do so." You are the doctor. Which makes more sense?

Diet **A** is obviously better but hard to get people to stay on it. This is one of the characteristics of ITT: It always makes the better diet look worse than it is. In the manuscript, I made several arguments trying to explain that there are two factors, only one of which (whether it works) is clearly due to the diet. The other (whether you follow the diet) is under control of other factors (whether WebMD tells you that one diet or the other will kill you, whether the evening news makes you lose your appetite, etc.). I even dragged in a geometric argument because Newton had used one in the *Principia*: "a 2-dimensional outcome space where the length of a vector tells how every subject did ... ITT represents a projection of the vector onto one axis, in other words collapses a two dimensional vector to a one-dimensional vector, thereby losing part of the information." Pretentious? *Moi*?

## WHY YOU SHOULD CARE -SURGERY OR MEDICINE?

Does your doctor actually read these academic studies using ITT? One can only hope not. Consider the analysis by David Newell of the Coronary Artery Bypass Surgery (CABS) trial. This paper is fascinating for the blanket, tendentious insistence, without any logical argument, on something that is obviously fundamentally foolish [106]. Newell considers that the method of

"the CABS research team was impeccable. They refused to do an 'as treated' analysis:' We have refrained from comparing all patients actually operated on with all not operated on: This does not provide a measure of the value of surgery."

You read it right. The results of surgery do not provide a measure of the value of surgery. So, in the **CABS** trial, patients were assigned to be treated with Medicine or Surgery. The actual method used and the outcomes are shown at **Table 22-2** below.

| **Survivors and deaths after allocation to surgery or medical treatment** | | | | |
|---|---|---|---|---|
| | Allocated medicine | | Allocated surgery | |
| | Received surgery | Received medicine | Received surgery | Received medicine |
| Survived 2 years | 48 | 296 | 354 | 20 |
| Died | **2** | **27** | **15** | **6** |
| Total | 50 | 323 | 369 | 26 |

TABLE 22-2 Results of the CABS trial from Newell [106].

The ITT analysis was described by Newell as having been "used correctly." Looking at the table, you see that a 7.8% mortality was found in those *assigned* to receive medical treatment (29 deaths out of 373), and 5.3% mortality for assignment to surgery (21 deaths of 371). If you look at the *outcomes* of each treatment as actually used, it turns out that medical treatment led to 33 deaths or a rate = 9.5% (33/349), while among those who actually underwent surgery, the mortality rate was only 4.1% (17/419). Mortality was less than half in surgery compared to medical treatment. Making such a simple statement, that surgery was better than medicine, Newell says, "would have wildly exaggerated the apparent value of surgery."

The "apparent value of surgery?" "Apparent?" Common sense suggests that appearances are not deceiving. If you were one of the 33-17 = 16 people who were still alive, you would think that it was the theoretical report of your death that had been exaggerated. The thing that is under the control of the patient and the physician, and which is not a feature of the particular modality, is getting the surgery actually implemented. Common sense dictates that a patient is interested in surgery, not the effect of being *told* that surgery is good. The patient has a right to expect that if they comply with the recommendation for surgery, the physician would try to avoid any mistakes from previous studies where the patient did not receive the operation. In another defense of ITT, Hollis [107] has the somewhat cryptic statement: “Most types of deviations from protocol would continue to occur in routine practice." This seems to be saying that the same number of people will always forget to take their medication and surgeons will continue to have exactly the same scheduling problems as in the CABS trial. ITT assumes that practical considerations are the same everywhere and that any practitioner is locked into the same ability or lack of ability as the original experimenter in getting the patient into the OR.

One might also ask what happens when two studies give different values from ITT analysis. In the extreme case, one might suggest that if the same operation were recommended at a hospital in Newcastle-upon-Tyne as opposed to a battlefield in Iraq, the two ITT values would be different. Which one is the appropriate one to be attributed to that surgical procedure?

What is the take home message? One general piece of advice that I would give based on this discussion in the medical literature: don’t get sick.

## WHY YOU SHOULD CARE -VITAMIN E SUPPLEMENTATION

A clear cut case of how off-the-mark ITT can be is a report on the value of antioxidant supplements. The Abstract of the paper concluded that "there were no overall effects of ascorbic acid, vitamin E, or beta carotene on cardiovascular events among women at high risk for CVD." The conclusion that there was no effect of supplements was based on an ITT analysis but, on the fourth page of the paper, is this remarkable effect of not counting subjects who didn’t comply:

> "Noncompliance led to a significant 13% reduction in the combined end point of CVD morbidity and mortality ... with a 22% reduction in MI ..., a 27% reduction in stroke ... a 23% reduction in the combination of MI, stroke, or CVD death."

The media universally reported the conclusion from the Abstract, namely that there was no effect of vitamin E. This conclusion is correct if you think that you can measure the effect of vitamin E without taking the pill out of the bottle or, as in the old joke about making a really dry martini, you don't remove the cap from the Vermouth bottle before pouring. Does this mean that vitamin E is really of value? The data would certainly be accepted as valuable if the statistics were applied to a study of the value of, say, replacing barbecued pork with whole grain cereal. Again, "no effect" was the answer to the question: "What happens if you are told to take vitamin E?", but it still seems most reasonable that the "effect of a vitamin" means, to most people, what happens when you actually take the vitamin.

## THE ITT CONTROVERSY

Advocates of ITT see its principles as established and may dismiss a common sense approach as naïve. They usually say that removing non-compliers introduces bias by destroying the original randomization. In this, they are confusing the process of randomization with the criteria for inclusion. If you excluded people with diabetes from your study and only found out when the study started that one of the subjects actually had diabetes, like the tainted juries in courtroom dramas, you would be required to remove them anyway. You would not have included them if their diabetes came out in the *voir dire*, so you can't include them now. Of course, if you don't know whether or not subjects have complied, you have to include everybody but that is what was always done because you have no choice. That is not the issue here. What happens when you know who did and who didn't comply?

The problem is not easily resolved; statistics is not axiomatic, there is nothing analogous to the zeroth law (the idea of thermal equilibrium on which thermodynamics rests). All statistics rests on interpretation and intuition. If this is not appreciated, if you do not go back to consideration of exactly what the question is that you are asking, it is easy to develop a dogmatic approach and insist on a particular statistic because it has become standard.

As I mentioned above, I had a good deal of trouble getting my original paper published and one anonymous reviewer said that "the arguments presented by the author may have applied, maybe, ten or fifteen years ago." This criticism reminded me of Molière's *The Doctor in Spite of Himself*:

> Sganarelle is disguised as a doctor and spouts medical double-talk with phony Latin, Greek and Hebrew to impress the client, Geronte, who is pretty dumb and mostly falls for it but:
>
> **Geronte:** ...there is only one thing that bothers me: the location of the liver and the heart. It seemed to me that you had them in the wrong place; the heart is on the left side but the liver is on the right side.
>
> **Sgnarelle:** Yes. That used to be true but we have changed all that and medicine uses an entirely new approach.
>
> **Geronte:** I didn't know that and I beg your pardon for my ignorance.

In the end, it is reasonable that scientific knowledge be based on real observations. This has never before been thought to include data that was not actually in the experiment. I doubt that *nous avons changé tout cela.*

## FOSTER, ET AL: OUTCOMES AFTER 2 YEARS

Described in Chapter 4 as the "shot heard 'round the world," Gary

Foster's 2002 study of low-carbohydrate diets found that, after one year, the diet was substantially better than a low-fat diet for markers of cardiovascular disease. The study, however, emphasized that, on weight loss, the low-carbohydrate diet was better at six months but that the diets were "the same at one year." This, of course, was an effect, of dwindling adherence in both the intervention and control groups although, in fact, Figure 4-3 showed that the lipid markers were noticeably better on the low-carb arm even at 1 year.

A follow-up to the landmark one-year study, "Weight and Metabolic Outcomes After 2 Years on a Low-Carbohydrate Versus Low-Fat Diet," published in 2010 [77], had a surprisingly limited impact. What was wrong? The first paper was revolutionary and, in the current one, the authors explicitly addressed the need for including a "comprehensive lifestyle modification program" since the original was criticized for simply giving the people on the Atkins diet a copy of the popular book. So what could be wrong? The conclusion was the same. The low-carbohydrate arm had better outcomes for most CVD risk factors although, again, there was no difference in weight loss after 2 years. As stated in the conclusion "neither dietary fat nor carbohydrate intake influenced weight loss when combined with a comprehensive lifestyle intervention." This is, after all, still the party line and should have been well-received by establishment nutrition. That should have been a big win for the only-calories-count crowd. Why was there so little impact? In fact, the paper is still rarely cited.

**Annals of Internal Medicine** | ARTICLE

**Weight and Metabolic Outcomes After 2 Years on a Low-Carbohydrate Versus Low-Fat Diet**

**A Randomized Trial**

**Gary D. Foster, PhD; Holly R. Wyatt, MD; James O. Hill, PhD; Angela P. Makris, PhD, RD; Diane L. Rosenbaum, BA; Carrie Brill, BS; Richard I. Stein, PhD; B. Selma Mohammed, MD, PhD; Bernard Miller, MD; Daniel J. Rader, MD; Babette Zemel, PhD; Thomas A. Wadden, PhD; Thomas Tenhave, PhD; Craig W. Newcomb, MS; and Samuel Klein, MD**

Background: Previous studies comparing low-carbohydrate and low-fat diets have not included a comprehensive behavioral treatment, resulting in suboptimal weight loss.

Objective: To evaluate the effects of 2-year treatment with a low-carbohydrate or low-fat diet, each of which was combined with a comprehensive lifestyle modification program.

Design: Randomized parallel-group trial. (ClinicalTrials.gov registration number: NCT00143936)

Setting: 3 academic medical centers.

Patients: 307 participants with a mean age of 45.5 years (SD, 9.7 years) and mean body mass index of 36.1 kg/m$^2$ (SD, 3.5 kg/m$^2$).

toms, bone mineral density, and body composition throughout the study.

Results: Weight loss was approximately 11 kg (11%) at 1 year and 7 kg (7%) at 2 years. There were no differences in weight, body composition, or bone mineral density between the groups at any time point. During the first 6 months, the low-carbohydrate diet group had greater reductions in diastolic blood pressure, triglyceride levels, and very-low-density lipoprotein cholesterol levels, lesser reductions in low-density lipoprotein cholesterol levels, and more adverse symptoms than did the low-fat diet group. The low-carbohydrate diet group had greater increases in high-density lipoprotein cholesterol levels at all time points, approximating a 23% increase at 2 years.

FIGURE 22-2 Cover page of Foster, *et al*, reference [77].

It is likely that the *zeitgeist* is different from what it was 8 years ago. Strict scientific standards have suffered tremendous blows. The willingness to disregard the results of big expensive experiments and to ignore common sense is now much more widespread. Everybody knows that in a big comparison trial, the low-carbohydrate diet will win in some way and that it is likely that the authors will try to put a negative spin on things. As Elizabeth Nabel put it after the embarrassing WHI Failure: "Nothing's changed." Low-fat is still the name of the game and the phrase is common in the USDA guidelines and hence in the school lunch program of the Healthy Hunger-Free Kids Act [108] endorsed by Michelle Obama. Press releases on such government programs quote a progression of "suits" with maudlin expressions of optimism about how well what I call "Fruits 'N Vegetables" are doing in improving obesity. There are numerous disclaimers about good fats, bad fats so that you can't really hold them to anything. However, since Foster's first study, numerous low-carb trials have showed it to be superior to any competition. Foster's study was, thus, not the challenge that the original was. But, in fact, it should have been given some attention, at least because it was a follow-up to the landmark first paper. In my opinion, it should have gotten more attention because it reached some kind of new low in misleading statements. It was the conclusion that "neither dietary fat nor carbohydrate intake influenced weight loss."

I admit that I had not read Foster's paper very carefully before making the pronouncement that it was not very good. I was upbraided by a student for such a rush to judgment. I explained that that is what I do for a living. I explained that I usually don't have to spend a lot of time on a paper to see the general drift — I could easily see a couple of errors in methodology, which I describe below but I was probably not totally convincing. So I read the paper, which is quite a bit longer than usual. The main thing that I was looking for was information on the nutrients that were actually consumed since it was their lack of effect that was the main point of the paper. The problem is that people feel that they can call anything that they want a low-carbohydrate diet and, of course, people really believe that "assigned to a low-carbohydrate diet" is the same thing as consuming a low-carbohydrate diet.

## "Any Reasonably Intelligent High School Student."

In a diet experiment, the food consumed should be right up front but I couldn't find it at all. Foster's paper is quite long with a tedious Appendix on the lifestyle intervention but I read the whole thing carefully. I really did. The data weren't there. I was going to write to the authors when I found out — I think through somebody's blog — that this paper had been covered in a story in the *Los Angeles Times*. As reported by Bob Kaplan:

> Of the 307 participants enrolled in the study, not one had their food intake recorded or analyzed by investigators. The authors did not monitor, chronicle or report any of the subjects' diets. No meals were administered by the authors; no meals were eaten in front of investigators. There were no self-reports, no questionnaires.
>
> The lead authors, Gary Foster and James Hill, explained in separate e-mails that self-reported data are unreliable and therefore they didn't collect or analyze any.

I confess to feeling a bit shocked. I don't like getting scientific information from the *LA Times*. How can you say "neither dietary fat nor carbohydrate intake influenced weight loss" if you haven't measured fat or carbohydrate? If you think that self-reported data is not good, then you can't make judgments about what was consumed. And, in fact, the whole nutrition field runs on self-reported data. Is all that stuff from the Harvard School of Public Health, all those epidemiology studies that rely on food records, to be chucked out?

(Personally, I would say yes, but not for that reason).

What would have happened if the authors had actually measured the relevant data, if they asked what people eat, as Kaplan put it "the single most important question ... that any reasonably intelligent high school student would ask?" It's not just bad experimental design. It is a question of what is on their mind. Do they not know that it is totally inappropriate to say that fat or carbohydrate are not important if they haven't measured it? They may be so biased that they don't see what is going on. As I mentioned in Chapter 4, in the first paper, Foster said in public that he set out to trash the Atkins diet. Not a good way to do science. You are supposed to try to trash your own theory and show that it survives.

## BACK TO INTENTION-TO-TREAT

Foster's paper is some kind of low point in bias. It also shows how misleading ITT can be. Chastised for jumping to conclusions, I re-read the paper carefully and the Figures in the paper caught my eye. The title of **Figure 2**: "Predicted absolute mean change in body weight ...." Predicted? That sounds strange. What about the data? The figure shows no difference in change in body weight between groups. It happens. Usually, the low-carb diet does quite a bit better but no guarantee of that. Figure 3 from the paper (my **Figure 22-3**), however, indicates changes in triglycerides for the 3, 6, 12 and 24 month time periods.

Reduction in triglycerides is virtually the hallmark of low-carbohydrate diets. Almost everybody on such a diet lowers their triglycerides (mine fell to half of the original value). In **Figure 22-3**, the difference between the two diets (shown by the double-headed arrow) was quite large at 3 or 6 months, the usual result. However, as the experiment continued, after 12 months, triglyceride values got closer and actually came together after 24 months.

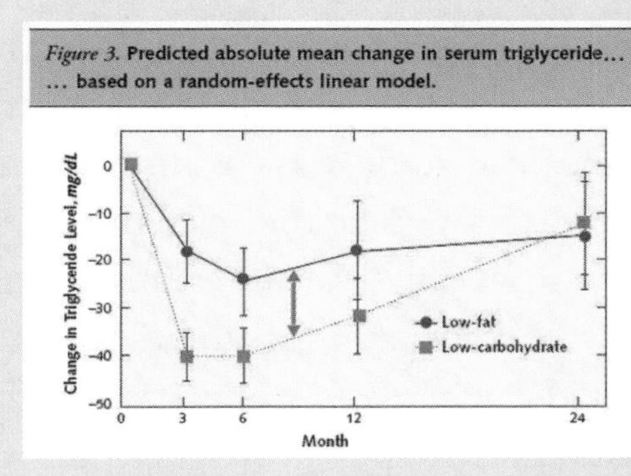


Figure 22-3. Figure 3 from Foster, *et al.* [77] The double-headed arrow represents the difference between the change in triglycerides on the two indicated arms of the study. The distance shown by the arrow is plotted on the Y axis of Figure 22-4.

This seemed strange so I realized I had to find out where "predicted" came from and that meant reading the Methods section and particularly the Statistical Analysis on how the data had been handled. In general, you usually only read the Methods section in detail if you think that there was a problem, or if a new method has been introduced, or if you want to repeat the author's experiment yourself. Large studies like this usually have a statistician and they use standard methods whose details may or may not be understood by a non-statistician (that's me) and frequently not by most of the authors. They are usually accepted at face value and it is assumed that authors have adequately explained to the statistician what the question is that they want to address. As I kept ploughing through the statistical section, I found it increasingly tedious and difficult to read until I hit this passage (I've **highlighted** the key words):

> The previously mentioned longitudinal models preclude the use of less robust approaches, such as **fixed imputation** methods (for example, last observation carried forward or the analysis of participants with complete data [that is, complete case analyses]). These alternative approaches assume that **missing data** are unrelated to previously observed outcomes or baseline covariates, including treatment (that is, **missing completely at random**).

Missing data? Missing completely at random? What's going on here? In a nutshell, this is another implementation of ITT. In the study, the authors used "data" from people who dropped out of the experiment. To do this, all they had to do was "assume that all participants who withdraw would follow first the maximum and then minimum patient trajectory of weight." Whatever this means, if anything, the key words are "withdraw" and "assume." In other words, this is really a step beyond ITT where you would include, for example, the weight of people who showed up to be weighed but had not actually followed one or another diet. Here, nobody showed up. There is no data. A pattern of behavior is assumed and data is — let's face it — made up.

The world of nutrition puts big demands on irony and tongue-in-cheek but the process in Foster's paper suggests that the results could, in theory, be fit to a model for a three-year study, or a ten-year study. As people dropped out you could "impute" the data. In some sense, you could do without any subjects at all. Nutrition experiments are expensive; think of the money that could be saved if you didn't have to put anybody on a diet and you could make up all the data. This is a joke.

## THE DIET OR THE LACK OF COMPLIANCE?

It is odd that ITT is controversial, by which I mean that it is odd that it exists at all. A reasonable way to deal with dropouts, however, that would satisfy everybody is simply to publish both the ITT data and the data that includes only the compliers, the so-called "per protocol" group, that is, the group that were actually in the experiment. This is what was done in the Vitamin E study described above. There, it made the authors' point of view look bad, but they did the right thing. Such data are missing from Foster's paper. Given the high attrition rate, one could guess that the decline in performance in both groups was due to including "data" from the large number of people who failed to complete the study. We do know this number, the number of people who dropped out. That's in the paper. So we can do something with Foster's data. To find out whether the decline in performance is due to including the made-up data from the drop outs, we can plot the difference in triglycerides between the two groups (the double-headed arrow in **Figure 22-3**, above), for each time point, against the number of people who discontinued treatment.

**Figure 22-4** gives you the answer. You can see a direct correlation between the number of dropouts and the group differences. "Decreases in triglyceride levels were greater in the low-carbohydrate than in the low-fat group at 3 and 6 months but not at 12 or 24 months" was almost surely due to the fact that the differences were diluted by people who weren't on the low-carbohydrate diet, or any diet; ITT, or whatever this was, always makes the better diet look worse than it is.

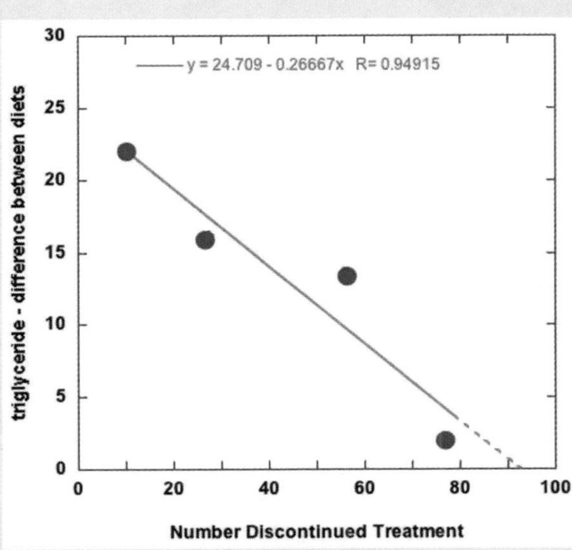


Figure 22-4. The differences in the reduction in TAG (vertical axis) between the low-carbohydrate and low-fat arms as a function of the number of subjects who dropped out of the study. The TAG differences were measured from the double-headed arrow shown in Figure 23-3. Data from Foster et al.[77].

This serves as an example of a case where correlation strongly implies causality. The declining difference between the triglyceride values of the two protocols is unlikely to be due to anything that people ate — if they had stayed with their diet, triglycerides would have been much lower on low-carb — but rather to whether they stayed with the diet. The association is *testing* that hypothesis. In understanding the impact of this kind of experiment, the take-home message is that ITT and imputing data will reduce the real effect of the intervention. In a diet experiment, the nature of the diet and compliance may be related — if the diet is unpalatable, people might not stay on it — but you have to show this. "Might" is not data. Along these lines, however, it is likely that the major reinforcer, the major reason people will stay on a diet, is that it works. In any case, one cannot assume that the two are linked without specifically testing the idea.

## SUMMARY

Intention-to-treat comes from the realization that, in some experiments, you don't know who followed the protocol and who didn't. In a clinic, you may write a prescription and not know if it's been filled. In this case, you have no choice but to include everybody's performance. The mechanical application of the idea in situations where you *do* know who complied and who didn't is another misunderstanding and dogmatic application of statistics.

ITT usually makes the better diet look worse than it actually is. Awareness of whether this method has been used is important for evaluating a scientific publication. In combination with the previous errors in the practice of current nutrition, things look grim for getting much information. The next chapter summarizes the various sources of error and suggests that the medical nutrition literature is deeply flawed and the product of poor methodology and poor scientific thinking. Because of the applications in health and disease, it becomes important to find a dispassionate body which can provide real peer review. Whether such a group can be found in the current social situation remains unknown. Some of the problems that they would have to deal with are summarized in the next chapter.

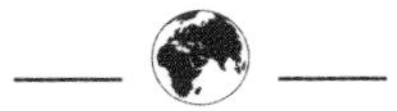

# Chapter 23

# The Fiend That Lies Like Truth

I pull in resolution and begin
To doubt th'equivocation of the fiend
That lies like truth.
— William Shakespeare, *Macbeth.*

Errors, inappropriate use of statistics and misleading presentations are everywhere in the medical literature. Specific examples were described in previous chapters. Let me summarize these and offer a few principles for dealing with the deficiencies. I think that you will need them.

## THE FIRST PRINCIPLE: TEACH ME

You have a right to demand, and the author of a scientific paper has an obligation to provide, a clear explanation of what the results of their study really mean. A good test of whether or not the authors are holding up their end of the arrangement is the number and clarity of the figures. Visual presentation is almost always stronger than long tabulation of numbers. This principle is simultaneously so reasonable and, at the same time, so widely violated that a whole book has been written on how scientific papers need more figures instead of these dense tables [109]. The tables make papers hard to read and ensure that the popular press will have to take the authors' conclusion at face value.

Scientific publication is changing, and increasingly, as more and more journals become open access and available on line, results of scientific studies will be universally available. An advantage to an open access on-line journal is that there is no longer a limit on pages or number of figures. Neither is there an extra charge to the authors for color. (In open-access, the author generally has to pay for the publication; that's why it is free to you). Whether authors will take advantage of this opportunity is unknown. Whatever the journal, however, clear presentation of the results is still the Golden Rule of Statistics: Let us see the data completely and clearly and in as many figures as it takes.

## SCIENCE, BUT NOT ROCKET SCIENCE

"Eating breakfast reduces obesity" is not a principle from quantum electrodynamics. Most of us know whether or not eating breakfast makes us eat more or less during the day. And your first reaction that eating anything is good for losing weight is appropriate and relevant. You don't need to have a physician, one who may have never studied nutrition, to tell you that your perception is right or wrong. A degree in biochemistry is not required to understand the idea that adding sugar to your diet will increase your blood sugar. And the burden of proof is on anybody who wants to say that sugar is okay for people with diabetes. Anything is possible but we start from what makes sense. Of course, there is technically sophisticated science and there are principles that require expertise to understand, but you should not assume this is the case. How do you deal with publications that are trying to snow you or that have a hard sell?

## BE SUSPICIOUS OF SELF-SERVING DESCRIPTIONS

If the paper is about a diet that is described as "healthy," your appropriate answer would be "that's for me to decide." That the media can refer to "healthy" is bad enough but in a scientific paper, it has to be considered an intellectual kiss of death. Nothing that you read after that can be taken at face value. If we knew what was healthy we would not have an obesity epidemic and we would not need another paper to describe it.

Guidelines, data or analyses that describe themselves as "evidence-based medicine," are likely to be deeply flawed. By analogy with a court of law, there must be a judge to decide admissibility of evidence. You can't pat yourself on the back and expect to be considered impartial. And the courts have ruled that testimony by experts has to make sense. Credentials are not enough. As in the first principle, experts have to be able to explain things to the jury.

Be suspicious if the authors tell you how many other people agree with their position. Science does not run on "majority rules" or consensus.

## LEAPING TALL BUILDINGS

As indicated in Chapter 16, the new grand principle of doing science is: *habeas corpus datorum*, let's see the body of the data. If the conclusion is non-intuitive and goes against previous work or common sense, then the data must be strong and clearly presented.

As usually described: If you say you can jump over the chair, I can cut you a lot of slack. If you say you can jump over the building, I need to see you do it. And my daughter, at age nine, suggested an additional requirement. In a discussion of superheroes, I pointed out that Superman used to be described as being "able to leap tall buildings in a single bound." She pointed out that if you try to leap tall buildings, you only *get* a single bound. You can't say your hundred million dollar, eight-year long random control trial was not a fair test. The fat-cholesterol-heart hypothesis was sold as an absolute fact. None of the big clinical trial should have failed. Not one. In the end, almost all of them failed. One failure should have done it.

"Let's see the body of the data," that is, show me what was done before you start running it through the computer. Statistics may be important, but in a diet experiment, where one has to assume that even a well-defined population is heterogeneous, you want to see what all the individuals did.

The compelling work of Nuttall and Gannon, showing that diabetes can be improved even in the absence of weight loss, is increased in impact by the presentation of the individual performance. **Figure 23-1** illustrates the benefits of a low-carbohydrate diet. Not only is there general good response in reduction of blood glucose excursions but all but two of the individual subjects benefitted substantially and all but one got at least somewhat better.

## UNDERSTAND OBSERVATIONAL STUDIES

The usual warning offered by bloggers and others is that association does not imply causality, that observational studies can only provide hypotheses for future testing. A more accurate description, as worked out in Chapter 17, is that observational studies do not *necessarily* imply causality. Sometimes they do. The association between cigarette smoke and lung disease has a causal relation because the associations are very strong and because the underlying reason for making the measurement was based on basic physiology, including the understanding of nicotine as a toxin.

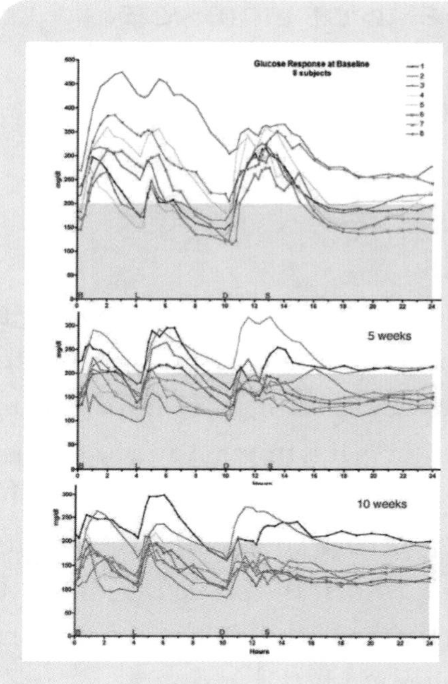


FIGURE 23-1. 24-hour responses for 8 individual subjects on diet of 30% bioavailable glucose. Letters: Breakfast, Lunch, Dinner, and Snack.

In this sense, observational studies *test* hypotheses rather than generating them. There are any number of observations of different phenomena but when you try to make a specific comparison, you usually have an idea in mind, conscious or otherwise. When a study tries to find an association between egg consumption and diabetes, it is testing the hypothesis that eggs are a factor in the generation of diabetes. There *is* a hypothesis. It is just not a sensible one. It is not based on any sound fundamental scientific principle. It is true, however, that if you do find a strong association with an unlikely hypothesis (definition of intuition) then you have a new plausible hypothesis but that is true of all experiments. And it must be further tested.

It is important to question the hypothesis being tested. If the Introduction section to the published study says eggs have been associated with diabetes, you can at least check whether the reference is to an experimental study rather than to the previous recommendations of some health agency.

## META-ANALYSIS AND THE END OF SCIENCE

> Doctors prefer a large study that is bad to a small study that is good.
>
> — *Anon.*

While intention-to-treat is the most foolish activity plaguing modern medical literature, the meta-analysis is the most dangerous. In a meta-analysis you pool different studies to see if more information is available from the combination. As such, it is inherently suspicious: if two studies have different conditions, the results cannot sensibly be pooled. If they are very similar, you have to ask why the results from the first study were not accepted. And, if the pooled studies give a different result than any of the individual studies, the authors are supposed to point out what the original study did wrong.

Simply adding more subjects is not usually considered a guarantee of reliability although papers in the medical literature frequently cite the large number of subjects as one of their strengths. If a meta-analysis is good for anything, which is questionable, it is for the originally intended role of evaluating small under-powered studies where you hope that putting them together might point you to something that you didn't see. It is a kind of "Hail Mary," last ditch play. It was not intended for appropriately powered studies with a large number of subjects.

A number of important meta-analyses have examined the effect of saturated fatty acids (SFA) on cardiovascular risk. One such, from Jakobsen, is shown in **Figure 23-2**. It is usually described as showing a small benefit in replacing SFA with PUFA and an increase in risk if the SFA is replaced with carbohydrate (CHO). Examination of the figure, however, reveals that almost all of the included studies failed to show any significant effect of replacing saturated fat. (The statistical rule is that if the error bar (horizontal line) crosses 1.0 (even odds) then there is no effect of the intervention) and yet the authors came up with an answer. How is this possible? It is the consequence of group-think. If everybody, the editors, the reviewers, assumes that a meta-analysis is an acceptable method, then peer review will be meaningless.

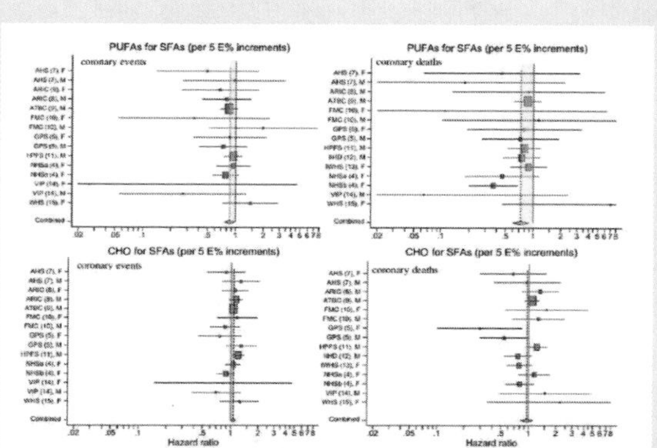


Figure 23-2. Hazard ratios for coronary events and deaths in different studies in the meta-analysis of Jakobsen, *et al.* [6]. Green: lower risk if SFA is substituted by indicated nutrient. Red: increased risk by substitution for SFAs. Figure redrawn from reference [6].

One of the benefits, conscious or unconscious, that keeps the practice going is that it is perfect for current medical research. With meta-analysis, no experiment ever fails, no principle is ever disproved—sugar causes heart attacks, cholesterol causes heart attacks, red meat causes heart attacks and statins prevent heart attacks — it doesn't matter how many studies show no effect. One winner and you can do a meta-analysis. Just one more expensive trial and we'll show that saturated fat is bad. And you don't even have to explain what the other guy did wrong as you might in a real experiment.

The idea that simply adding more subjects will improve reliability is not reasonable. Most of us think that if the phenomenon has big variability, then mixing studies will reduce predictability although it may sharpen statistical significance. There is a specific treatment, called the Bonferroni correction, to take account of the fact that as *n* gets larger, the mathematical difference between experimental and controls will sharpen, which is recognized as misleading. And again, in science, it is expected that if your results contradict previous experiments, you will provide evidence as to the cause of the differences. What did previous investigators do wrong? And do those investigators now agree that you've improved things? Probably not, if you don't ask them.

## BE SUSPICIOUS OF GRAND PRINCIPLES:

"Random controlled trials are the gold standard." "Metabolic Ward Studies are the gold standard." "Observational studies are only good for generating hypotheses." Such grand principles are unknown in the physical sciences where the method that we choose depends on the question that we want to answer. You do not need to carry out a long-term trial to see if a treatment is appropriate for an acute condition. You do not need a random-controlled study to find out whether penicillin is effective for treating gram-positive infections. Penicillin is a drug and you may have to do a random-controlled trial to determine safety but, at the efficacy end, if the results are clear-cut, only a small number of tests is necessary. How many? It depends on how many people recover spontaneously. A statistician can do that for you if you ask the question appropriately.

The random-controlled trial as a gold standard has really never recovered from Smith and Pell's landmark paper "Parachute use to prevent death and major trauma related to gravitational challenge: systematic review of randomised controlled trials" [110]. They concluded that: "the effectiveness of parachutes has not been subjected to rigorous evaluation by using randomised controlled trials ..."

Described as both funny and profound, the paper included all the relevant information (making fun of the excessive statistical detail in the literature):

> "We chose the Mantel-Haenszel test to assess heterogeneity, and sensitivity and subgroup analyses and fixed effects weighted regression techniques to explore causes of heterogeneity. We selected a funnel plot to assess publication bias visually and Egger's and Begg's tests to test it quantitatively."

Smith and Pell pointed out that there were only two solutions to the problem of a lack of random controlled trials:

> "The first is that we accept that, under *exceptional* circumstances, *common sense* might be applied when considering the potential risks and benefits of interventions (My *emphasis*).
>
> The second is that we continue our quest for the holy grail of exclusively evidence based interventions and preclude parachute use outside the context of a properly conducted trial."

In the end, the authors suggested that

> "those who advocate evidence based medicine and criticise use of interventions that lack an evidence base ... demonstrate their commitment by volunteering for a double blind, randomised, placebo controlled, crossover trial."

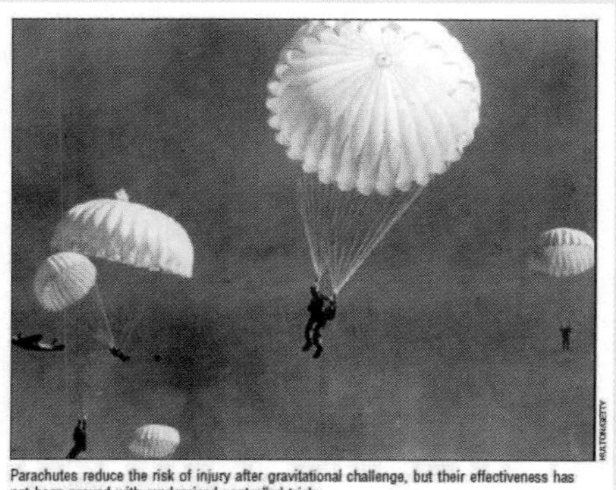

Parachutes reduce the risk of injury after gravitational challenge, but their effectiveness has not been proved with randomised controlled trials

Figure 23-2. The original figure from Smith and Pell [110].

## SUMMARY

The multiple faults that are commonly found in the medical literature have made it tough going and, more often than not, readers will not be happy with the latest study showing that processed food or one or another of the usual suspects will kill you. Armed with a few principles you can understand what is explicitly wrong with these studies that go so strongly against common sense. Failure to show individual data, the use of questionable practices like intention-to-treat and meta-analyses and most of all, failure to actually apply common sense, are the things to look for. There is the barrier of accepting that the medical literature could be so pervasively bad. It will be hard to accept that the Harvard School of Health, that the Best and the Brightest could be making elementary mistakes. There are, however, many precedents.

Easy to forget, though, is that it's about food. Beyond therapy, we like food. Don't forget taste. And even if you insist on food as medicine, it is likely that there was real biologic benefit in the tastes that we have evolved. Easy to forget that it's about taste. That's next.

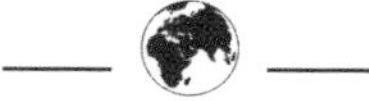

# Part 3

---

# Food And Eating

---

# Chapter 24

# Chemistry And Food -The Recipes -

---

## "NOTHING TO EAT ON A LOW-CARB DIET."

Two practical objections to low-carbohydrate diets that are frequently put forward are that there are limited choices and that the foods that are allowed are inherently expensive. In fact, if you stick a pin in the *Larousse Gastronomique*, the classic French encyclopedic guide to food, you will probably be 3 recipes away from a low-carb dish. There is not much to the idea that everything has to be between two slices of bread or accompanied by a side of fries. If you want to replace the carbs with something you may have to learn how to cook. If you are trying to lose weight, you might want to see how far you can get by simply removing the carbohydrate without replacement. This will reduce cost and not require learning to cook new dishes.

There are now numerous excellent low-carbohydrate cookbooks, e.g. Judy Barnes Baker's *Nourished* and Dana Carpender's *500 Low Carb Recipes* and a very large number of websites. I will describe a few principles and give you some basics to get you started but there are thousands on the internet and many traditional recipes are inherently low-carb. It is low-fat that is the new idea, increasingly recognized as a fad, commonly by those who forget that they were once the strongest supporters.

## CHEMISTRY IS EASY

> What is accomplished by fire is alchemy — whether in the furnace [chemistry] or in the kitchen stove. And he who governs fire is Vulcan, even if he be a cook or a man who tends the stove [chemist].
>
> — Paracelsus

Chemistry is about change, that is, it is about cooking, about fire, just as Paracelsus described it. He was a sixteenth century doctor and an alchemist. He had one foot in the medieval world and one foot in modern science and he was something of a madman. He recognized that cooking and chemistry were the same thing and he saw that it was all about fire and transformation.

## CHEMISTRY AND FOOD

Chemistry is easy. At least compared to physics. There is only one force, the electromagnetic force — that means two kinds of electric charge, plus and minus, and opposite charges attract while like charges repel. (No gravitation because atoms are too small and the two strange nuclear forces don't enter into it). In the world of chemistry, almost everything follows from that basic idea. As applied to cooking, it means there are roughly two kinds of things in the world: hydrophilic (water-like) and hydrophobic (water-fearing, that is, fat-like). The first is like water or salt which dissolves freely in water, has separation of charge, that is, is polar. Cooking is frequently challenged with the problem of "oil and water don't mix," that is, how to keep the sauce from separating. Physical agitation, as in homogenized milk, or chemical emulsifying agents like, egg yolk in mayonnaise, are some of the answers.

Learning low-carbohydrate cooking is largely learning how to cook vegetables. Most of us know how to cook a steak. In cooking vegetables, the major problem is dealing with water. If you look at dried vegetables, you see that some are very small and you can appreciate that they originally contained a huge amount of water. If you want to fry vegetables, you usually need very high heat for a short period of time or the internal water will not be driven off fast enough and you will wind up boiling the vegetables and they will be soggy. This is why serious amateur cooks buy restaurant stoves or restaurant stoves retrofitted for consumers, like Wolf® or Viking®. They are capable of much higher heat than standard consumer stoves and are really worth it if you can afford them.

If you don't salt and extract the water from cabbage before making coleslaw, when you do add mayonnaise, the oil-water interface may cause the water to come out of the cabbage and the product will, again, be soggy. Also, many vegetables, like cauliflower or spaghetti squash, have a subtle taste which will be diluted by the water after steaming or boiling them. It is good to squeeze the water out of these before serving or further processing them.

Vegetables and leafy greens are the main thing that people add back to low-carb diets, at least according to our survey of the Active Lower Carber Forums, an online support group [18]. Cooking vegetables can seem like a big task and, like all such tasks, will give rise to substantial procrastination. Although it only takes 10 minutes to core and steam cauliflower, it can take days to getting around to setting knife to food. For procrastination in general, I recommend timing the steps. The actual time is always less than you think. Most of the recipes below are for vegetables and most start from scratch.

## HOW TO BOIL WATER

It is always better not to take too much for granted. It frequently seems that you have to learn everything. After you teach a dog to fetch a stick, you have to teach them to let go. So, on boiling water, it may be helpful to know that people do ask questions. If you are going to ingest the water directly as in coffee or soup, you generally want to start with cold water since it has fewer dissolved minerals from pipes. If you are just boiling eggs, it doesn't matter. Cover the pot until it boils. To keep it boiling at lowest heat, remove the cover.

## HOW TO BOIL EGGS

There are some very elaborate ways to boil eggs in order to make them easy to peel but the simplest is to just put the cold or room temperature eggs into boiling water. One or two may crack. Eat those first. You can use water that is just below boiling (add cold water after it boils) but the idea is that the sudden change in temperature allows the shell and the attached membrane to separate from the white of the egg. Hard-boiled eggs are one of the staples of low-carbohydrate life style. For traveling, it is the easiest thing to carry along. (The little packets of mayonnaise that are in your workplace cafeteria also help).

## WORLD'S MOST REGAL RECIPE

Low-carb diets may or may not be expensive. It's usually meat that's on sale and even Brussels sprouts can be expensive if you buy them fresh. (In New York, just before St. Patrick's Day, corn beef *and* cabbage are very cheap). But let's get this one out of the way. You can make an expensive dish. Here's a regal recipe from the court of Louis XVIII:

> Take three veal chops. Tie them together and broil them. Eat the middle one.

## LE STEAK HACHÉ

It is worth the trouble to chop your own hamburger. I find the best cut is chuck although you can obviously experiment to find personal taste. Chuck is also called blade steak or seven-bone steak in some places; if you know what a shoulder blade looks like, you will recognize the cross section.

Analogous to James Bond, you want it chopped, not ground. Easiest is the knife blade of a food processor rather than meat grinder which tends to give you the smooth paste-like texture — one reason you don't want to buy ground beef at the supermarket. (We don't even want to think about the others). The meat should really be like chopped steak. Julia Child recommended two perfectly balanced chef 's knives. (Don't you love recipes like that?)

1. Unless it's a very lean cut, remove all visible fat (the marbling will provide sufficient fat for taste).

2. Chop roughly by hand into small pieces and then chop in the food processor until uniformly chopped but not smooth. The key is to have some texture. If you overdo it, you can use it for meat loaf.

Making it this way will show you why they invented hamburger.

## LA FLEUR DE BAS-CARBS

Cauliflower is a staple of low-carbohydrate diets. It is not carbohydrate-free but the total amount of carbohydrate is relatively low. It can be used as a substitute for potato. Jay Wortman's captivating documentary *My Big, Fat Diet* [111], about a First Nations (Canadian analog of Native Americans) community whose life style was turned around by low-carb eating, describes how local stores could not keep cauliflower adequately stocked.

## Recipe 1. Steamed cauliflower

It takes about 1 minute to core a cauliflower. Make a cone-shaped hole. Put the cauliflower, core side down, in a pot with 1 inch of boiling water. You do have to remember to turn the stove off after 7 or 8 minutes but you can do something else while it's cooking. (It's done when you can stick a fork in it easily). You now have something you can use immediately — top with cheese, make into mashed, or refrigerate for later preparation.

## Recipe 2. Faux mashed

Cauliflower "mashed potatoes" is as good as most real mashed. It is different than the best. If you have to have that, you may have to count carbs or calories. I personally don't think of faux mashed as a substitute for potatoes but rather as a vegetable purée.

Steam or boil the cauliflower for slightly longer than you might for other recipes. Purée the cauliflower (easiest in a food processor). I prefer to add butter and salt and eat as cauliflower puree but you can use it as mashed potatoes adding more butter, sour cream or whatever you would do to mashed potatoes. The taste is best if you squeeze the water out of the cauliflower with your hands or using that low-tech cooking device that most of us never have or can't find; the cheesecloth.

Beyond eating it as simple purée, because it is less heavy than potatoes, you can use it to stuff peppers.

## Recipe 3. Home-fries

Home-fries pretty much by definition don't have a recipe beyond frying the cauliflower and breaking it up in the pan or wok as you go. Like home-fried potatoes, cooking time will be reduced if you steam or boil first, slightly less than you would do for straight cauliflower.

Use any of the usual additions that you would for regular home-fries; onion, pepper and left-overs.

### Recipe 4. Deep-fried flowerets

A staple of Arabic cooking, it is the single easiest recipe in the world. Heat the oil (350-375 oC) and drop in the separated flowerets. Cook until slightly browned, about 5 minutes, salt and, if possible eat immediately. If you have the kind of set-up where guests are close to the cooking area, this is the best fried food for a party. As with any deep-fried food, the secret is to keep constant high temperature, which keeps the food from becoming greasy. This means start with the food at room temp and cook in small batches — you can serve each batch while you wait for the oil to re-equilibrate.

## A SELECTION OF EASY VEGETABLE RECIPES

### Recipe 1. Spaghetti squash

Easiest method: cut the squash in half the long way. Place cut side down in a baking dish (both sides if smaller squash and they fit). Add about ½ inch of water. Cover with plastic wrap. Microwave for 20-23 minutes for half large squash or 23-26 minutes for both halves of a smaller squash. When done, scrape out the seeds leaving as much of the interior as you can and scrape out the remainder into a bowl and season with butter and salt. Depending on the age of the squash, you may need to squeeze out the water for better taste.

While some people use the squash as a substitute for pasta, I find that it has a very delicate nutty taste that does not stand up to tomato or other strong flavors. One good variation is cooked shrimp with dried seaweed.

## Recipe 2. Sautéed cucumbers

I'm not a big fan of cucumbers but this is an elegant side dish. Cut the cucumber the long way. Scoop out the seeds and cut on the diagonal to make crescent shape slices about ⅛ inch think. Sauté in butter until the slices are translucent.

## Recipe 3. Microwave Italian Style Broccoli

Americans tend to under-cook vegetables because our parents or grand-parents over-cooked them. For straight broccoli, the Italians are best. There is a mixture of water, garlic and oil which is cooked for the right time in a frying pan. The method keeps structure of the broccoli while bringing out the taste. If you go to a good Italian restaurant or order broccoli when traveling in Italy, you will see. An approximation is to slice the whole vegetable the long way, arrange in a baking dish with the flowerets pointing into the center (microwaves cook from the perimeter). Add a small amount of water (half-cup for whole broccoli). Add chopped garlic and olive oil. Microwave on high for 5-8 minutes depending on amount and freshness.

## Recipe 4. Hearts of Palm

Easy dish for variety using bottled hearts of palm. Drain the stalks and slice the long way. Fry in butter to drive off residual liquid. They are slightly sour and while they are cooking, sprinkle with sucralose or other sweetener. It doesn't take much so you can use sugar if you want. Also, black pepper helps.

## Recipe 5. Stuffed Peppers

The trick to cooking with peppers is that they have an outer membrane that is unappetizing and indigestible. The best way to remove them is to burn them off in a gas flame. Put the whole pepper on a skewer and hold it over a high flame allowing it to char. You can frequently find bottled roasted peppers that are whole and can be used for stuffing. Spaghetti squash is a good stuffing. Top with cheese and bake for 20-30 minutes.

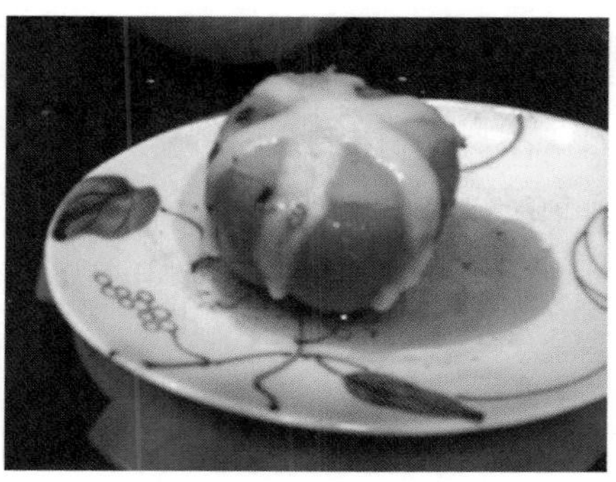

## THE SAUCES -MAYONNAISE

Mayonnaise is one of the things that you give up on a low-fat diet but it is traditional in French and other cooking. The commercial mayonnaise is, in my opinion, very good but not comparable to home-made and some people don't like it because it is high in the kind of fat called omega-6 which we probably get too much of.

Home-made mayonnaise is more like a real sauce while store-bought is a day-to-day condiment. There are many methods and most are difficult but there is one fool-proof, quick way that involves only three really important principles. Violate these and you will have a much harder time.

1. Use an immersion (stick) blender.
2. Everything at room temperature.
3. If you add lemon juice, add it after making the mayonnaise. (The acid my make it harder to thicken).

Before you start, you can rub the mixing bowl with garlic. Best is to use the jar that you are going to store it in; make sure the neck of the jar is big enough for the blender). If you use a lot of garlic (4-6 depending on taste) this is called aiöli (*pr.* Eye-o-lee), which is a well-known variation.

The oil: light olive oil may be best; virgin olive oil will have very strong taste you may not like. I use 1:1 light olive oil and avocado oil (if you can find it) or peanut oil (because I like the taste but, as above, people don't always like vegetable oils).

Add one or two tablespoons of wine vinegar in the jar with salt and pepper. Small amount of prepared brown mustard (I use ®Gulden's). Add one egg yolk or whole egg (room temp) and 1 cup oil. Put the immersion blender at the bottom of the jar and turn the blender on. As it emulsifies, move the blender up and down until you have a uniform mixture.

Useful trick for thicker mayonnaise: crack the uncooked egg, stir it as for scrambled eggs and put it in the freezer. The next day, take it out and allow it to come to room temperature. For unknown reasons, it will now thicken much better. This is done in making commercial mayonnaise where they use fewer eggs. There is no reason to avoid cholesterol but commercial mayonnaise has less cholesterol than you might think for this reason.

## ALL-PURPOSE SAUCE

There are many variations of mayonnaise — obviously you can add anything you like — but common ones add some kind of tomato or aromatic relish. Russian dressing is mixture of mayonnaise and ketchup pretty much *verboten* with store-bought ketchup because of the added sugar. Adding store-bought salsa to mayonnaise produces a quick all-purpose sauce that can be used as salad dressing or served with fish or beef.

Classic French Remoulade is mayonnaise seasoned with chives, herbs and other aromatic stuff. There are numerous recipes. Like many New Orleans adaptations, the term *Remoulade* in Cajun cooking can mean anything and there are many variations with the characteristic multiple ingredients and overdoing everything. *Laissez rouler les bons temps.*

## AVOCADO

The secret to avocado is salt. If you serve it in slices, salt the slices and let them stand for a while. The secret to guacamole is restraint. Rub the bowl with garlic, salt the avocado and mash. (Don't overdo it, there should be some pieces). Depending on your taste, you can add other things but nothing tastes better than simple.

## A MEDITERRANEAN INTERLUDE

Mediterranean Diets are very popular and are considered to be some kind of ideal, because they are not explicitly low-fat (most of the time) while still allowing you to avoid saying low-carbohydrate. They are evocative of picnics in the verdant hills of Italy, but their real advantage is that nobody is sure what they are and hence they can be used to push your favorite diet recommendations.

What follows is a version of my blogpost. At the time, I had written of Mediterranean diets that "... nobody is sure what they are and hence there are no long term trials of the type that makes low-fat diets look so bad, as in the Women's Health Initiative." Well, there is at least one study claiming that one or another version of the diet would prevent heart disease. The paper [112] "*Primary Prevention of Cardiovascular Disease with a Mediterranean Diet*" was the most widely accessed paper at the New England Journal of Medicine. The data are shown in **Figure 24-1** with a calculation of the effect.

Table 3. **Outcomes According to Study Group.***

| End Point | Mediterranean Diet with EVOO (N=2543) | Mediterranean Diet with Nuts (N=2454) | Control Diet (N=2450) |
|---|---|---|---|
| event frequency | 3.8 % | 3.5 % | 4.4 % |
| Person-yr of follow-up | 11,852 | 10,365 | 9763 |
| Primary end point‡ | | | |
| No. of events | 96 | 83 | 109 |

Figure 24-1. Outcome data from the MEDIPREV trial [112] with approximate calculation of event frequency.

A sign of the continuing state of poor science in nutrition, the paper shows little effect of a Mediterranean diet while claiming that it will prevent heart attacks. In fact, it is not clear from the paper what people really ate beyond adding nuts or EVOO (whose meaning is left as a puzzle for the reader).

As described on one of the Greek food sites "anyone visiting Greece would wonder exactly what is meant by the Mediterranean diet, for while those of us outside the Med have been eating more whole grains, extra virgin olive oil and fresh vegetables .... as the Greeks become more affluent they eat more meat." I haven't been in Greece for many years but I remember quite a bit of meat even twenty years ago. Of course, affluence is a sometime thing in Greece as elsewhere but I'll offer my own view of Mediterranean eating.

## TOURNEDOS ROSSINI

Start with Giochinno Rossini. It is generally known that his life as a composer included significant time for food. He retired in his forties and devoted the rest of his life to cooking and eating. (William Tell was his last opera). Rossini said that he had only cried twice as an adult. The first time was when he heard Paganini play the violin and the second, when a truffled turkey fell in the water at a boating party.

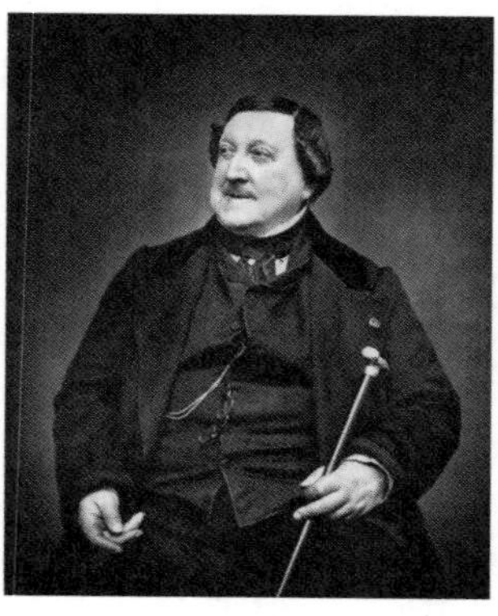

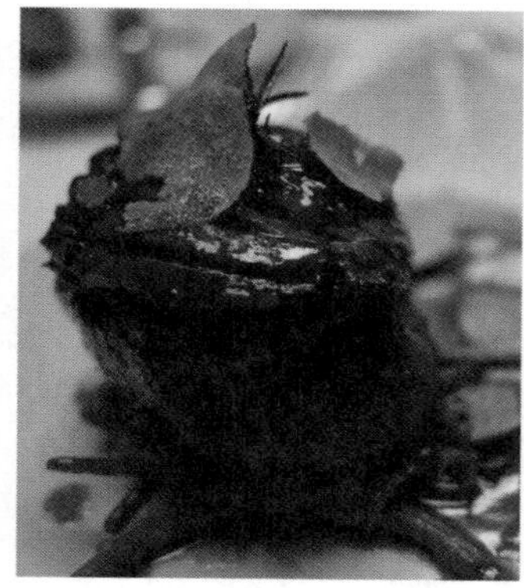

Giachino Rossini, photo by Carjat, 1865. Tournedos Rossini

Rossini's later life was spent more or less in seclusion so there is some uncertainty about his gastronomic experiences. It is not even clear whether Tournedos Rossini was made by him or for him. In fact, it is not even clear where the name Tournedos comes from. Derived from *tourner en dos*, turning to the back, it may refer to the method of cooking or possibly that the presenter had to turn his back during the preparation so as not to let anyone see the secret of the final sauce. The recipe, although simple in outline, has expensive ingredients and the final sauce will determine the quality of the chef. It simply involves frying a steak and then putting a slab of pate de foie gras with truffles on top and adding the sauce, based on a beef reduction.

1. Sauté the 4 center-cut filets mignons, chain muscle removed, 6 ounces in the 2 tablespoons (30 milliliters) clarified butter or vegetable oil on both sides until rare.
2. Remove excess fat with paper towel and place on heated plates.
3. Place warm *paté de foie gras* slices on each tournedo.
4. Cover with *Périgueux* Sauce.
5. Bring 1½ cups (375 milliliters) of *demi-glace* to slow simmer. Add 5 tablespoons (75 milliliters) of truffle essence and 2 ounces (50 grams) of either chopped or sliced truffles. Off heat and cover with tight-fitting lid, allow truffles to infuse into the sauce for at least 15 minutes. (The sauce using truffles sliced into shapes rather than pieces is called *Périgourdine*).
6. Finish with a little truffle butter.

## LARDO DI COLONNATA

Not really a make-at-home item, this traditional creation from Tuscany captures the care in processing that makes Italian food

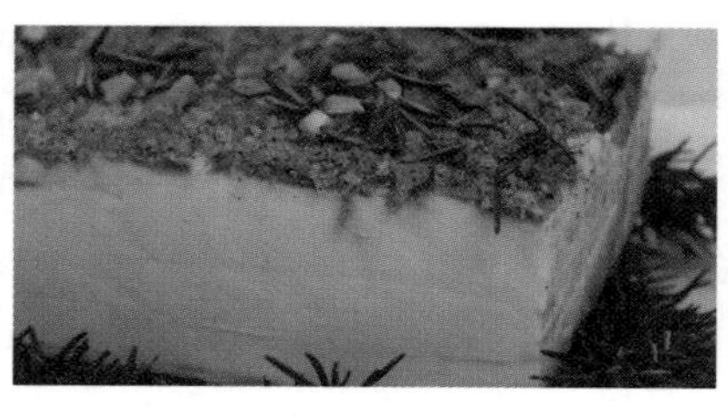

famous. The original curing method supposedly goes back to the year 1000 and has been handed down from generation to generation. The lard, of course, comes from pigs that have not undergone the genetic transformation that American pigs have. In any case, you will need marble tubs which you should keep in the basement assuming that there are no caves in your neighborhood. You rub the tubs with garlic and then layer the pork lard and cover with brine, add sea salt and spices and herbs. You continue with additional layers until the tub is full and then cover with a wooden lid. Curing time is about 6 to 10 months.

## GREEK BARBECUE

A sign of affluence, or at least an interest in food, is the availability of festive holiday foods all year. The most popular food for Easter is whole lamb roasted on a spit. The recipe is simple, if not convenient for the small family.

"You will need 1 whole lamb, skinned and gutted..." Seasoning can be simple, salt and pepper or the lamb can be basted with *ladolemono*, a mixture of lemon juice, olive oil and oregano.

Lamb on the spit "is especially popular [at Easter] because it follows 40 days of fasting for lent and people are definitely ready for some meat, though not everyone fasts the entire forty days." This reminds me of little known angle on the Seven Countries study.

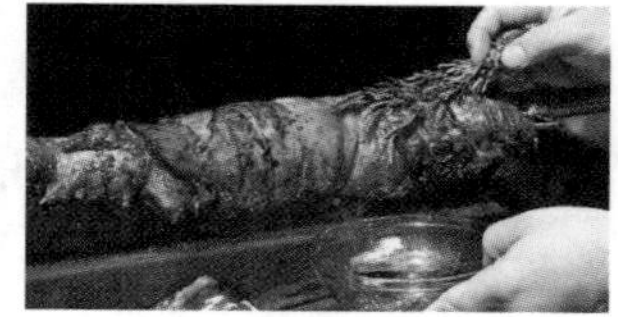

## ANCEL KEYS AUF NAXOS

The idea of a Mediterranean diet derives, in some way, from Ancel Keys's Seven Countries study. He discovered that the two countries with the highest consumption of fat, had the lowest incidence of cardiovascular disease (Crete) and the highest (Finland), and he attributed this to the type of fat, olive oil for Crete and animal fat for Finland. It was later pointed out that there were large differences in CVD between different areas of Finland that had the same diet. This information was ignored by Keys who was also a pioneer in this approach to conflicting data. As mentioned in Chapter 3, there was the additional problem that Keys collected data on Crete during Lent. Further revelations described in *The Big Fat Surprise* suggest that the Seven Countries Study and the fruit of that poisoned tree were largely the triumph of Keys's imagination over reality [11].

## KOKORETSI

Leopold Bloom ate with relish the inner organs of beasts and fowls. He liked thick giblet soup, nutty gizzards, a stuffed roast heart, liver slices fried with crust crumbs, fried hencod's roes.

> Most of all he liked grilled mutton kidneys which gave to his palate a fine tang of faintly scented urine.
>
> — James Joyce, ***Ulysses***.

Along with Greek Barbecue, it is traditional at Easter to serve *kokoretsi*, which is made from the internal organs of the lamb. Liver, spleen, heart, glands are threaded onto skewers along with the fatty membrane from the lamb intestines. When the skewer is full, the lamb intestines are wrapped around the whole creation. It is then barbecued over low heat for about 3-5 hours.

One of the regrettable aspects of the decline in food in the United States is the general disappearance of organ meats. The Paleo movement, however, may help with this.

Organ meats were once very popular; the quotation above is

probably the second most widely quoted passage from James Joyce's *Ulysses*. Because of various ethnic influences, organ meats were probably more popular in New York than in America (which begins somewhere in New Jersey). Entries on the internet, including Jimmy Moore 's confrontation with beef tongue are, to me, quite remarkable in that corned, (as in corned beef), tongue was once a staple of my diet.

When I was in grade school, there were many weeks where I would bring tongue sandwiches on Silvercup bread for lunch every day. Silvercup, made in Queens was the New York version of Wonder Bread. The Silvercup sign is still a fixture of the New York landscape — it is now the site of Silvercup Studios, the major film and television production company that kept the name when it bought the building in 1983 after the baking company folded. (You name the TV show, it was probably produced at Silvercup).

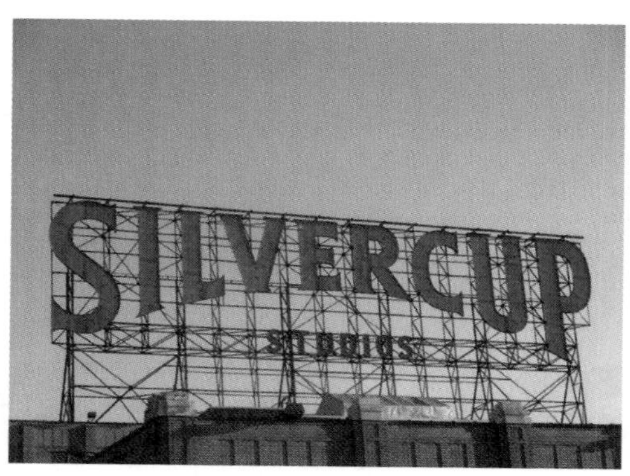


Of course, everybody draws the line somewhere. Although I used to eat with my friends at *Puglia*, the Little Italy restaurant that specialized in whole sheep's head, I passed on this delicacy mostly because of the eyeballs. Also, although you gotta' love the euphemism "Rocky Mountain Oysters," bull testicles don't do it for me, at least if I know for sure in advance. (I don't really mind, in retrospect, if the folk-myths about the tacos that I ate outside the bullring in Mexico City were really true).

## Digression on the Etymology of Food Words

Whether it is the steak itself or the cook whose back is turned in Tournedos, it is generally difficult to find the etymology of food words, although some are obvious. The conversion of Welsh Rabbit to Welsh Rarebit is surely an attempt to be more politically correct and avoid Welsh profiling. One disagreement that I remember from when I was in college is now settled. There were many ideas about the origin of the word pumpernickel. One of my favorites was that Napoleon had said that it was "*pain pour Nicole*" (his horse). Great but not true. It is now agreed that it comes from the Old German, *pampern*, to fart and *Nickel* meaning goblin, along the lines of Saint Nick for Santa Claus. So pumpernickel means Devil's Fart presumably due to the effect of the unprocessed grain that gives it its earthy quality. Which reminds me of the ADA's take on fiber that I quoted in one of my blogposts: "it is important that you increase your fiber intake gradually, to prevent stomach irritation, and that you increase your intake of water and other liquids, to prevent constipation." Foods with fiber "have a wealth of nutrition, containing many important vitamins and minerals." In fact, fiber "may contain nutrients that haven't even been discovered yet!" (Their exclamation point).

In Brooklyn, the Mediterranean diet means Italian sausage, largely from Southern Italy. I had always assumed that *Soppresata* (pronounced, as in Naples, without the final vowel) was so-called because it was super-saturated with fat, but since first writing this in a blogpost, my Italian friends have suggested that it comes from Soppressata, that is "pressed on," but this is also unconfirmed. There are many varieties but supposedly the best is from Calabria. For something like this, with so

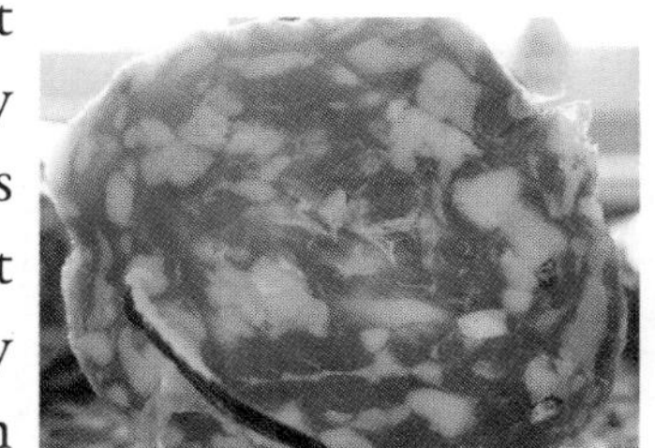

many varieties which each cook is sure is the best, there is no exact recipe, but you can get started with this from About.com Italian Food.

6.6 pounds (3 kg) of pork meat — a combination of loin and other lean cuts
1 pound (500 g) lard (a block of fat)
1 pound (500 g) pork side, the cut used to make bacon Salt, pepper
Cloves, garlic and herbs (rosemary, lemon peel, parsley, etc.)
½ cup *grappa* (I think that you could also use brandy if you want)

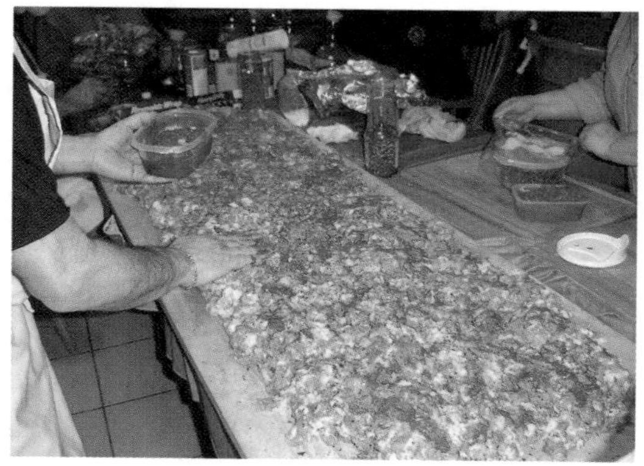

The basic idea is to remove all the gristle, and chop it with the lard and the pork side. About.com recommends a meat grinder but I suspect that the knife blade of a food processor is better. Then, wash the casing well in vinegar, dry it thoroughly, and rub with a mixture of well ground salt and pepper. "Shake away the excess, fill the casing, pressing down so as to expel all air, close the casing, and tie the salami with string. Hang for 2-3 days in a warm place, and then for a couple of months in a cool, dry, drafty spot and the *sopressata* is ready." At exactly what moment these simple, natural ingredients turn into processed red meat is unknown.

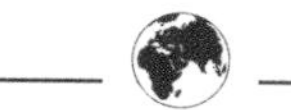

# Part 4

---

# The World Turned Upside Down

---

# Chapter 25

# The Second Low-Carb Revolution

The LEO Conference, held in Gothenburg, celebrates non-conformity in science. The 2008 meeting honored Uffe Ravnskov, the arch cholesterol skeptic [22, 27]. Speakers before me quoted Max Planck as saying that if you really wanted to introduce a new idea in science, you had to wait for the old generation to die out. When I spoke [113], I suggested that, since I was in that generation, we might want to do it a little sooner.

Coincidentally, it was in Sweden that we saw one of the key battles of the second low-carbohydrate revolution. Dr. Annika Dahlqvist lives in Njurunda, Sundsvall. She described, on her blog [114], how she discovered that a low-carbohydrate diet would help in her own battle with obesity and various health problems that included enteritis (irritable bowel syndrome or IBS), and gastritis, fibromyalgia, chronic fatigue syndrome and insomnia and snoring (the last two probably constitute the original "double whammy"). Recommending low-carbohydrate diets for her patients and publicly advertising her ideas drew a certain amount of media attention leading to

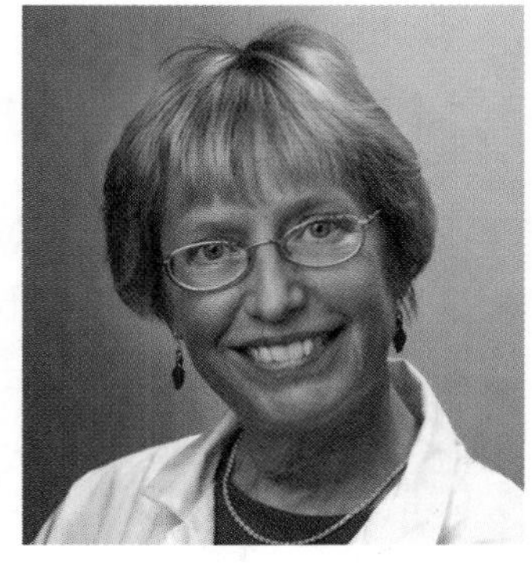

a run in with the authorities. In November 2006, she lost her job at Njurunda Medical center. Ultimately exonerated in January 2008, the National Board of medicine found that a low-carbohydrate diet was "consistent with good clinical practice." This was the likely prelude to the announcement in 2013 that the SBU (Swedish Council on Health Technology Assessment) endorsed low-carbohydrate diets for weight loss. The SBU is charged by the government with assessing health care treatments. While their statements were far from enthusiastic, it was one of a number of events in 2013 and 2014 that indicated the fall of the low-fat paradigm and greater or lesser acceptance of carbohydrate restriction.

The changes go on as I write this. We are still some distance from "Yorktown" and there is very strong resistance from the loyalists. The switch from demonizing fat to demonizing sugar is a mixed blessing; the same poor science is used to show how bad sugar is and starch is criticized only if it is "refined." Oddly, a major factor in the revolution is the recognition that, after all these years, the statins are not penicillin. They may, in fact, do more harm than good in many people who have not had a cardiovascular event.

## THE BIG PICTURE

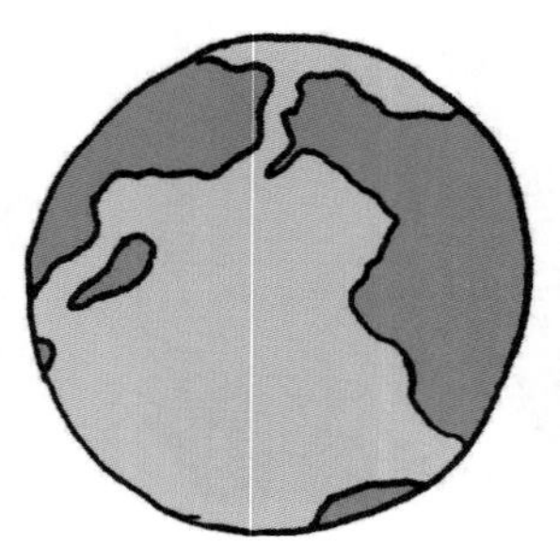

We are in the middle of a change in scientific thinking and one can anticipate a certain amount of chaos. For the individual dieter, however, the big picture is simple: If you have a weight problem, your best bet is to try a low-carbohydrate diet. Other dietary approaches may work but they don't have the backing of the science and they're less reliable. If you have diabetes, it is the first thing to try. More to the point, the recommendations of health agencies for high levels of carbohydrate, indeed, the necessity for any significant level of carbohydrate at all, are wrong.

Many people discover this for themselves — "I went to this conference and they had a buffet and I really pigged out on lobster and roast beef all weekend but somehow I didn't gain any weight." Nobody says that about the pasta buffet. The studies from Volek's lab described in Chapter 9 are classic and compelling but, in fact, almost every comparison of diets in the scientific literature shows that low-carbohydrate diets are more effective for weight loss and most other metabolic disturbances. The rationale is that dietary carbohydrate is the major stimulus for secretion of insulin which is a generally anabolic (building up) hormone. Chapter 14 explained how it is possible to lose more weight calorie-for-calorie on a low-carb diet — the bottom line is that insulin slows the break down (lipolysis) of fat and if you come in with another meal before the system has had a chance to deal with stored fat, it will accumulate. Also, on a low-carbohydrate diet, for whatever reasons, your appetite goes down. Most people find it easier to adhere to a carbohydrate-restricted diet than to any other.

The real plus for low-carbohydrate diets is anecdotal: It changes your interaction with food. For people with a weight problem, every meal is a battle. At every meal you're trying to make sure you don't cross some line of calories, fat, whatever. If you make a substantial cut in the amount of carbohydrates that you eat, even if you are not overly careful, even if you spend a couple of days at the conference buffet, you are unlikely to gain any weight. You lose a substantial part of your obsession with and anxiety about food.

If you don't have a weight problem, and you are in good health, you may not have to change your diet. You may feel better with fewer carbohydrates in your diet but there is no ideal diet, no perfect diet that we evolved to eat. The paleo diet, based on what kinds of foods were assumed to be available as we evolved, is part of the current diet scene, but we really evolved to be adaptable to different nutritional environments. It is good to know that you don't have a biological need for any carbohydrate and that the opposite of lowering fat is not eating all the fat in sight. It might well be, as critics of low-carbohydrate diet say, that the recommended strategy include assurances that "you can eat all the fat that you want," but the emphasis is really on "want." Fat is filling. How much do you want? It is important to stress that the low-fat idea was not originally instituted to deal with obesity but rather to prevent heart disease (which it didn't) and it always had a moralistic overtone. It was somebody's idea of what we should have been eating during the millennia in which haute cuisine evolved and the period in which people perfected sausages and other food in ethnic cuisines. The low-fat idea was the work of puritans. It gave rise to the obesity epidemic and the fact that many people did *not* get fat is only a testament to the adaptability of humans in dealing with all kinds of food.

## "SUDDENLY LAST SUMMER." TRIUMPH OF LOW-CARB

My blogpost hit it pretty well and I repeat it here:

It was in July of 2012 that I suddenly realized that we had won, at least scientifically. It was now clear that we had a consistent set of scientific ideas that supported the importance of insulin signaling in basic biochemistry and cell biology and that there was a continuum with the role of dietary carbohydrate restriction in obesity, diabetes, or for general health. The practical considerations, how much to eat of this, how much to eat of that, were still problematical but now we had the kernel of a scientific principle. In fact, it was not so much that we had the answer as that we had the right question. In science, the question is frequently more important than the answer. Of course, winning wasn't the original idea. When my colleagues and I got into this, about ten years ago, coming from basic biochemistry, we hadn't anticipated that it would be such a battle, that there would be so much resistance to what we thought was normal scientific practice.

Surprisingly, it was cancer studies that showed us how it all fit together. The locale was the conference in Washington, D.C. called "Metabolism, Diet and Disease." The first day of the conference would probably be more accurately described as Metabolism, Drugs and Cancers. A surprising thread in the various talks — surprising to me — was the interaction between obesity and cancer. Figure 25-1 shows how strong this is.

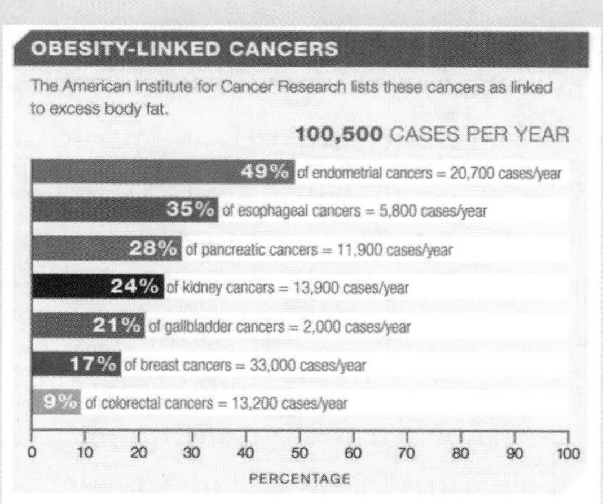


FIGURE 25-1. Correlation of Obesity and Cancer Data from the American Institute for Cancer Research.

Less surprising, because of the numerous studies, was the effect of calorie restriction, the apparent basis for the connection between obesity and cancer: reducing calories has been shown to reliably increase longevity and to control cancer in animals. An additional thread was that the hormone insulin popped up as a major player in various experiments in cancer. The identification of downstream signaling elements — the compounds and proteins that transmit the information about cell stimulation to the interior of the cell

— were important results and, again, they frequently pointed to the components of insulin pathways and even to an association between cancer and diabetes. This was not new to me — outstanding experiments had pointed the way to the critical role for insulin and I always wondered why the connection to dietary carbohydrate was not made. In any case, the second day of the conference included presentations on dietary carbohydrate restriction. Although not listed on the organizing committee, Gary Taubes had been one of the organizers and deserves credit for a program with both cancer people and low-carbohydrate people.

My colleague Dr. Eugene Fine presented a poster at the Washington conference. Many conferences have poster sessions in which presenters pin typically 4 x 6 foot posters to easels and participants can discuss the subject matter with the presenter. Posters don't always have a big impact and we are grateful to Gary Taubes for making Gene's poster known to the main speakers. The work, now published in the journal *Nutrition* [13], describes a small study conducted with ten seriously ill cancer patients. The study had the modest goal of showing that a ketogenic diet was a safe and feasible regimen and, in fact, the patients did well and six of ten had stable disease or partial remission. By itself, this study would usually been considered only a small step forward, but, in fact, it was a key link in tying together the field of carbohydrate restriction and the field of cell signaling in normal and cancer cells. An experiment such as this is difficult to do — patients need to have refused or failed chemotherapy, that is, for patients to agree to experimental nutrition approaches, they usually have exhausted the traditional regimens. One way to look at the significance is that, given what we know about insulin and what we know about low-carbohydrate diets, the experiment should have been done twenty years ago. There were simply two lines of thought that had to be brought together.

Now in hindsight, it seems that workers in carbohydrate restriction should have paid more attention to downstream cell signaling; we thought that the role of insulin in system biochemistry made it clear that carbohydrate restriction was built on a solid foundation. The resistance to the idea seemed incomprehensible and parochial but this conference made it clear that there was more that was needed to make a consistent biological story. It became clear that there was a conceptual barrier to acceptance of carbohydrate restriction beyond the traditional resistance to anything associated with the Atkins diet. There was a mindset that prevented adequate synthesis of all the information.

## Targeting Cancer Through Insulin Inhibition

Much of the valuable work on cell biology was informed by an approach to disease that tended to downplay the biochemistry at the upstream-stimulus level, namely, what you eat. The major goal was to characterize the individual components in the inner working of the cell and to search for those components that were specifically malfunctioning in pathological states. These agents, primarily proteins, could then be targeted with drugs, either directly or indirectly, sometimes through their synthesis at the genomic level. With the important observation that calorie restriction could ameliorate or prevent cancer, a link with obesity was established and, in some way, excess calories became interchangeable with weight gain. The obesity-cancer link became a serial link and it was assumed, as it is assumed in nutrition, that preventing obesity was part of preventing associated pathologies. In this way, successes of carbohydrate restriction in improving cardiovascular risk factors, for example, have frequently been dismissed as due to the attendant weight loss. This, despite the evidence that the improvements in risk factors or other outcomes persist even in the absence of weight loss or even when benefits were demonstrated in eucaloric trials.

The rationale, then, was that calorie restriction, the recognized approach to obesity, would point to those intracellular components that could be targeted for drug development. In many cases, this was a conceptual error. In nutrition, it is likely that the doctrine of "a calorie is a calorie" is the single greatest impediment to understanding. The identification of obesity with excess calories, and the failure to look beyond this effect, that is, the failure to ask how the separate nutrients, carbohydrate, fat and protein individually affected cellular metabolism and how these effects interacted — there is, after all, no calorie receptor — compromised otherwise sophisticated and informative experiments. Similarly, we and other workers in carbohydrate restriction failed to see how important it was to look at downstream cellular signaling.

Gene's study treated ten seriously ill cancer patients with low-carbohydrate ketogenic diets and showed that it was a safe and feasible regimen for such patients. The rationale followed from the fact that rapidly growing tumors have a requirement for glucose (cannot metabolize fat or ketone bodies) but simply reducing carbohydrates to give the host an advantage was unlikely to be effective since blood glucose is regulated to stay fairly constant and the cancers are also good at getting whatever glucose is there, over-express GLUT1 receptors, the non-insulin-dependent glucose receptor.

Ketosis, the state associated with very low energy or very low-carbohydrate intake, held some promise. Fine's hypothesis was that if we think of cancer in terms of genetics, we could think of cancer cells as having evolved through the life of the individual, an individual whose systemic environment, in a modern setting, would be unlikely to have any significant level of ketosis, that is, would be unlikely to provide any selective pressure for the adaptation to use of ketone bodies as a fuel source. The host, on the other hand, was well-adapted to this substrate — it is unlikely that our ancestors regularly had three squares a day. Some fraction of cancer lines, then, might not deal well with a ketotic environment.

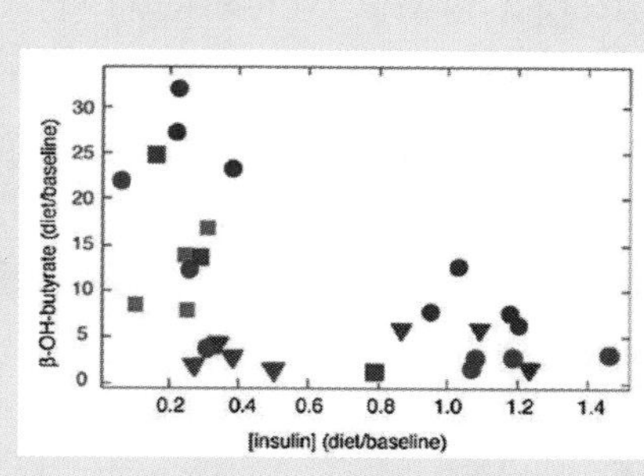


FIGURE 25-2. Ketonemia versus insulinemia: the lowest insulinemia correlated with the highest ketonemia levels. Uniquely colored symbols represent values for each patient.

In the experiment, it turned out that those patients who became stable or showed partial remission had the highest level of ketone bodies. **Figure 25-2** shows individual time points with different symbols for each patient. As expected, there was a correlation between ketone bodies and insulin levels.

Although this was a small sample, **Figure 25-3A** shows that the patients were divided in terms of outcome into those who had progressive disease or those who became stable or showed partial remission. The level of ketone bodies was the best predictor of this outcome. **Figure 25-3B shows, on the other hand, that improvements did not depend on** calories or weight loss. Patients who demonstrated stable disease or partial remission had a three-fold higher average ketotic response compared to those with continued progressive disease. In distinction, both groups showed similar calorie deficits or, as shown, degree of weight loss, suggesting that the well-established benefits in caloric restriction reflect an underlying mechanism beyond the energy itself.

## SUMMARY

A small study in advance cancer patients might be considered only a minor step forward but, in fact, it ties into a vast area of research on the downstream signaling in both cancer and normal cells — that is, the changes in the cell following stimulation by an external food or hormones. Of particular interest is the well-known effect of calorie restriction. It was widely understood that dietary calorie restriction would have a therapeutic effect on animals with cancer and, in addition, reducing calories was the only way to prolong life in animals. Studies following this idea showed that it was an insulin pathway that was involved. Gene Fine's study nailed the link for us. It is an encouraging situation, because if this is the worst of times in nutrition, it is also the golden age of biology and bringing all of the science to bear on the problem has great promise indeed.

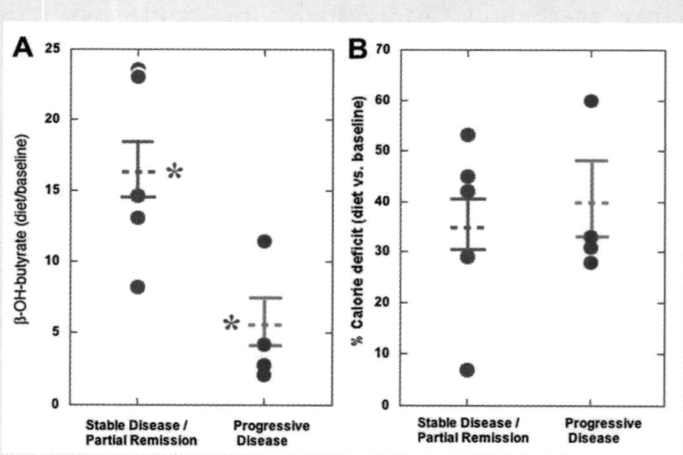


FIGURE 25-3. **A.** Ketosis versus disease progression. Patients who demonstrated stable disease or partial remission had much greater ketotic response compared to those with progressive disease.
**B.** Calorie deficit *vs.* outcome: the stable disease/partial remission and progressive disease groups showed no difference in calorie reduction.

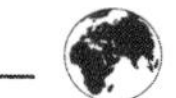

# Chapter 26

# Summary And The Second Revolution

## WHERE ARE WE NOW?

The low-carbohydrate revolution of 2002 was precipitated by the popular exposés of the low-fat-diet-heart hypothesis and its failed tests. The well-armed forces mustered by diet-heart fared poorly in the early confrontations with the actual experimental evidence. The loose band of revolutionaries let them set up the battle as they chose. Without laboring the analogy, the literature was along the lines of wartime reports and as in many revolutions, success was short-lived, done in largely by resistance from the medical and nutritional community. Scientific developments, however, have continued to reinforce the idea that control of metabolism by insulin and other hormones is the key factor in weight loss, diabetes and the metabolic syndrome. Now classic, well-controlled experiments nailed the idea. Carbohydrate restriction is the best treatment for all of the features of metabolic syndrome and, consistent with the nature of a disease of carbohydrate intolerance, carbohydrate restriction is the "default" treatment for diabetes (the one to try first). At the same time, tests of the diet-heart hypothesis continue to be done and continue to "underwhelm." Bias against publishing studies of low-carbohydrate diets may also be as strong as ever. A low-carbohydrate paper submitted to *New England Journal of Medicine*, *British Medical Journal* or other major journals will be treated with superficial politeness but palpable disdain.

For the scientist and consumer alike, the situation has become more confusing, more ambiguous. A major factor appears to be a near disintegration of standards. Epidemiologic studies trying to show the risks in saturated fat (good fats-bad fats), in red-meat, in sugar (good carbs-bad carbs) continue to proliferate. In the absence of critical peer review, they are accepted for publication and their conclusions are presented at face value in the media, notably online medical publications which distill their essence for physicians. The same journals and sometimes the same popular medical sites publish papers describing how bad the obesity epidemic is and directly, or by implication, blame the patient. These same journals also ironically publish articles describing the breakdown in standards in the medical literature.

The effects of carbohydrates *per se* are generally ignored. If they are mentioned at all, it is always to point out the dangers in their "refined" state. Wild, exaggerated effects are attributed to sugar but these are seen as separate from carbohydrates and the lipophobes seem to have maintained control of the market — low-fat products are the major form of every kind of product in the supermarket including "half and half." And yet, there is a sense that it is all over. The accumulating failures of low-fat and the popular books and articles are finally taking their toll. The publication in May of 2014 of Nina Teicholz's *The Big Fat Surprise* [11] may be the second low-carb revolution's *Common Sense* but whatever it is that deals the death blow, the nutritional establishment has cracked. Squabbling among themselves is a sure sign. Walter Willett, head of the Harvard School of Public Health calling for retraction of a published paper is embarrassing to us all (http://bit.ly/ 1znPrs8).

## THE FUTURE

> "... it is, perhaps, the end of the beginning."
>
> — Winston Churchill.

Nutrition, however serious a health issue, is not at the same moral level as civil rights but it is clear that, paraphrasing Martin Luther King on Jim Crow:

Low-fat is dead. It is just a question of how long and expensive you want to make the funeral. Continual failures of large trials and what must be reasonably seen as a refusal to accept outcomes, in combination with the success of alternative approaches, control of metabolism through the glucose-insulin axis makes a new method of thinking inevitable.

Surprisingly, the key scientific focus of the second low-carbohydrate revolution may be cancer. It has long been recognized that total caloric restriction, at least in animals, was of benefit in slowing progression of disease and extending life. While this led to the questionable paradigm of identifying calories with obesity and identifying obesity, in turn, as stimulating physiologic effects, the primary observation is real and the study of downstream cell signaling that follows from it has been very productive. The extent to which the effects of calorie restriction are due to the *de facto* reduction in carbohydrate is an important question not yet fully examined. The picture of the internal workings of the cell has, in any case, pointed to the critical role of insulin.

Research in carbohydrate restriction has probably under-estimated the importance and value of detailed downstream stimulus-response coupling in cells, while cell biology has been remiss in insufficient attention to the nature of upstream signaling, that is, the effect of diet. It is not calories but carbohydrate that stimulates insulin release and obesity is largely a response, not a stimulus. In addition, ketone bodies, originally considered primarily a marker for fat breakdown is now understood to be a more global cell signal. The possibility of cancer treatment based on the theory that tumors may be more poorly adapted to use this energy source (because of their evolution within the lifespan of the individual) [13] is one specific approach tested in a small pilot study. More generally, the long-overdue tests of carbohydrate restriction as a cancer therapy may be the important battleground in the second low-carbohydrate revolution. The new scientific paradigm may also be better received in the area of oncology due to the failure to otherwise contain the disease. In obesity, diabetes and metabolic diseases, it may be necessary to clear out the backlog of biased, unscientific and statistically flawed studies that have so far impeded progress. New standards will have to be implemented to improve the future literature. Scientific truth is its own justification but in this area, relief of much human suffering makes it of importance in the society at large. Progress may be slow but it is necessary that the nutrition world be turned upside down.

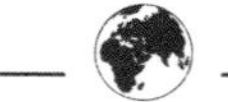

# Acknowledgements

Two people, Monika Hendry and Paula Nedved, have made this book possible. Their continual encouragement, their probing questions and excellent proof-reading abilities kept the book alive through periods in which there were many doubts and discouragements. I am also grateful to Prof. Wendy Pogozelski for Chapter 11 and for enthusiasm about the final product. Insofar as this book is scientifically accurate it is due to my interactions with my colleagues, Drs. Eugene J. Fine, Frederick Sacks, Jeff S. Volek, Eric C. Westman, Jay Wortman, Steve Phinney and many others who have for so long tried to be loyal opposition to the medical and nutritional monarchy. Thanks also to members of the Nutrition and Metabolism Society and Facebook friends, especially the pseudonymous Amanda B. Wreckondwith, who have provided continued encouragement. I am grateful to the State University of New York Downstate Medical Center who has given me the freedom to work and think outside the box.

# Bibliography


1. Pogozelski W, Arpaia N, Priore S: **The Metabolic Effects of Low-carbohydrate Diets and Incorporation into a Biochemistry Course.** *Biochemistry and Molecular Biology Education* 2005, 33:91-100.
2. Feinman RD, Makowske M: **Metabolic Syndrome and Low-carbohydrate Ketogenic Diets in the Medical School Biochemistry Curriculum.** *Metabolic Syndrome and Related Disorders* 2003, 1:189-198.
3. Makowske M, Feinman RD: **Nutrition education: a questionnaire for assessment and teaching.** *Nutr J* 2005, 4(1):2.
4. Hu FB, Stampfer MJ, Manson JE, Rimm E, Colditz GA, Rosner BA, Hennekens CH, Willett WC: **Dietary fat intake and the risk of coronary heart disease in women.** *N Engl J* Med 1997, 337(21): 1491-1499.
5. Pollan M: **In defense of food: an eater's manifesto.** New York: Penguin Press; 2008.
6. Jakobsen MU, O'Reilly EJ, Heitmann BL, Pereira MA, Balter K, Fraser GE, Goldbourt U, Hallmans G, Knekt P, Liu S *et al*: **Major types of dietary fat and risk of coronary heart disease: a pooled analysis of 11 cohort studies.** *Am J Clin Nutr* 2009, 89(5):1425-1432.
7. Siri-Tarino PW, Sun Q , Hu FB, Krauss RM: **Meta-analysis of prospective cohort studies evaluating the association of saturated fat with cardiovascular disease.** *Am J Clin Nutr* 2010, 91(3): 535-546.
8. Siri-Tarino PW, Sun Q , Hu FB, Krauss RM: **Saturated fat, carbohydrate, and cardiovascular disease.** *Am J Clin Nutr* 2010, 91(3): 502-509.

9. American Diabetes Association: **Nutrition Recommendations and Interventions for Diabetes-2008.** *Diabetes Care* 2008, 31(Suppl 1):S61-S78.
10. American Diabetes Association: **Nutrition Recommendations and Interventions for Diabetes-2013.** *Diabetes Care* 2013, 36(Suppl 1):S12-S32.
11. Teicholz N: **The Big Fat Surprise. Why Butter, Meat & Cheese Belong in a Health Diet.** New York: Simon & Schuster; 2014.
12. Reaven GM: **Role of Insulin Resistance in human disease.** Diabetes 1988, 37:1595-1607.
13. Fine EJ, Segal-Isaacson CJ, Feinman RD, Herszkopf S, Romano MC, Tomuta N, Bontempo AF, Negassa A, Sparano JA: **Targeting insulin inhibition as a metabolic therapy in advanced cancer: a pilot safety and feasibility dietary trial in 10 patients.** *Nutrition* 2012, 28(10):1028-1035.
14. Kannel WB, Gordon T: **The Framingham Study: diet and regulation of serum cholesterol, Section 24.** In: *The Framingham Study: An Epidemiological Investigation of Cardiovascular Disease.* edn. Edited by Kannel WB, Gordon T. Washington, DC; 1970.
15. Hahn F, Eades MR, Eades MD: **The slow burn fitness revolution : the slow motion exercise that will change your body in 30 minutes a week, 1st edn.** New York, NY: Broadway Books; 2003.
16. Westman EC, Phinney SD, Volek J: **The new Atkins for a new you: the ultimate diet for shedding weight and feeling great forever.** New York: Simon & Schuster; 2010.
17. Eades MR, Eades MD: **Protein Power.** New York: Bantam Books; 1996.
18. Feinman RD, Vernon MC, Westman EC: **Low carbohydrate diets in family practice: what can we learn from an internet-based support group.** *Nutr J* 2006, 5:26.
19. Somers S: **Suzanne Somers' eat great, lose weight,** 1st edn. New York: Crown; 1997.
20. Atkins RC: **Dr. Atkins' New Diet Revolution.** New York: Avon Books; 2002.

21. Keys A: **Diet and blood cholesterol in population survey–lessons from analysis of the data from a major survey in Israel.** *Am J Clin Nutr* 1988, 48(5):1161-1165.
22. Ravnskov U: **The Cholesterol Myths: Exposing the Fallacy that Cholesterol and Saturated Fat Cause Heart Disease.** Washington, DC: NewTrends Publishing, Inc.; 2000.
23. Taubes G: **Good Calories, Bad Calories.** New York: Alfred A. Knopf; 2007.
24. Colpo A: **The Great Cholesterol Con**: Lulu Press; 2006.
25. Keys A: **Coronary heart disease in seven countries.** 1970, 41 (Suppl):1-211.
26. Taubes G: **The Soft Science of Dietary Fat.** *Science* 2001, 291:2536-2545.
27. Ravnskov U: **Cholesterol - friend or foe?** *Scand Cardiovasc J* 2007: this volume.
28. Sarri K, Kafatos A: **The Seven Countries Study in Crete: olive oil, Mediterranean diet or fasting?** *Public Health Nutr* 2005, 8(6):666.
29. Forsythe CE, Phinney SD, Feinman RD, Volk BM, Freidenreich D, Quann E, Ballard K, Puglisi MJ, Maresh CM, Kraemer WJ *et al*: **Limited effect of dietary saturated fat on plasma saturated fat in the context of a low carbohydrate diet.** *Lipids* 2010, 45(10):947-962.
30. Forsythe CE, Phinney SD, Fernandez ML, Quann EE, Wood RJ, Bibus DM, Kraemer WJ, Feinman RD, Volek JS: **Comparison of low fat and low carbohydrate diets on circulating Fatty Acid composition and markers of inflammation.** *Lipids* 2008, 43(1):65-77.
31. Volek JS, Fernandez ML, Feinman RD, Phinney SD: **Dietary carbohydrate restriction induces a unique metabolic state positively affecting atherogenic dyslipidemia, fatty acid partitioning, and metabolic syndrome.** *Prog Lipid Res* 2008, 47(5): 307-318.
32. McLaughlin T, Reaven G, Abbasi F, Lamendola C, Saad M, Waters D, Simon J, Krauss RM: **Is there a simple way to identify**

**insulin-resistant individuals at increased risk of cardiovascular disease?** *Am J Cardiol* 2005, 96(3):399-404.

33. Wills G: **Lincoln at Gettysburg : the words that remade America.** New York: Simon & Schuster; 1992.

34. Brillat S, Fisher MFK: M. F. K. Fisher's translation of **The physiology of taste : or, Meditations on transcendental gastronomy**, 1st Harvest/HBJ edn. New York: Harcourt Brace Jovanovich; 1978.

35. Taubes G: **What if It's All Been a Big Fat Lie?** *New York Times Magazine* 2002.

36. Naughton T: **The McGovern Report**. In.; 2007.

37. Foster GD, Wyatt HR, Hill JO, McGuckin BG, Brill C, Mohammed BS, Szapary PO, Rader DJ, Edman JS, Klein S: **A randomized trial of a low-carbohydrate diet for obesity.** *N Engl J Med* 2003, 348(21): 2082-2090.

38. Volek JS, Feinman RD: **Carbohydrate restriction improves the features of Metabolic Syndrome. Metabolic Syndrome may be defined by the response to carbohydrate restriction.** *Nutr Metab (Lond)* 2005, 2:31.

39. Leren P: **The Oslo diet-heart study. Eleven-year report.** *Circulation* 1970, 42(5):935-942.

40. Leren P, Helgeland A, Hjermann I, Holme I: **The Oslo study: CHD risk factors, socioeconomic influences, and intervention.** *Am Heart J* 1983, 106(5 Pt 2):1200-1206.

41. Paul O, Lepper MH, Phelan WH, Dupertuis GW, Macmillan A, Mc KH, Park H: **A longitudinal study of coronary heart disease.** *Circulation* 1963, 28:20-31.

42. Howard BV, Manson JE, Stefanick ML, Beresford SA, Frank G, Jones B, Rodabough RJ, Snetselaar L, Thomson C, Tinker L *et al*: **Low-fat dietary pattern and weight change over 7 years: the Women's Health Initiative Dietary Modification Trial.** *JAMA* 2006, 295(1):39-49.

43. Howard BV, Van Horn L, Hsia J, Manson JE, Stefanick ML,

Wassertheil-Smoller S, Kuller LH, LaCroix AZ, Langer RD, Lasser NL *et al*: **Low-fat dietary pattern and risk of cardiovascular disease: the Women's Health Initiative Randomized Controlled Dietary Modification Trial.** *JAMA* 2006, 295(6):655-666.

44. Tinker LF, Bonds DE, Margolis KL, Manson JE, Howard BV, Larson J, Perri MG, Beresford SA, Robinson JG, Rodriguez B *et al*: **Low-fat dietary pattern and risk of treated diabetes mellitus in postmenopausal women: the Women's Health Initiative randomized controlled dietary modification trial.** *Arch Intern Med* 2008, 168(14):1500-1511.

45. Brehm BJ, Seeley RJ, Daniels SR, D'Alessio DA: **A randomized trial comparing a very low carbohydrate diet and a calorie-restricted low fat diet on body weight and cardiovascular risk factors in healthy women.** *J Clin Endocrinol Metab* 2003, 88(4):1617-1623.

46. Nordmann AJ, Nordmann A, Briel M, Keller U, Yancy WS, Jr., Brehm BJ, Bucher HC: **Effects of low-carbohydrate vs low-fat diets on weight loss and cardiovascular risk factors: a meta-analysis of randomized controlled trials.** *Arch Intern Med* 2006, 166(3):285-293.

47. Borghjid S, Feinman RD: **Response of C57Bl/6 mice to a carbohydrate-free diet.** *Nutr Metab (Lond)* 2012, 9(1):69.

48. Ahren B, Scheurink AJ: **Marked hyperleptinemia a er high-fat diet associated with severe glucose intolerance in mice.** *Eur J Endocrinol* 1998, 139(4):461-467.

49. Winzell MS, Ahren B: **The high-fat diet-fed mouse: a model for studying mechanisms and treatment of impaired glucose tolerance and type 2 diabetes.** *Diabetes* 2004, 53 Suppl 3:S215-219.

50. Klein S, Wolfe RR: **Carbohydrate restriction regulates the adaptive response to fasting.** *Am J Physiol* 1992, 262(5 Pt 1):E631-636.

51. Borsheim E, Cree MG, Tipton KD, Elliott TA, Aarsland A, Wolfe RR: **Effect of carbohydrate intake on net muscle protein synthesis during recovery from resistance exercise.** *J Appl Physiol* 2004, 96(2): 674-678.

52. Harper HA: **Review of Physiological Chemistry**, 8th edn. Los Altos, CA: Lange Medical Publications; 1961.
53. Martin DW, Mayes PA, Rodwell VW, Granner K: **Harper's review of biochemistry**, 20th edn. Los Altos, Calif.: LANGE Medical Publications; 1985.
54. Bray GA: **The epidemic of obesity and changes in food intake: the Fluoride Hypothesis.** *Physiol Behav* 2004, 82(1):115-121.
55. Young FG: **Claude Bernard and the discovery of glycogen; a century of retrospect.** *British medical journal* 1957, 1(5033):1431-1437.
56. Cahill GF, Jr.: **Starvation in man.** *N Engl J Med* 1970, 282(12):668-675.
57. Stanhope KL, Schwarz JM, Keim NL, Griffen SC, Bremer AA, Graham JL, Hatcher B, Cox CL, Dyachenko A, Zhang W *et al*: **Consuming fructose-sweetened, not glucose-sweetened, beverages increases visceral adiposity and lipids and decreases insulin sensitivity in overweight/obese humans.** *J Clin Invest* 2009, 119(5):1322-1334.
58. Lanaspa MA, Ishimoto T, Li N, Cicerchi C, Orlicky DJ, Ruzycki P, Rivard C, Inaba S, Roncal-Jimenez CA, Bales ES *et al*: **Endogenous fructose production and metabolism in the liver contributes to the development of metabolic syndrome.** *Nature communications* 2013, 4:2434.
59. Taubes G, Couzens CK: **Big Sugar's Sweet Little Lies**. In: *Mother Jones* 2012.
60. Lin J, Yang R, Tarr PT, Wu PH, Handschin C, Li S, Yang W, Pei L, Uldry M, Tontonoz P *et al*: **Hyperlipidemic effects of dietary saturated fats mediated through PGC-1beta coactivation of SREBP.** *Cell* 2005, 120(2):261-273.
61. Volek JS, Phinney SD, Forsythe CE, Quann EE, Wood RJ, Puglisi MJ, Kraemer WJ, Bibus DM, Fernandez ML, Feinman RD: **Carbohydrate Restriction has a More Favorable Impact on the Metabolic Syndrome than a Low Fat Diet.** *Lipids* 2009, 44(4):297-309.

62. Raatz SK, Bibus D, Thomas W, Kris-Etherton P: **Total fat intake modifies plasma fatty acid composition in humans.** *J Nutr* 2001, 131(2):231-234.

63. Westman EC, Vernon MC: **Has carbohydrate-restriction been forgotten as a treatment for diabetes mellitus? A perspective on the ACCORD study design.** *Nutr Metab (Lond)* 2008, 5:10.

64. Rizza RA: **Pathogenesis of fasting and postprandial hyperglycemia in type 2 diabetes: implications for therapy.** *Diabetes* 2010, 59(11):2697-2707.

65. Westman EC, Yancy WS, Jr., Humphreys M: **Dietary treatment of diabetes mellitus in the pre-insulin era (1914-1922).** *Perspect Biol Med* 2006, 49(1):77-83.

66. Jenkins DJ, Kendall CW, McKeown-Eyssen G, Josse RG, Silverberg J, Booth GL, Vidgen E, Josse AR, Nguyen TH, Corrigan S *et al*: **Effect of a low-glycemic index or a high-cereal fiber diet on type 2 diabetes: a randomized trial.** *JAMA* 2008, 300(23):2742-2753.

67. Westman EC, Yancy WS, Mavropoulos JC, Marquart M, McDuffie JR: **The Effect of a Low-Carbohydrate, Ketogenic Diet Versus a Low-Glycemic Index Diet on Glycemic Control in Type 2 Diabetes Mellitus.** *Nutr Metab (Lond)* 2008, 5(36).

68. Yancy WS, Jr., Foy M, Chalecki AM, Vernon MC, Westman EC: **A low-carbohydrate, ketogenic diet to treat type 2 diabetes.** *Nutr Metab (Lond)* 2005, 2:34.

69. Stratton IM, Kohner EM, Aldington SJ, Turner RC, Holman RR, Manley SE, Matthews DR: **UKPDS 50: risk factors for incidence and progression of retinopathy in Type II diabetes over 6 years from diagnosis.** *Diabetologia* 2001, 44(2):156-163.

70. Reaven G: **Syndrome X: 10 years a er.** *Drugs* 1999, 58 Suppl 1:19-20; discussion 75-82.

71. Reaven GM: **The Insulin Resistance Syndrome: Definition and Dietary Approaches to Treatment.** *Annu Rev Nutr* 2004.

72. Reaven GM: **The metabolic syndrome: requiescat in pace.** *Clin*

*Chem* 2005, 51(6):931-938.

73. Yancy WS, Jr., Provenzale D, Westman EC: **Improvement of gastroesophageal reflux disease after initiation of a low-carbohydrate diet: five brief case reports.** *Altern Ther Health Med* 2001, 7(6):120, 116-129.

74. Skinner BF: **About behaviorism**, 1st edn. New York,: Knopf; distributed by Random House; 1974.

75. Feinman RD, Fine EJ: **Nonequilibrium thermodynamics and energy efficiency in weight loss diets.** *Theor Biol Med Model* 2007, 4:27.

76. Hirsch J, Hudgins LC, Leibel RL, Rosenbaum M: **Diet composition and energy balance in humans.** *Am J Clin Nutr* 1998, 67(3 Suppl):551S-555S.

77. Foster GD, Wyatt HR, Hill JO, Makris AP, Rosenbaum DL, Brill C, Stein RI, Mohammed BS, Miller B, Rader DJ *et al*: **Weight and metabolic outcomes after 2 years on a low-carbohydrate versus low-fat diet: a randomized trial.** *Ann Intern Med* 2010, 153(3):147-157.

78. Gannon MC, Nuttall FQ: **Control of blood glucose in type 2 diabetes without weight loss by modification of diet composition.** *Nutr Metab (Lond)* 2006, 3:16.

79. Feinman RD, Fine EJ: **Perspective on Fructose.** *Nutr Metab (Lond)* 2013, 9.

80. Bray GA, Smith SR, de Jonge L, Xie H, Rood J, Martin CK, Most M, Brock C, Mancuso S, Redman LM: **Effect of dietary protein content on weight gain, energy expenditure, and body composition during overeating: a randomized controlled trial.** *JAMA* 2012, 307(1):47-55.

81. Ioannidis JP: Meta-research: **The art of getting it wrong.** *Res Synth Meth* 2010, 1:169-184.

82. Ioannidis JP, Tatsioni A, Karassa FB: **Who is afraid of reviewers' comments? Or, why anything can be published and anything can be cited.** *Eur J Clin Invest* 2010, 40(4):285-287.

83. Ziliak ST, McCloskey DN: **The cult of statistical significance : how the standard error costs us jobs, justice, and lives.** Ann Arbor: University of Michigan Press; 2008.
84. Wainer H: **Medical Illuminations.** Oxford, UK: Oxford University Press; 2014.
85. Norman GR, Streiner DL: **PDQ statistics**, 3rd edn. Hamilton, Ont.: B.C. Decker; 2003.
86. Appel LJ, Sacks FM, Carey VJ, Obarzanek E, Swain JF, Miller ER, 3rd, Conlin PR, Erlinger TP, Rosner BA, Laranjo NM *et al*: **Effects of protein, monounsaturated fat, and carbohydrate intake on blood pressure and serum lipids: results of the OmniHeart randomized trial.** *JAMA* 2005, 294(19):2455-2464.
87. Watson JD, Crick FH: **Molecular structure of nucleic acids; a structure for deoxyribose nucleic acid.** *Nature* 1953, 171(4356): 737-738.
88. Weinberg S: **Dreams of a final theory,** 1st edn. New York: Pantheon Books; 1992.
89. Mukherjee S: **The emperor of all maladies : a biography of cancer,** Large print edn. Waterville, Me.: Thorndike Press; 2010.
90. Fanu L: **The Rise and Fall of Modern Medicine.** New York: Carroll & Graf; 1999.
91. Cahill LE, Chiuve SE, Mekary RA, Jensen MK, Flint AJ, Hu FB, Rimm EB: **Prospective study of breakfast eating and incident coronary heart disease in a cohort of male US health professionals.** *Circulation* 2013, 128(4):337-343.
92. Stein R: **Daily Red Meat Raises Chances Of Dying Early**. In: *The Washington Post.* Washington, D.C.; 2009.
93. Sinha R, Cross AJ, Graubard BI, Leitzmann MF, Schatzkin A: **Meat intake and mortality: a prospective study of over half a million people.** *Arch Intern Med* 2009, 169(6):562-571.
94. Layman DK, Boileau RA, Erickson DJ, Painter JE, Shiue H, Sather C, Christou DD: **A reduced ratio of dietary carbohydrate**

**to protein improves body composition and blood lipid profiles during weight loss in adult women.** *J Nutr* 2003, 133(2):411-417.

95. Layman DK, Evans E, Baum JI, Seyler J, Erickson DJ, Boileau RA: **Dietary protein and exercise have additive effects on body composition during weight loss in adult women.** *J Nutr* 2005, 135(8):1903-1910.

96. Thorpe MP, Jacobson EH, Layman DK, He X, Kris-Etherton PM, Evans EM: **A diet high in protein, dairy, and calcium attenuates bone loss over twelve months of weight loss and maintenance relative to a conventional high-carbohydrate diet in adults.** *J Nutr* 2008, 138(6):1096-1100.

97. Douglas P-J, Eric W, Richard DM, Robert RW, Arne A, Margriet W-P: **Protein, weight management, and satiety**. *The American Journal of Clinical Nutrition* 2008, 87(5):1558S-1561S.

98. Douglas P-J, Kevin RS, Wayne WC, Elena V, Robert RW: **Role of dietary protein in the sarcopenia of aging.** *The American Journal of Clinical Nutrition* 2008, 87(5):1562S-1566S.

99. Pan A, Sun Q , Bernstein AM, Schulze MB, Manson JE, Stampfer MJ, Willett WC, Hu FB: **Red meat consumption and mortality: results from 2 prospective cohort studies.** *Arch Intern Med* 2012, 172(7): 555-563.

100. Pan A, Sun Q , Bernstein AM, Schulze MB, Manson JE, Willett WC, Hu FB: **Red meat consumption and risk of type 2 diabetes: 3 cohorts of US adults and an updated meta-analysis.** *The American journal of clinical nutrition* 2011, 94(4):1088-1096.

101. Pan A, Sun Q , Bernstein AM, Manson JE, Willett WC, Hu FB: **Changes in Red Meat Consumption and Subsequent Risk of Type 2 Diabetes Mellitus: Three Cohorts of US Men and Women.** *JAMA internal medicine* 2013:1-8.

102. Feinman RD: **Red meat and type 2 diabetes mellitus.** *JAMA internal medicine* 2014, 174(4):646.

103. Hainer V, Stunkard A, Kunesova M, Parizkova J, Stich V, Allison

DB: **Atwin study of weight loss and metabolic efficiency**. *Int J Obes Relat Metab Disord* 2001, 25(4):533-537.

104. Ebrahim S, Smith GD, May M, Yarnell J: **Shaving, coronary heart disease, and stroke: the Caerphilly Study.** *Am J Epidemiol* 2003, 157(3):234-238.

105. Djoussé L, Gaziano JM, Buring JE, Lee IM: **Egg consumption and risk of type 2 diabetes in men and women.** *Diabetes Care* 2009, 32(2): 295-300.

106. Newell D: **Intention-to-Treat Analysis: Implications foQuantitative andQualitative Research**. *International Journal of Epidemiology* 1992, 21(5):837-841.

107. Hollis S, Campbell F: **What is meant by intention to treat analysis? Survey of published randomised controlled trials.** *BMJ* 1999, 319(7211):670-674.

108. Program USNSL: **Comparison of Current NSLP Elementary Meals vs. Proposed Elementary Meals.** www.whitehouse.gov/sites/default/files/cnr_chart.pdf

109. Wainer H: **Medical illuminations : using evidence, visualization and statistical thinking to improve healthcare,** First edition. edn. Oxford, United Kingdom ; New York, NY, United States of America: Oxford University Press; 2014.

110. Smith GC, Pell JP: **Parachute use to prevent death and major trauma related to gravitational challenge: systematic review of randomised controlled trials.** *BMJ* 2003, 327(7429):1459-1461.

111. Wortman J: ***My Big, Fat Diet***. (2008) www.mybigfatdiet.net.

112. Estruch R, Ros E, Martinez-Gonzalez MA: **Mediterranean diet for primary prevention of cardiovascular disease.** *The New England journal of medicine* 2013, 369(7):676-677.

113. Feinman RD, Volek JS: **Carbohydrate restriction as the default treatment for type 2 diabetes and metabolic syndrome.** *Scand Cardiovasc J* 2008, 42(4):256-263.

114. Dahlqvist A: *Dr Annika Dahlqvists LCHF-blogg*. vol. 2014; 2014.

115. Volek JS, Phinney SD: **The Art and Science of Low-Carbohydrate Living** Charleston, S.C. Beyond Obesity; 2011.

# APPENDIX

## BLOGPOST "FROM A FUTURE HISTORY OF DIABETES"

I don't believe in time travel, of course, so when somebody sent me the following article that was supposed to be a chapter from a Study of the History of Diabetes from 2019, I didn't think about it much. Then I read an article about a woman who had been charged with neglect in the death of her son from complications due to diabetes. It seems she "was trying to live by faith and felt like God would heal him." For some reason, that made me think of the Future History, so here it is.

### Chapter IV. ACCORD to The Court

We have seen how, early in the history of medicine, diabetes was recognized as a disease of carbohydrate intolerance and how, until the discovery of insulin, removing carbohydrate from the diet became the major treatment (Chapters I and II). We chronicled the shift away from this medical practice under the influence of low-fat recommendations and the ascendancy of pharmacology that followed the discovery of insulin. Nonetheless, it persisted in the popular mind that you don't give candy to people with diabetes, even as health agencies seemed to encourage sucrose (sugar) consumption.

The rather sudden reappearance of carbohydrate restriction, the so-called modern era in diabetes treatment, is usually dated to 2008, the precipitating event, publication of the ACCORD study in which a group undergoing "intensive treatment" to lower blood glucose showed unexpected deaths [1]. ACCORD concluded that, "These findings identify a previously unrecognized harm of intensive glucose lowering in high-risk patients with type 2 diabetes." The intensive treatment turned out to be intensive pharmacologic therapy and this flawed logic lead to a popular uprising of sorts, a growing number of patients claiming that they had been hurt by intensive drug treatment and typically that they had only been able to get control of their diabetes by adherence to low-carbohydrate diets. Blogs compared the ACCORD conclusion to an idea that alleviating headaches with intensive aspirin led to bleeding and we should therefore not treat headaches.

The conflict culminated in the large judgment for the plaintiff in *Cedric Banting v. American Diabetes Association* (ADA) in 2017, affirmed by the Supreme Court in 2015. Dalton Banting, coincidentally a distant relative of the discoverer of insulin, was an adolescent with diabetes who took prescribed medications and followed a diet consistent with ADA recommendations. He experienced worsening of his symptoms and ultimately had a foot amputated. At this point his parents found a physician who recommended a low-carbohydrate diet which led to rapid and sustained improvement. The parents claimed their son should have been offered carbohydrate-restriction as an option. The case was unusual in that Banting had a mild obsessive-compulsive condition, expressed as a tendency to follow exactly any instructions from his parents or other authority figures. Banting's lawyers insisted that, as a consequence, one could rely on his having complied with the ADA's recommendations. Disputed by the defense, this was one of several issues that made *Banting* famous for vituperative courtroom interactions between academics.

Banting was a person with type 2 diabetes. Unlike people with type 1 diabetes, he was able to produce insulin in response to dietary (or systemic) glucose but his pancreas was progressively dysfunctional and his body did not respond normally, that is, he was insulin-resistant. Although most people with type 2 diabetes are at least slightly overweight, Banting was not, although he began gaining weight when treated with insulin.

The phrase "*covered with insulin ...*" rocked the court: the president of the ADA, H. Himsworth, Jr., was asked to read from the 2008 guidelines [2]: "Sucrose-containing foods can be substituted for other carbohydrates in the meal plan or, if added to the meal plan, covered with insulin or other glucose lowering medications."

> Jaggers (attorney for Banting): "Are there other diseases where patients are counseled to make things worse so that they can take more drugs?"

> Himsworth: "We only say 'can be.' We don't necessarily recommend it. We do say that 'Care should be taken to avoid excess energy intake.'"

It soon became apparent that Himsworth was in trouble. He was asked to read from the passage explaining the ADA's opposition to low-carbohydrate diets:

"Low-carbohydrate diets might seem to be a logical approach to lowering postprandial glucose. However, foods that contain carbohydrate are important sources of energy, fiber, vitamins, and minerals and are important in dietary palatability."

> Jaggers: "Important sources of energy? I thought we wanted to avoid excess energy," and "would you say that taking a vitamin pill is in the same category as injecting insulin?"

Finally,

> Jaggers: "Dr. Himsworth, as an expert on palatability, could you explain the difference between Bordelaise sauce and Béarnaise sauce?" [laughter]

Damaging as this testimony was, the tipping point in the trial is generally considered to have been the glucometer demonstration. Banting consumed a meal typical of that recommended by the ADA and glucometer readings were projected on a screen for the jury, showing, on this day, so-called "spikes" in blood glucose. The following day, Banting consumed a low-carbohydrate meal and the improved glucometer readings were again projected for the jury. Defense argued that one meal did not prove anything and that one had to look at the whole history of the lifestyle intervention but was unable to show any evidence of harm from continued maintenance of low blood sugar despite testimony of several expert witnesses. In the end, the jury agreed that common sense overrides expert testimony and that Banting should have been offered the choice of a carbohydrate-restricted diet.

*Banting* was held in New York State which adheres to the *Frye* standard: in essence, the idea that scientific evidence is determined by "general acceptance." The explicit inclusion of common sense was, in fact, a legal precedent [3]. The Supreme Court ultimately concurred and held that the more comprehensive standards derived from *Daubert v. Merrill-Dow*, could sensibly be seen to encompass common sense.

The final decision in Banting lead to numerous law suits. The ADA and other agencies changed their tactics claiming that they never were opposed to low-carbohydrate diets and, in fact, had been recommending them all along [4]. This is discussed in the next chapter.

**References**

1. Gerstein, H. C. *et al.*, Effects of intensive glucose lowering in type 2 diabetes. *N Engl J Med* 358 (24), 2545 (2008).
2. American Diabetes Association, Nutrition Recommendations and Interventions for Diabetes–2008. *Diabetes Care* 31 (Suppl 1), S61 (2008).
3. Berger, M, Expert Testimony: The Supreme Court's Rules Issues in Science and Technology (2000).
4. American Diabetes Association, Nutrition Recommendations and Interventions for Diabetes–2018. *Diabetes Care* 36 (Suppl 1), S12 (2018).

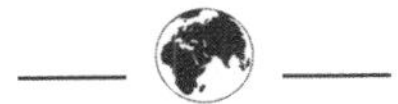

# INDEX

In this index, *b* denotes text box, *f* denotes figure, and *t* denoted table. **Bolded** page numbers indicate photos.

## E

## H

## K



## L

**N**

**P**

## Q



## R

## S

**W**

**Y**